Children and Young People's Nursing
at a Glance

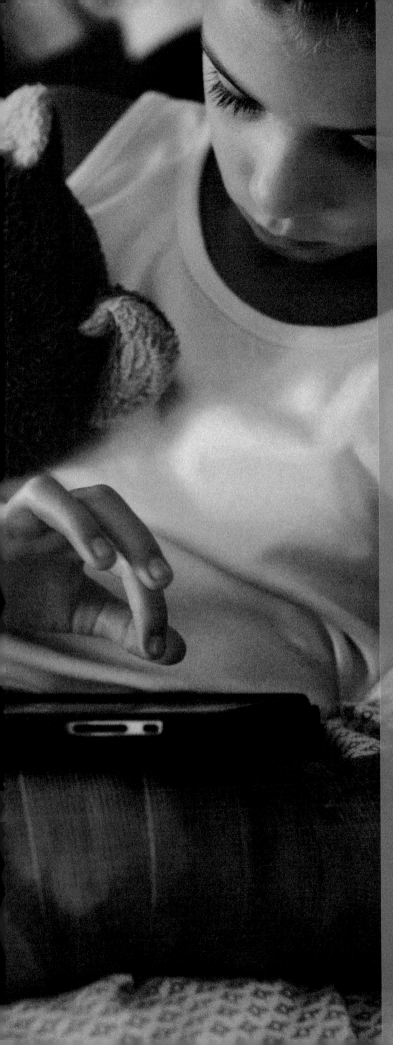

Children and Young People's Nursing

at a Glance

Second Edition

Edited by

Elizabeth Gormley-Fleming
Associate Director Academic Quality
Assurance
Centre for Academic Quality Assurance
and Children's Nursing Team
School of Health and Social Work
University of Hertfordshire
Hatfield, UK

Sheila Roberts
Senior Lecturer in Children's Nursing
School of Health and Social Work
University of Hertfordshire
Hatfield, UK

Series Editor: Ian Peate

WILEY Blackwell

This second edition first published 2023
© 2023 by John Wiley & Sons Ltd

Edition History
John Wiley & Sons Ltd (1e, 2015)

The right of Elizabeth Gormley-Fleming and Sheila Roberts to be identified as the authors of the editorial material in this work has been asserted in accordance with law.

Registered Offices
John Wiley & Sons, Inc., 111 River Street, Hoboken, NJ 07030, USA
John Wiley & Sons Ltd, The Atrium, Southern Gate, Chichester, West Sussex, PO19 8SQ, UK

For details of our global editorial offices, customer services, and more information about Wiley products visit us at www.wiley.com.

Wiley also publishes its books in a variety of electronic formats and by print-on-demand. Some content that appears in standard print versions of this book may not be available in other formats.

Library of Congress Cataloging-in-Publication Data
Names: Gormley-Fleming, Elizabeth, editor. | Roberts, Sheila, (Senior
    lecturer in children's nursing) editor.
Title: Children and young people's nursing at a glance / edited by
    Elizabeth Gormley-Fleming, Sheila Roberts.
Other titles: At a glance series (Oxford, England)
Description: Second edition. | Hoboken, NJ : Wiley-Blackwell, 2023. |
    Series: At a glance | Includes bibliographical references and index.
Identifiers: LCCN 2022032478 (print) | LCCN 2022032479 (ebook) | ISBN
    9781119830665 (paperback) | ISBN 9781119830801 (adobe pdf) | ISBN
    9781119830825 (epub)
Subjects: MESH: Pediatric Nursing | Handbook
Classification: LCC RJ245 (print) | LCC RJ245 (ebook) | NLM WY 49 | DDC
    618.92/00231–dc23/eng/20220826
LC record available at https://lccn.loc.gov/2022032478
LC ebook record available at https://lccn.loc.gov/2022032479

Cover image: © Rebecca Nelson/Getty Images
Cover design by Wiley

Set in 9.5/11.5 pt Minion Pro by Straive, Pondicherry, India

Printed and bound by CPI Group (UK) Ltd, Croydon, CR0 4YY

C9781119830665_100523

Contents

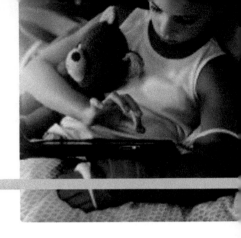

Part 1

Part 2

Contributors

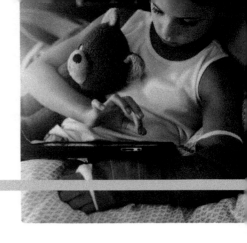

Alison Jithoo [Chapters 124, 126]
Senior Lecturer for Child Nursing
Liverpool John Moores University

Andrea Cockett [Chapters 79, 95, 98]
Deputy Head at School of Nursing
Kingston University

Angela Ryan [Chapter 55]
Nurse Tutor in Centre of Children's Nurse Education
Children's Health, Ireland

Beckie Giacopazzi [Chapter 19]
Acting Superintendent Radiographer, Great Ormond Street
Hospital for Children NHS Foundation Trust, London

Caroline Boyle [Chapter 32]
Programme Lead and Specialist Practitioner Community
Children's Nursing at School of Nursing and Allied Health
Liverpool John Moores University

Elizabeth Gormley-Fleming [Chapters 1–6, 8–18, 20,
21, 23, 24, 26–28, 30, 34–38, 40–44, 46, 50, 53, 54, 57,
59–63, 65, 66, 68, 70–75, 77, 80–83, 85–94, 96, 97,
99–101, 103–115, 117–123, 125, 127, 129]
Associate Director Academic Quality Assurance
Centre for Academic Quality Assurance and Children's
Nursing Team, School of Health and Social Work, University
of Hertfordshire

Emmie Hopkinson [Chapters 45, 51, 52]
Children's Nursing Student
Kingston University

Fearghal Lewis [Chapter 102]
Lecturer Children's Nursing
Queen's University Belfast

Frances Howlin [Chapter 56]
Emeritus Assistant Professor Children's Nursing
UCD School of Nursing, Midwifery and Health Systems
University College Dublin
and
Community RGN, Health Service Executive
Balally Primary Care Centre Dublin South East Clonskeagh
Dublin

Gayle Le Moine [Chapter 78]
Senior Lecturer in Children's Nursing
School of Nursing in Midwifery and Social Work, Canterbury
Christ Church University

Jillian Quinn [Chapter 22]
Airway Clinical Nurse Specialist
Children's Health Ireland (CHI)
Crumlin, Dublin, Ireland

Julia Petty [Chapters 47–49, 52]
Associate Professor (learning and teaching) / Senior Lecturer
Children's Nursing, School of Health and Social Work,
University of Hertfordshire

Julie Brown [Chapters 76, 84]
Lecturer Children's Nursing
Queen's University Belfast

Karen Grant [Chapter 25]
Associate Director of Nursing
Unplanned Care, Isle of Wight NHS Trust

Kath Evans [Chapters 7, 33, 69]
Director, Children's Nursing/Chair of the Children's Board
Barts Health and Nursing & Academic Fellow
School of Health Sciences
City University and Children & Young People's Clinical Lead
North East London Integrated Care System and Participation
Clinical Champion for NHS England
London BCYP Transfromation Programme

Katy Weaver [Chapter 31]
Learning Disability Play Nurse Specialist (Healthcare Play
Specialist), Royal Alexandra Children's Hospital, University
Hospitals Sussex NHS Foundation Trust

Laura Schwartz [Chapters 39, 116]
Senior Lecturer in Children's Nursing in the School of Nursing
Allied Health Liverpool John Moores University

Lisa Whiting [Chapter 29, 64]
Professional Lead in Children's Nursing and Associate
Professor [Research], School of Health and Social Work,
University of Hertfordshire

Owen Arthurs [Chapter 19]
Professor of Radiology, Great Ormond Street Hospital for
Children NHS Foundation Trust, London

Patricia McNeilly [Chapters 76, 84, 102]
Senior Lecturer in Children's Nursing
Queen's University Belfast

Sheila Roberts [Chapters 29, 64, 67]
Senior Lecturer in Children's Nursing, School of Health and
Social Work, University of Hertfordshire

Siobhan Fitzgerald [Chapter 22]
Clinical Nurse Specialist in Airway Management
ENT Department in Children's Health Ireland
Crumlin, Dublin, Ireland

Vanessa Keane [Chapter 58]
Lead Practice Educator for Nursing and Non-Medical
Education, Great Ormond Street Hospital for Children NHS
Foundation Trust and Fellow for Higher Education Academy

Preface

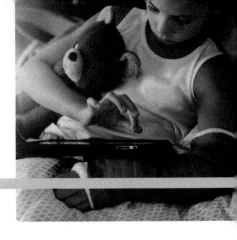

We are very pleased that the second edition of this textbook has been commissioned. This highlights the usefulness of this text to children's nurses, nursing associates, and students who are working towards registration. As with the first edition, the primary focus remains unchanged; that is, to illuminate the best clinical practice for children's and young people's nurses.

Feedback from students and colleagues is that they like the approach taken in this series, important information is easily accessible, and is presented in a concise format with appropriate visuals. Building on the excellent first edition, we have retained this format and added key points to each chapter.

The content of this textbook has been comprehensively reviewed for this second edition against contemporary evidence-based practice guidelines and consideration given to the changing landscape of children's and young people's health and societal changes. The Nursing and Midwifery Council (2018) Standards Framework for nurse education and the Code for professional standards have been considered in this second edition and underpin much of the content.

Children's and young people's nurses are committed to providing safe and effective care that is based on evidence. This textbook aims to provide a useful reference on the clinical care needs of neonates, children, and young people, considering policy, skills, and the practice of children's nursing in today's healthcare environment. It is also a useful text to others who work with children and young people in the delivery of healthcare.

Some chapters required extensive review and new chapters have been included in this edition. It was also interesting to see that some practices in children's nursing have not changed or advanced since the first edition was published.

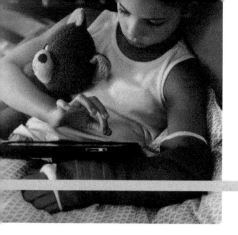

Acknowledgements

We wish to acknowledge the contribution of all the original authors and editors. We did make every effort to locate you. It was great that some of you were able to contribute to this second edition and for this we are very grateful. Some of you have gone on to other lives and some of you were willing, but the pressures of the pandemic did not permit you to update your chapters as your clinical or academic lives were rightly the priority. We were delighted to welcome on board new authors. To all of you, original, existing and new authors, this text would not have reached this stage without you. Thank you.

Our world continues to be in turmoil, we are coming out of a pandemic and the impact of this will be felt for many years by everyone. We must remember that we have all played a part in this: in the clinical setting, delivering education remotely or studying towards registration. We should congratulate ourselves and each other for continuing to make the care of children our first priority.

On a personal note, thank you to my family for your patience as ever, Kieran, Kate and Eilis.

Elizabeth Gormley-Fleming and Sheila Roberts

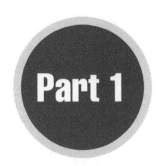

Part 1

Chapters

1 Assessment of the child and young person

Figure 1.1 Assessment of the child and young person.

Assessment is the gathering of information and formulation of judgements in partnership with the child and family. It is a continuous, dynamic process and includes the physiological, physical, psychological, social, and spiritual aspects of the child and the effect that their health problem is having on their development and family life. Accurate assessment of the infant or child is essential to the delivery of safe and effective care. Depending on the child's presenting condition, a focused assessment may be required in the case of the seriously ill child, necessitating prioritization of care until the child's condition is stable.

Assessment leads to the identification of health problems and the development of care plans.

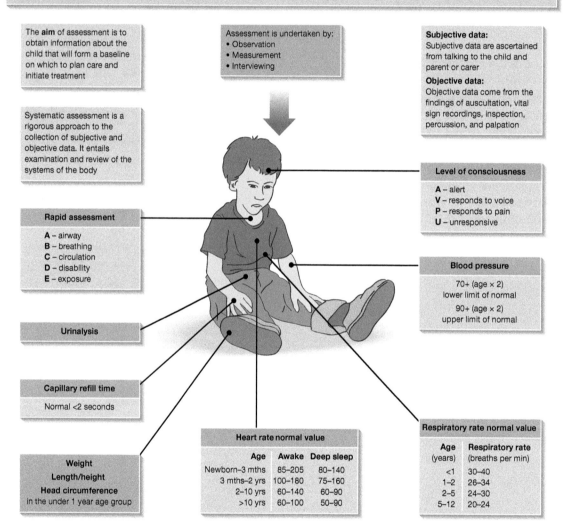

The **aim** of assessment is to obtain information about the child that will form a baseline on which to plan care and initiate treatment

Systematic assessment is a rigorous approach to the collection of subjective and objective data. It entails examination and review of the systems of the body

Assessment is undertaken by:
- Observation
- Measurement
- Interviewing

Subjective data:
Subjective data are ascertained from talking to the child and parent or carer

Objective data:
Objective data come from the findings of auscultation, vital sign recordings, inspection, percussion, and palpation

Level of consciousness

A – alert
V – responds to voice
P – responds to pain
U – unresponsive

Rapid assessment

A – airway
B – breathing
C – circulation
D – disability
E – exposure

Blood pressure

70+ (age × 2)
lower limit of normal

90+ (age × 2)
upper limit of normal

Urinalysis

Capillary refill time

Normal <2 seconds

Weight
Length/height
Head circumference
in the under 1 year age group

Heart rate normal value		
Age	Awake	Deep sleep
Newborn–3 mths	85–205	80–140
3 mths–2 yrs	100–180	75–160
2–10 yrs	60–140	60–90
>10 yrs	60–100	50–90

Respiratory rate normal value	
Age (years)	Respiratory rate (breaths per min)
<1	30–40
1–2	26–34
2–5	24–30
5–12	20–24

Box 1.1 HEADSSS tool

HEADSSS is an interview prompt tool used specifically to assess the health needs of young people. It may be used as a self-assessment tool as well as by healthcare professionals. It has been successful in identifying concerns that require further interventions. The acronym stands for:
H – home
E – education and employment
A – activities
D – drugs/drink
S – sex
S – self-harm, depression, and suicide
S – safety (relationships, **online)**

Key points
- Use a recognized framework when assessing the child or young person, as this will enable a systematic and thorough approach.
- Assessment is an ongoing process and will take place at many points in the child's or young person's clinical journey.
- Age- and development-appropriate questions and tools should be used.

Children and Young People's Nursing at a Glance, Second Edition. Edited by Elizabeth Gormley-Fleming and Sheila Roberts.
© 2023 John Wiley & Sons Ltd. Published 2023 by John Wiley & Sons Ltd.

Introduction

Assessment is a key component of nursing practice and is required for planning and implementing child- and family-centred care (Figure 1.1). Registered nurses must be proficient in assessment at the point of registration. They need to be able to prioritize the physical, social, behavioural, cognitive, spiritual, and mental health needs of the child/young person. Partnership working with the child and family is required as their needs and preferences must be given due regard. The nurse needs to utilize this information when prioritizing and planning child-centred evidence-based care to meet the patient's needs. Assessment is the collection of data, both subjective and objective, which aims to achieve a complete picture of the child's health status. Good assessment is a combination of the interpretation of physical data and the information gained from observation of the child and family and from listening to them. Assessment tools may be used for aspects of the assessment, such as pain, nutrition, or wound assessment.

Interviewing – history taking

Gaining the trust of the child and family is an essential element in developing an effective therapeutic relationship. Introducing yourself to the child and family with explanations of expected outcomes will put the child and family at ease. Age-appropriate language should be used. Questions should be directed at both the child and the parent. Young people should have an opportunity to talk in private if they wish and the HEADSSS tool is commonly used when history taking in this age group (Box 1.1).

When taking a history, a structured approach should be used. This needs to include:
- Presenting complaint.
- History of presenting complaint.
- Past medical history (birth and neonatal history in infants and young children), immunizations, illnesses, and hospitalizations.
- Allergies.
- Current medication.
- Developmental history.
- Family history.
- Social history – nursery, school, HEADSSS tool.

Observation – subjective data

Subjective data are what the child and parent say along with the visual information gained from the initial encounter with the child and family or while obtaining objective data (physical examination and recording of vital signs). This includes noting:
- Their colour: are they pale, mottled, cyanosed, jaundiced, flushed.
- Behaviour: alert, crying, agitated, combative, lethargic, drowsy, distressed.
- Mental health and wellbeing status, HEADSSS assessment for young people (Box 1.1).
- Interaction with parents/carers/strangers.
- Interaction with environment, wanting to play or sleepy.
- Position: normal, floppy, or stiff.
- The general appearance of the child, e.g. unkempt or clean.
- Obvious birthmarks, bruises, or rashes.
- Dysmorphic features.

Measuring – objective data

All infants, children, and young people require a baseline physical assessment. This is a multifaceted process and some aspects are common to all children who require assessment of their health status. The physical assessment is concerned with the analysis and interpretation of data. Privacy and dignity should be maintained during this process. Consent should be obtained prior to undertaking a physical assessment.

Physical assessment includes:
- Basic physical recordings of temperature, pulse rate, respiratory rate, oxygen saturation, and blood pressure.
- Respiratory assessment, rate of breathing, depth of breathing, noise of breathing, presence of cough, chest movement, nasal flaring, use of other accessory muscles, child's colour, ability to speak/feed, position of the child, peak flow, and oxygen saturation level.
- Heart rate including pulse volume.
- Capillary refill time.
- Neurological status using Glasgow Coma Scale or AVPU (Alert, Voice, Pain, Unresponsive).
- Level of hydration: obvious signs of dehydration include sunken anterior fontanelle, dull sunken eyes, dry oral mucosa, lethargy, weak cry, decreased urinary output.
- Weight.
- Height/length.
- Head circumference.
- Skin assessment using recognized pressure risk assessment tool.
- Urinalysis.
- Blood glucose if required.

All findings need to be documented, as they are a legal record of the nursing assessment, the foundation on which care is planned and the basis of communication with the multidisciplinary team. A more focused nursing assessment may be required of a specific body system relating to the presenting problem or other concerns noted. This may be uni- or multisystem. Clinical judgement will determine where the focus of assessment will be.

Approach to assessment

The approach taken to assessment will impact on the success and ease of actually undertaking the physical assessment. The children's nurse should consider the following:
- Age and development stage of the child.
- Undertaking examination of the least intrusive areas first and painful, sensitive areas last.
- Their own behaviour and showing respect for the child's culture and personal preference.
- Clustering their assessment with other areas of care so as to avoid unnecessary disruption, but also being aware of the clinical needs of the child against their need to rest.
- Identifying what parts of the assessment should be carried out before the child is likely to become upset and cry, e.g. chest auscultation, heart sounds.
- Encouraging the child and family to voice any concerns or questions.

Evaluation

Evaluation requires the children's nurse to ensure the correct information has been collected, and that it is accurate and documented. Abnormal findings should be acted on straightaway. The children's nurse will need to process the information, both objective and subjective, and utilize this to draw on their problem-solving and critical thinking skills to plan person-centred, evidence-based nursing interventions.

Summary

Assessment is a dynamic, continuous process that needs to include the child's and parent or caregiver's perspectives. Evidence-based and best practice approaches should always be used when assessing the child or young person. Observation is as essential as physical assessment, and good communication skills are important too.

2 SBAR framework

Figure 2.1 Example of an SBAR template.

SBAR template	
S	Situation
B	Background
A	Assessment
R	Recommendation

Figure 2.2 Readback: This is when the receiver of the information provides a summary for the giver. The receiver should follow the SBAR tool for this readback summary.

Situation	• My name is...... I am a ...... on Ward ..... • I am calling about (patient). in Bed two in Bay four. She has become........ • Her vital signs are....... • Her PEWS is ....
Background	• Why was the patient admitted? • When was the patient admitted, past medical history • Their condition changed in the last .... • What procedures have they had? • Laboratory tests and results. • Current medication • Allergies • Vital signs and PEWS • Pain score • IV lines
Assessment	• Action taken (oxygen commenced, infusion stopped) • Clinical impression • I am very concerned • I am not sure what the problem is but i am now very concerned
Recommendation	• What do you need: e.g. I want you to come and review the patient immediately... • What action do you want now, e.g. stop intravenous fluids/perform ECG/repeat blood gas

Box 2.1   SBAR tool/framework

S – Situation
B – background
A – Assessment
R – Recommendation

Box 2.2   Risk areas in communication

- Shift to shift – continuity of care and ongoing assessment
- Across professions – own 'language', variation in communication, own hierarchies
- Department level – patients may pass through many departments during their hospitalization
- Care settings – hospital to hospital, hospital to community; variation in communication styles, quality of information, cultures
- Patient needs – level of complexity of needs requiring more information to be communicated
- Out of hours – nights, weekends
- Poor or absent records
- Confidence level of staff – may be reluctant to ask more senior staff for help
- Interruptions at handovers

Children and Young People's Nursing at a Glance, Second Edition. Edited by Elizabeth Gormley-Fleming and Sheila Roberts.
© 2023 John Wiley & Sons Ltd. Published 2023 by John Wiley & Sons Ltd.

What is the SBAR tool?

SBAR (Box 2.1) is a structured communication tool that enables healthcare staff to share focused, clear, and concise information effectively with one another. Originally developed for use in the military, it quickly became recognized as an effective means of improving patient safety. It is acknowledged that miscommunication contributes significantly to patient harm.

The SBAR tool consists of four standardized prompt questions. These standardized prompts permit all healthcare staff to communicate effectively and with confidence. They should enable the receiver to be given clear information, reduce the need for repetition, and lower the likelihood of errors. The SBAR tool can be used in a variety of settings, clinical and non-clinical, and by all healthcare staff. The mnemonic may be used on cards, notepads, and patient records as a reminder to staff that this is the standard method of communication (Figure 2.1). The giver of the information should always ask the receiver to repeat the information to affirm their understanding (Figure 2.2)

When should SBAR be used?

The SBAR tool organizes relevant information in a coherent manner with the most important points clearly identifiable. The role of the giver of information and the receiver are clear when using this tool. The giver of information must ensure that they have formulated their thinking, have a comprehensive understanding of their patient/service user, and have all the required and relevant information to hand. The receiver of the information should know what to expect and avoid asking any questions when information is being shared. The benefit of this is that staff will be able to make prompt assessment as the information is received.

When can SBAR be used?

The SBAR tool can be used in any clinical or managerial setting. It can be employed as a uni- or multidisciplinary communication tool. It is primarily used to escalate clinical problems that require urgent attention. It is also utilized to facilitate efficient patient handover between clinical teams. It can be used for verbal and written exchanges, so is an effective framework for email communication

How can SBAR help with communication?

Strong links between good communication and good clinical outcomes have been recognized. Poor communication is frequently the cause of patient dissatisfaction. This includes inadequate written and verbal communication, both of which are cited as the root cause of serious error. The use of the SBAR tool helps prevent any breakdown in communication. The healthcare team can develop a shared understanding of the communication required for the critical exchange of information. Good transfer of care-related information relies consistently on good communication.

There are a number of stages in a patient's journey where communication can go wrong (Box 2.2).

Communication barriers do exist in healthcare, where there are various disciplines operating within complex environments. Hierarchy, ethnic background, and gender are considered to be some of these barriers. The SBAR tool provide a means of having a common language between all disciplines and removes hierarchy.

The use of the SBAR tool avoids the sharing of vague and assumptive information. It is direct and is a call to action. The giver of information is required to prepare and think prior to communicating, and to be confident and assertive as they are required to make a recommendation.

Scenario

Apply the SBAR tool to the following scenario:

Kate, a 4-year-old female, was admitted to the Children's Ward, 10B, two days ago. She has been diagnosed with a left lower lobe pneumonia. She had oxygen saturations of 89% on admission, respiratory rate 48 breaths/min, heart rate 120 bpm and a temperature of 38.9 °C. She has been requiring oxygen via face mask overnight. She has been prescribed intravenous antibiotics, nebulized salbutamol, and oral paracetamol. She has started drinking a little. You go to her room to assess her after handover. You notice she is 'working hard' to breathe. Her saturations are 88%, respiratory rate 58 breaths/min, heart rate 160 bpm. She is pale and drowsy. Her PEWS (Paediatric Early Warning Score) is now 5. You recommence her oxygen via face mask. You now want the paediatrician to come and see her urgently. Think about how you would present Kate using the SBAR tool, before reading what follows.

Situation

My name is Sue, I am a staff nurse on Ward 10B. I am calling you about Kate, who has increased work of breathing. Her oxygen saturations dropped to 88% in room air, she has a heart rate of 160 and a respiratory rate of 58 bpm. Her PEWS is 5. She is pale and has intercostal recession. She is lethargic.

Background

Kate is a 4-year-old who was admitted two days ago. She was diagnosed with left lower lobe pneumonia. She has been receiving intravenous antibiotics, nebulized salbutamol, and oral paracetamol. She had been responding well and her PEWS was 1 when last recorded two hours ago. Oxygen therapy was discontinued yesterday. She has been drinking adequately and is eating small amounts.

Assessment

I have sat her up and recommenced her oxygen, 5 L via a face mask. I have put her back on cardiac and respiratory monitor. She sounds as if she has a lot of secretions and is making attempts to cough. I am worried about her as her response to oxygen was slow.

Recommendation

I would like you to come and review Kate. Is there anything else I can do in the meantime?

Summary

When using the SBAR tool the practitioner should aim to:

- Communicate effectively
- Identify priorities
- Utilize decision-making strategies
- Develop problem-solving skills
- Be confident and assertive

Key points

- The effective use of this tool requires practice.
- The use of the SBAR tool helps prevent any breakdown in communication.
- Patient safety is enhanced when this tool is used.

3 The nursing process/care process

Figure 3.1 Planning care using the nursing process and nursing models.

What is nursing theory?

- Nursing theory is the cognitive knowledge and understanding that is used by practitioners to help them deliver the best possible care based upon best evidence
- Nursing theory is partly drawn from a range of subjects from the arts and science domains that can be applied to the practice of nursing

Key point
Nursing theory is knowledge that comes from experiential learning and research and is used by the nurse to guide practice

What are nursing models?

- Nursing models are a combination of theories and concepts that provide a framework to assess, plan, implement, and evaluate care
- Many nursing models proposed by theorists
- Most common are those that include 'activities of daily living'
- Casey's partnership model is based upon the notion of partnership with the family, where parents or carers provide care until the child or young person is mature enough to do it themselves

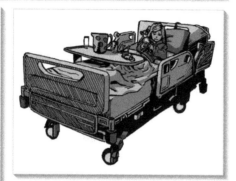

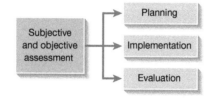

Subjective and objective assessment → Planning

Implementation

Evaluation

What is the nursing process?

- The nursing process is a framework for organizing individualized nursing care
- Involves four stages: assessment, planning, implementation, and evaluation (APIE)
- An essential component is that goals or objectives are measurable to enable care to be evaluated and improved upon: subjective, objective, assessment, planning, implementation, evaluation (SOAPIE)

Key point
The involvement of children and families in planning and implementation of care is recognized by professional bodies as vital in the formation of effective partnership with families and children in the provision of care and healthcare services

Benefits of care plans

- Improved quality of care
- Improved communication
- Evidence-based practice
- Reduce risk of litigation
- Standardized care
- Continuity of care
- Patient and staff satisfaction

The nursing process is a way of thinking about nursing in a logical and problem-solving manner

- It is a framework for organizing individualized nursing care and promotes continuity of care
- The nursing process has four stages:
  – assessment, planning, implementation, and evaluation

Nursing has a theoretical base that has many elements, including physiology, psychology, pathology, pharmacology, and sociology. To deliver quality care to patients that is focused, safe, and organized, that care needs to be planned. Documenting the plan of care for a patient and its implementation ensures continuity of care and provides a legal document demonstrating that care has been delivered. Care can be organized using the nursing process and nursing models can help focus care to meet the specific needs of patients. Multiple staff, registered nurses, healthcare support workers, nursing associates, and student nurses will be involved in the execution of this process, so an understanding of it is important in ensuring that the care delivered is of good quality.

What is nursing theory?

Nursing theory is the cognitive knowledge and understanding used by practitioners to help them deliver the best possible care based on best evidence. Nursing theory is partly drawn from a range of interconnected subjects from both the arts and sciences that can be applied to the practice of nursing. This knowledge comes from experiential learning and research and is part of the rich tradition linked to the development of nursing. The importance of children's and young people's nurses delivering care that is underpinned by evidence-based theory is a requirement of the Nursing and Midwifery Council (NMC 2018).

There are several models that are commonly used in the nursing of sick children and young people. The most common are 'activities of daily living' models, which include Henderson, Roper et al., and Orem. Casey's model for children's nursing is all about partnership and has become standard practice in UK children's units.

The central premise of these activities of daily living models is that normally people maintain their own functions in these areas, but in times of illness these may be compromised and the patient may require support from healthcare professionals. In the case of children, some activities of daily living such as keeping the body clean may be compromised simply by developmental age. This is why children's nurses have adopted Casey's theoretical framework based on the notion of partnership, and in turn on the philosophy of children's nursing and the notion of the indivisible family unit, where parents or carers provide essential care until the child is mature enough to do it themselves. Orem's model is sometimes called the self-care model and is orientated

Children and Young People's Nursing at a Glance, Second Edition. Edited by Elizabeth Gormley-Fleming and Sheila Roberts.
© 2023 John Wiley & Sons Ltd. Published 2023 by John Wiley & Sons Ltd.

Box 3.1 Child-/person-centred care

Child-/person-centred care means putting the child's needs as they define those needs at the centre of the care-giving process

There are six principles of child-/person-centred care:
- Respecting the individual and their family. It is important to get to know the patient as a person and recognize their uniqueness
- Treat with dignity, compassion, and respect
- Understand their goals and life experiences
- Gain their trust and maintain their confidentiality
- Empower by giving them responsibility for their health
- Work with the child and family to coordinate care

towards restoring an individual to a health status where self-care is possible. It is particularly useful in rehabilitation settings (e.g. after childhood head injury). The prevailing model currently is person-centred care (Box 3.1), which is based on the humanist principles of Carl Rogers.

What is the nursing/care process?

The nursing process is a framework for organizing individualized nursing care. It involves four stages: assessment, planning, implementation, and evaluation (APIE). The intention of the nursing process is to enable continuity of care by thorough documentation of information, to provide continuous observations, and to ensure effective interventions. There has been some criticism of the nursing process approach to care, as it potentially imposes rigid constraints on practice, and may be seen as cumbersome and outdated. A number of factors have been recognized as inhibiting the use of the nursing process, namely, lack of knowledge, high workloads, and lack of training and education. Adequate time must be devoted to this important part of the caring process and the delivery of safe effective nursing care.

Care plans provide an excellent means through which the rights of children and their families can be respected. They enable children and families to be fully informed and to share in decision making about their care. The involvement of children and families in the planning and implementation of care is recognized as vital in the formation of effective partnerships in the provision of care and healthcare services.

The NMC requires nurses to respect the patient or client as an individual and to recognize and respect the role of patients or clients as partners in the contribution they can make. This includes identifying their preferences regarding care (NMC 2018). The primary rationale for using the nursing process is the creation of a care plan that to determines the nursing care given to an individual patient. An essential component is that the goals or objectives of the care plan are measurable to enable care to be evaluated and improved upon.

The nursing process can be perceived as the cognitive vehicle for planning the coordination of care delivered to a patient. Universally, it is the language of nursing and wherever nurses work they will use the same basic steps constituting the nursing process, APIE or SOAPIE (see Figure 3.1). It is important to remember that patient care must be documented and that every child should have an individual plan of care that has been determined following a full nursing assessment.

Planning care

Nursing care has always been planned. Now the focus of care has changed from the completion of tasks to the provision of holistic care, where patients are viewed as individuals with diverse and individual needs. Delivery of person-centred care is a core skill required by all registered nurses and nursing associates. Person-centred care means putting the person's needs (as they define those needs) first, and this may mean prioritizing their needs above those identified by the healthcare provider. Planning care should involve, where possible, the child and family to uphold the overarching family-centred care philosophy of children's and young person's nursing. Planning care involves reviewing all of the identified needs or patient problems and prioritizing them.

Maslow's hierarchy of human needs can help nurses plan nursing care objectively. Clearly, if a child has compromised respiratory efforts, this must be prioritized before planning dietary intake, for example. Care plans are frameworks through which nurses apply the nursing process in addressing the needs of their patients. A nursing care plan is a written statement of the patient's nursing problems and the measures that will be used to effect a solution or mediate these problems.

Care pathways involve the multidisciplinary team in the treatment and management of a patient and provide a programme of evidence-based care delivery. They provide care that is focused, cost-effective, and collaborative. For each clinical problem, the essential steps involved in the care of the patient are set out and planned with regard to that individual's expected progress. The pathways provide a plan of desired patient outcomes, linked to an estimated time frame and the resources available. They can assist in the application of national evidence-based guidelines into local practice. Care pathways have the advantage of improving teamwork, reducing duplication of documentation, and providing continuous records of care for a patient. When using care pathways or predetermined core care plans, it is important that they are still be individualized. When planning care, nurses must ensure that the goals of care are achievable and aligned to the goals of the child or young person themselves.

Summary

The nursing process can be applied in any nursing healthcare situation and offers a cognitive toolkit to assess, plan, implement, and evaluate care. It is easy to use because it is systematic. However, in practice it requires a number of nursing skills: a good understanding of how health problems can impact on an individual child with reference to pathophysiology and social science; excellent interpersonal skills of communication with well-developed listening skills; and technical proficiency in delivering care based on best evidence that is person centred.

Key points
- All nurses from the point of registration must be proficient in assessing, planning, delivering, and evaluating evidence-based person-centred care.
- The concept of child/person centred care continues to evolve.

4 Person-/child-centred care and nursing models

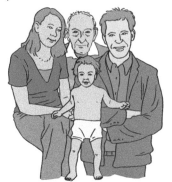

Figure 4.1 How to implement nursing models in practice.

Ways in which personal use of nursing models can be developed

- Used as part of preceptorship, clinical supervision to explore nursing actions in more depth
- Development of a personal toolkit using a range of nursing models
- Incorporated into reflective practice

Use of nursing models in practice settings

- As part of the philosophy of care
- As part of multidisciplinary working
- In conjunction with care pathways and guidelines
- As a framework for care planning

Figure 4.2 Suggested activities.

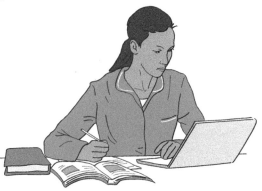

2. Find out a bit more about the three nursing models and compare this with your reflection. Think of ways in which your newly gained knowledge could enhance your practice

1. Reflect on a shift, referring to the three nursing models outlined in this chapter:
   – i.e. is there any indication of use of any of these?

3. Find out about two other nursing models not mentioned in this chapter. What are their strengths and how could they be used to develop your practice?

Nursing models are theoretical frameworks, the first of which was developed in the 1950s to provide guidance on the delivery of nursing care (Figure 4.1). There are many different types; however, they all provide direction on how to implement care for an individual. A nursing model contains concepts, processes, and goals that guide care delivery. They are seen by some as being too traditional and not always suited to contemporary care provision; this is because of the continuing drive towards evidence-based practice, which is often based on hard scientific facts. Person-/child-centred care is now a recognized goal for all children and young people.

Models are extremely important in the development of nursing practice, providing direction to children's and young people's nurses when planning, implementing, and evaluating care. They can be utilized in all settings where children and young people receive care. All nursing models have a focus on meeting the needs of an individual; however, the way in which this is defined varies considerably. The models most frequently used are discussed here, but there are many others that can also be considered that assist in providing high-quality care that meets the needs of the child and family. Nurses may find that they draw on more than one nursing model in their practice. In contemporary children's nursing practice, the nurse is required to understand and apply a person-centred approach to nursing care at assessment, planning, and decision making, and to be able to set goals when working with the child, family, communities, and populations (Figure 4.2).

Nursing models used in children's and young people's nursing

The partnership model, which was developed in the UK by Anne Casey in the 1980s, is the one that is most closely identified with children and young people. Unlike many nursing models, it was developed for this specific group, its main focus being the concept of family-centred care. Roper et al. created the activities of daily living conceptual model, which uses 12 activities of living as the central component with five underpinning factors: biological, psychological, socio-cultural, environmental, and politico-economic. Orem's self-care model is based on meeting the self-care needs that the person is unable to meet themselves. Each person has universal self-care requisites based on human functioning (e.g. a sufficient intake of food), developmental self-care requisites linked to their stage in life, and particular self-care requisites that arise from their health issue.

Person-/child-centred care is a more holistic approach to care delivery. It involves knowledge of the individual as a whole, involving them in assessing their own needs and in planning their own care. This humanistic approach permits equality between the nurse and the child and their family.

How nursing models can be used in practice

All nursing models have a theoretical base. By exploring these concepts, nurses can build on their knowledge to develop their expertise in becoming caring and compassionate practitioners. Nursing models are often incorporated into care planning. This can be implicit: the philosophy of the partnership model may be used to inform practice but not be directly visible in the care setting. In contrast, Roper et al.'s activities of daily living model is often easy to detect, for example in admissions documentation. This has led to criticism that it has been reduced to a tick-box approach, which detracts from a model that has a lot to offer in furthering our understanding of individualized care. It would be unusual to see Orem's self-care model being used directly in practice, but on closer inspection it is frequently integrated into the care plan, such as encouraging the child and family to take control of their health, which is part of the systems approach advocated by Orem.

With person-/child-centred care, caring is made central to nursing practice. The child and family are equal partners and not just passive recipients of care. This move has seen a shift from dependency to empowerment and respect for the choices and preferences of the child and the family. Founded on the principles of humanism, person- child-centred care is underpinned by four concepts:

- Respect for persons
- Right to self-determination
- Mutual respect
- Understanding

The core values that underpin person-centred care are identified in Box 4.1.

This model of care promotes the need for a trusting relationship to be developed with the child, family, and nurse so that self-esteem and self-efficacy can be achieved. A good starting point when embedding child-centred practice is to ask three quick questions:

Box 4.1 Core values that underpin person-/child-centred care

- Individuality
- Choice
- Privacy
- Independence
- Rights
- Empowerment
- Dignity
- Respect
- Partnership

Box 4.2 Implications for person-/child-centred care practice

- Treat the child as an individual and listen to their concerns and wishes. These may be different from those of their parents, but acknowledging the family is also important. Collaboration will lead to a positive experience for all parties.
- Do not dismiss the views or fears of the child – try to see their situation from their perspective and as they understand it. Open communication will lead to improved satisfaction, and reduced anxiety and apprehension.
- Include the child in planning their care to meet what they see as their needs. The care plan is led by the needs of the child, not by the needs of the service.
- Write care plans in the first person: 'I would like to have my dressing changed when I come before my physio', for example.
- Enable the family to support the treatments where possible. Recognize that relinquishing partial control to the parents/carers will empower them and enable them play an active role in their child's care.

- Why are you here?
- What do you think is going on with yourself/your child?
- What do you think is making you feel like this, giving you these symptoms?

The implications for children's nursing practice are outlined in Box 4.2.

Summary

Nursing models are theoretical frameworks. Individual practice can be enhanced by applying nursing models in all aspects of care. Evidence-based practice requires an individualized approach and use of nursing models can help to achieve this. Nurses should be encouraged to explore different nursing models and have a flexible approach towards combining them in practice. Proficiency is required by all children's nurses in working in partnership with children and their families to develop person-/child-centred care plans that consider their individual needs, circumstances, characteristics, and choices.

Key points

- Consider the views and needs of the child from their perspective when possible and be aware that these may conflict with those of the parent.
- Person-/child-centred care helps to guide clinical decision making.

5 The care plan

Box 5.1 Care plan framework.

Identified problem/need

- The need should have been clearly identified during the assessment.
- The problem/need should be individualized.
- The problem/need covered should be specific, so that if three needs or problems are identified during the assessment, there should ideally be three care plans.
- The child and their carers need to be involved in the identification of their needs – they are the 'expert' in how the illness makes them feel and the impact it has on the family unit.

Short-term goals

- Often used when a period of assessment is needed (e.g. the child is acutely unwell).
- Should be SMART (specific, measurable, achievable, realistic, and time-specific).
- Should be mutually agreed by and acceptable to the child and their carers.
- Should be clear and concise.

Long-term goals

- Should be SMART.
- Should be mutually agreed by and acceptable to the child and their carers.
- Should be clear and concise.

Interventions

- The child and their carers should work in collaboration with the nurse to ensure the interventions are individualized, specific, and meet the needs of the child.
- The practitioner leading on each of the interventions should be skilled and competent to carry them out.
- Interventions should be prioritized to meet the needs of the child and their carers.
- The interventions identified should have a theoretical base.
- The practitioner should consider cultural diversity as well as gender, age appropriateness, and religious beliefs when planning any intervention.
- The core principles of care, compassion, dignity, privacy, and quality should underpin clinical practices.

Evaluation

Remember that evaluation should happen continuously
It should include the child and their carers
It should provide clear evidence as to whether the interventions are making a difference
It should provide an overview of the child's condition in order to modify care

Review date

Essential in order to measure care outcomes in a timely manner

Box 5.2 Common care planning problems.

- **Incomplete initial assessments** – leading to gaps in care and increased levels of risk.
- **Unrealistic care planning** – could give false hope, or increased level of expectation about the child's outcome.
- **Lack of clear goals and vague interventions** – leading to difficulties in evaluating care.
- **Not individualized** – may lead to inappropriate clinical intervention.

Box 5.3 Example – care plan.

Scenario

Jane is 23 and has two children: James who is 4 years and Madelaine who is 18 months. Jane lives by herself with the children and has very little social or family support. Jane calls you and requests a Health Visitor meeting. You arrange to see her at the family home. When you arrive, Jane expresses her concern about James' sleep pattern. She is struggling to get him to bed before 11pm. When he is in bed, James takes a further 30–60 minutes to settle, often disrupting Madelaine. James gets angry at bedtime, he shouts, screams, and kicks so that Jane does not follow through any routine. James tells you that he hates bedtime and is old enough to stay up late to watch the television. He denies feeling tired. James is due to start school in September.

Identified problem/need

James lives with his mum and sister in the family home. He is 4 and is due to start school in September. James is not going to bed until 11pm most nights, and when he is in bed does not settle until 11.30pm–12am. Prior to bedtime James shouts, kicks, and screams, often disturbing his younger sister. James states he 'hates' bedtime and he is not tired.

Goals

To assess potential bio-psycho-social issues that may prevent James from wanting to go to bed.
For James to have an established sleep routine that ensures flexibility.

Interventions

- For James to be allowed to talk about bedtime – identifying any fears or concerns he may have about this aspect of his daily routine.
- To provide James with reassurance in relation to any issues identified, referring on to specialist services as required.
- To support Jane in purchasing aids/equipment that may support a new bedtime routine (e.g. new duvet cover of James' favourite cartoon character, night-time light, bedtime books).
- To ensure the bedroom environment is supportive of sleep.
- Discuss daytime routine with Jane and identify how James could increase his activity levels.
- To develop a bedtime routine with Jane – one that is consistent and appropriate for James' age.
- To support Jane in the implementation of the routine, providing guidance and positive feedback.
- Discuss the implications of the sleep routine on James' initial behaviours (e.g. Jane to expect that initially James will not like these changes to his bedtime routine).
- Discuss with Jane ways in which she can cope with the stresses of providing James with a boundaried approach to bedtime.
- Identify how James will be rewarded when small achievements are made.

Evaluation

I developed the care plan with James and his mum today, James' opinion was sought. He did not think he should be going to bed any earlier but did add that he would like to go to the park more often. Jane was in agreement. I have left a copy of the care plan with the family so Jane can read it and add any further comments. Jane has requested that we meet again in a week. An appointment has therefore been arranged for 8 July at 2.30pm.

Review

The care plan is to be reviewed after each visit.

Children and Young People's Nursing at a Glance, Second Edition. Edited by Elizabeth Gormley-Fleming and Sheila Roberts.
© 2023 John Wiley & Sons Ltd. Published 2023 by John Wiley & Sons Ltd.

Achildren and young people's nurse must work in partnership with the child and family to develop person-/child-centred care plans. Proficiency in planning person-/child-centred care is a requirement for all registered nurses. Care plans should shape how the child is cared for, and ensure that each clinical intervention undertaken is suitable, consistent, and needs led.

Care planning is a necessity within legislative practice; it is the framework that drives identification of the child's needs, highlights professional responsibilities, and requires clear evaluation of outcomes. Care planning is a continuous process, one that requires review and update dependent on the specific requirements of the child and their carers.

There are many clearly defined benefits to undertaking the care planning process: ensuring a personalized approach to the child and their carers; providing standardization of the child's care, thus reducing the risk of health inequality; ensuring the child's and their carers' voices are heard as part of the planning stage (this approach can increase compliance, and readily supports the maintenance of a therapeutic relationship); and, finally, facilitating care planning that is underpinned by choice. Providing suitable options to the child and their carers supports the notion of a mutually agreed plan of care.

Person-/child-centred care planning is thus intrinsically linked to the nursing process.

Assessment

The first stage of the nursing process is the assessment. Its aim is to collect and record information pertaining to the health status of the individual child and its effect on the family unit. A precise and comprehensive assessment should provide clear insights into the needs of the child, so that issues can be identified and informed interventions can be developed. Assessment should be a systematic process that utilizes both objective and subjective data. It should not be rushed, Communication and questioning styles need to be age appropriate.

Information from the child/young person should be obtained before that from parents/carers if possible. It is important that parents/carers have an equal opportunity to participate in this process, Information may also be obtained from other physical sources (e.g. referral letters), alongside visual observation and non-verbal communication.

What to assess

Knowing what to assess can sometimes be a challenge. Many organizations use specific assessment documentation or tools, which are often linked to a nursing model. The most common models utilized for this purpose are Roper et al.'s 12 activities of daily living, family-centred care, and Orem's self-care model (see Chapter 4). The paediatric assessment triangle is another tool that may be used to assess a child or young person.

In terms of assessment, it is important to ensure that any assessment of the child uses a holistic approach that encompasses elements such as biological health, psychological wellbeing, and social needs. It is important to understand the context in which children and their families normally live, their routines, and what types of coping mechanisms are utilized. Assessment of the impact the health issue is having on family relationships and the psychological health of carers is an important factor that can also impinge on the child's needs.

Using open questions can be helpful in obtaining information. The importance of observation and non-verbal clues are also implicit within the assessment process.

Planning

The care plan should be based on the evidence gained from the assessment; it should be specific and individualized (see Boxes 5.1 and 5.2).

Goals (either short or long term, or both) need to be developed that are mutually agreed and acceptable to the child. Planning care should not preclude the need to involve other professional groups, as their impact on the child's wellbeing may further support the identified need. The manner in which the overarching goals will be achieved should be developed within the intervention element of the care plan. Intervention should be aimed at resolving problems, maintaining care needs, or identifying any deterioration that may occur.

The practitioner needs to ensure that both the goals and interventions are written using an approach consistent with the SMART model (specific, measurable, achievable, realistic, time specific). Professional responsibility should be highlighted as part of the intervention development process, so identifying who will lead on a specific task in the child's care determines the need for clear communication of the care plan across the team.

Effective communication is an essential part of care planning. It is imperative that children and their carers are given opportunities to work with the nurse, making certain that they are active partners in the decision-making process. This will ensure that interventions are specific and that each child is treated as an individual.

Implementation

This is the third phase of the nursing process, but also an integral part of the care plan. In this phase the identified interventions are implemented. Those practitioners involved should have the skills and knowledge to deliver the care and assess the appropriateness of the planned intervention. It is imperative to continue working closely with the child and their carers and to provide clear choices where possible in terms of the planned interventions.

Evaluation

This stage is concerned with the outcome of the care plan. It should be an ongoing process that is led by the needs of the child and their response to any intervention. The practitioner should, through the evaluation of the care records, be able to identify changes in the child's wellbeing and, redefine the plan of care accordingly. Often the evaluation process is linked with a reassessment of the child's situation, which could lead to a new care plan being introduced or one being discontinued (if all needs have been met). Again, it is important that the child and their carers are involved, and that their opinions are valued and incorporated into future care decisions (see Box 5.3 for an example).

Documentation

Documentation underpins the success of the care plan process. All clinical records should be written in line with local policy and the Nursing and Midwifery Council's requirements. Practitioners should be encouraged to write the care plan documentation in a factual and objective manner, avoiding judgemental statements, abbreviations, and discriminatory language. Clear and concise documentation reduces the risk of clinical errors, mistakes, and complaints. The child and their carers should be able to access their care plan and review it with the nursing staff.

Key points
- Care should always be planned with the child's/young person's needs at the centre.
- Goals should be SMART.
- A framework or model should be followed to ensure a holistic plan of care is provided, taking into account the needs, preferences, and wishes of the child/young person and/or family/carers.

6 Record keeping

Children and Young People's Nursing at a Glance, Second Edition. Edited by Elizabeth Gormley-Fleming and Sheila Roberts.
© 2023 John Wiley & Sons Ltd. Published 2023 by John Wiley & Sons Ltd.

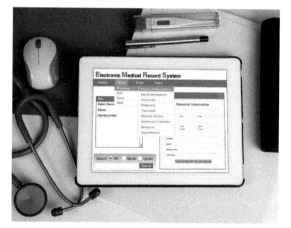

Figure 6.1 Electronic patient record. *Source:* Pandpstock001 / Adobe Stock.

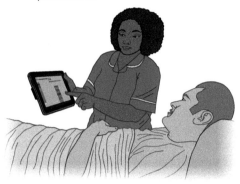

Figure 6.3 Electronic patient records in use at the point of patient care.

Figure 6.2 Principles and good practice in record keeping.

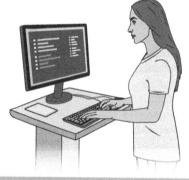

Records should be:
Clear
Intelligible
Accurate

Child/person-centred records:
Clearly record the expressed wishes and preferences of the child and/or their family/carers

Function of records:
Communication tool
Permanent record
Permit audit and research

Principles of good record keeping are:
- Accountability
- Transparency
- Integrity
- Protection
- Compliance
- Accessibility
- Retention
- Disposition

Records should:
- be contemporaneous – dated, timed, and signed
- be accurate, without falsifications
- have risk identified and action taken to mitigate risk and impact
- contain no unnecessary abbreviations, jargon, or speculation
- be kept securely
- collect, treat, and store all data and other findings as per local policy

NMC Code and record keeping:
'Keep clear and accurate records relevant to your practice'
- Priorities People
- Practise Effectively
- Preserve Safety
- Promote professionalism and trust

Introduction

Record keeping is an integral component of effective communication in nursing care and is necessary in promoting patient safety. Keeping detailed records about the conditions, treatments, and outcome of the treatments administered to the child and young people is an important skill. Electronic health records management systems are now widely implemented across healthcare settings (Figure 6.1). Records include electronic and handwritten documents, emails, text messages, photographs, consent forms, printouts, and videos. The principles of good record keeping are applicable to both digital and paper-based nursing records (Figure 6.2). As practice moves more towards electronic patient records, children's nurses must ensure they have the requisite IT skills and knowledge to maintain high standards of record keeping.

Good record keeping

The principles of good record keeping are:
- Accountability
- Transparency
- Integrity
- Protection
- Compliance

- Accessibility
- Retention
- Disposition

The purposes of record keeping are to:

- Act as a communication tool: the written record should be able to communicate the care given, the effectiveness of that care, and the status of the patient without further explanation.
- Demonstrate the decisions made that inform care delivery.
- Provide a permanent record of care given, decisions made, impact of care, and outcomes.

The patient's records are often the first port of call when complaints are made or investigations are required, so the children's nurse needs to consider if their records will hold up to legal challenge.

Children's nurses must be familiar with the Nursing and Midwifery Council's (NMC) Code of Conduct and the relevant areas that relate directly and indirectly to record-keeping practice. The following sections of the Code that make direct reference are as follows:

- Priorities People: refers to the need to get properly informed consent prior to care delivery and the need to document this.
- Practise Effectively: Keep clear and accurate records relevant to your practice. This section identifies six key areas of responsibility for the author of the record. These are:
  ○ Complete records in real time or as soon as possible after the event noting the time and date.
  ○ Any issues or risk identified should have the steps taken to ameliorate the issue/risk recorded and the impact of those actions taken.
  ○ Records must be accurate and factual with no falsification. If this is found not to be the case, then immediate action must be taken.
  ○ Any entry made in either a paper-based or electronic records system must be attributed to the author only.
  ○ Records should be clearly written, timed, and dated. Jargon, speculation, and abbreviations should be avoided.
  ○ Records must be stored securely, and the nurse must take the steps necessary to ensure this.

The indirect reference in this section of the code refers to the terms the nurse uses in their practice and advises that you should use terms that the people in your care, their families, and your colleagues can understand.

- Preserve Safety: This section advises of the need to document all events formally and take action as appropriate to resolve issues quickly.

The nursing record should reflect patient-centred care (Figure 6.3). Using the child's or young person's name is a good starting point.

The cost to the National Health Service of healthcare litigation in England is increasing and poor record-keeping is often cited: 'if it was not recorded it never happened'. Hence, nurses should ensure that their record keeping is meticulous.

Top tips for record keeping

- Do your records meet the CIA mnemonic? Are they:
  ○ Clear
  ○ Intelligible
  ○ Accurate?
- Avoid flowery language, adhere to the facts, and avoid personal comments. The nursing record should be sufficiently detailed, concise, and relevant. Use a systematic approach such as ABCDE

(Airway, Breathing, Circulation, Disability, Exposure) or SBAR (see Chapter 2) to help structure the record.

- Any decisions made based on clinical findings should be documented and the information given to the child and their family should also be recorded.
- Any discussions had with family/carers and other healthcare professionals should be documented and include the names of those involved in the discussion.
- Any consent obtained or refusal of consent for treatment should be documented clearly.
- Avoid using abbreviations unless they are approved by the relevant healthcare environment.
- Records should be contemporaneous – write as you go, do not leave writing your records until the end of the shift. If the nursing notes have to be written retrospectively, then this should be acknowledged.
- If records are handwritten, then they should be written in black or blue ink that is not erasable.
- Be objective and avoid speculation.
- If using paper-based records, errors should be scored through with a single line, dated, and signed.
- If a digital system is used, then the record must be traceable to the provider of care that is being documented.

Countersigning

- Record keeping can be delegated to healthcare support workers, student nurses, or nursing associates to allow care to be documented.
- As this is a delegated activity, the registered nurse must ensure the student nurse/nursing associate or healthcare support worker is competent to undertake the documentation of care,
- The registered nurse must countersign all documentation entries.

Nursing records are necessary to facilitate synchronous patient care, clinical audit, patient safety, and patient decision making, and in promoting continuity of care across interprofessional and interagency boundaries. Records show how decisions about the care of a child or young person were made and may be used in addressing complaints and in any subsequent legal processes. The nursing record will provide evidence if the standard of care is later questioned.

How long should records for children be kept?

In the case of children, personal injury claims are allowed up to 3 years after their majority (normally 18 years), although in all cases an individual judge may lengthen the period allowed.

Summary

Much potential litigation can be mitigated by clear and accurate record keeping. Importantly, the NMC makes it clear that it is a nurse's duty to keep up to date with, and adhere to, all relevant legislation and policies relating to record keeping.

Key points
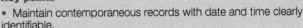
- Maintain contemporaneous records with date and time clearly identifiable.
- Be objective, avoid personal comments.
- Avoid abbreviations and keep language simple and straightforward.

7 Engagement and participation of babies, children, and young people in their care and in the design and delivery of health services

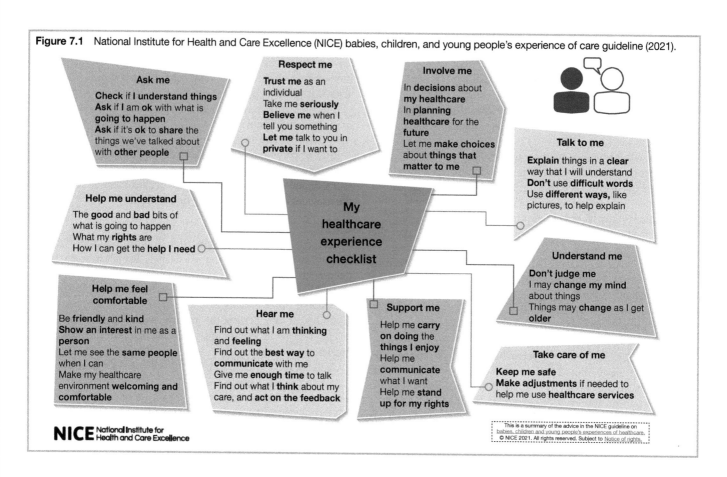

Figure 7.1 National Institute for Health and Care Excellence (NICE) babies, children, and young people's experience of care guideline (2021).

Introduction

Children and young people can provide a window into the National Health Service (NHS), sharing powerful insights of what it is like for them to use their local health services. 'I felt really scared,' said an 11-year-old describing his experience in an Emergency Department (ED) on a Friday night surrounded by intoxicated adults. Statements such as this reach right to the heart of how much further we still have to go in getting our services right for young people. No country has yet been successful in giving its citizens a truly central role in improving health and healthcare, preferring to rely on economic and professional levers, yet there is a shift to empowering citizens and as one-fifth of our population are babies, children, and young people, their voice cannot *not* be heard.

The recent landmark publication by the National Institute for Health and Care Excellence (NICE), the Guideline on 'Babies, Children, and Young People's Experience of Healthcare', provides evidence-based direction on the interventions required to improve

the experiences and outcomes of this population group, enabling us to meet the requirements of the NHS Constitution in ensuring the best possible experience of care for and with babies, children, and young people (Figure 7.1).

As active citizens, children and young people take actions and make contributions in everyday life that influence their personal circumstances and society. While their age and level of maturity are influential, all, whether a baby, toddler, a non-verbal child with complex needs, or an articulate young person, have a right to be listened to and to be active participants in decisions that affect them, the services they utilize, and their communities, as articulated clearly in the United Nations Convention of Rights of the Child. The NICE guidance states that all health organizations must demonstrate how they have listened to the voices of children and young people. We miss opportunities and do a great injustice to babies, children, and young people when as a society we fail to listen to their views, take on board their perspectives, and value their

Children and Young People's Nursing at a Glance, Second Edition. Edited by Elizabeth Gormley-Fleming and Sheila Roberts.
© 2023 John Wiley & Sons Ltd. Published 2023 by John Wiley & Sons Ltd.

contribution in shaping their care and in the role they play in informing the design and delivery of children's health services.

There are two fundamental levels of participation and involvement. The first and perhaps more important is individual engagement in their healthcare, in making choices, and in having a degree of control in decision making, according to their development stage. Frameworks such as 'Ask Three Questions', profiled in NICE's Making decisions about your care (https://www.nice.org.uk/about/what-we-do/our-programmes/nice-guidance/nice-guidelines/shared-decision-making), and health information specifically for children and young people advocated by the Patient Information Forum in its Children and Young People's Guide are resources to draw on. Continuously working to build our communication skills in engaging with children and young people, which the resource 'CYP Me First' advocates for, are helpful, as direct feedback from children and young people indicates that we don't always get communication with them right. Building children and young people's confidence in interactions with health professionals is also required as they prepare for transition into adult services, where self-advocacy skills are essential. The NICE Guidance on transition from children's to adults' services for young people using health or social care services offers direction on this (https://pifonline.org.uk/resources/publications/2020-guide-to-producing-health-information-for-children-and-young-people). The second level is more generic involvement as a service user or as a member of the public to inform the wider development of health services. Twenty-two focus groups with over 200 children between the ages of 4 and 14 years informed the development of the NICE Guidance on experiences of care [NG204]. This work confirmed their desire to be involved in decisions surrounding their personal care and also in the development of health services.

A recent publication entitled *Embedding Young People's Participation in Health Services* explores further individual and collective participation, analysing the impact of the NHS England Youth Forum, which brings together 25 young people annually from across the country to advise on the commissioning of health services. This forum demonstrates that children and young people want to be listened to, have their recommendations acted on, be informed of what happens as a result of their recommendations, and also meet with decision makers so the young people can explain why the recommendations may not have been taken on board. Children and young people value the opportunity to make a difference and see it as an opportunity to develop skills. High-quality, productive engagement results in the development of children and young people's self-confidence; it should be enjoyable, sociable, and fun.

Children and young people are key stakeholders in health and healthcare, not just beneficiaries or passive recipients of services. As health professionals, it is our responsibility to create the mechanisms to facilitate effective engagement of children and young people who are current and future consumers of healthcare to cultivate true participation and co-production across the NHS. If health services are to deliver high-quality, holistic care, the contributions of children and young people need to be harvested, valued, and acted on. Poor healthcare experiences increase the likelihood of unmet healthcare needs. Trauma from poor healthcare experiences is distressing and can have a powerful, long-lasting impact, including on confidence to seek healthcare, as fear and anxiety around accessing and receiving healthcare can be created. Children and young people's engagement and involvement will result in a much richer perspective that will assist in improved outcomes and enhanced services.

Practical hints and tips in achieving effective engagement and participation

• Put in place training programmes for staff to address principles of engagement and participation of children and young people in decisions about their individual care and in wider service enhancement programmes.
• Governance systems and policies need to be in place to ensure that engagement and participation are safe, meaningful, ethical, and systematic.
• Commit to gathering a diverse pool of children and young people. They are not a homogenous group and diverse needs, backgrounds, capabilities, and interests should be utilized.
• Consider collaborating with local authorities, as they have statutory youth councils that can be helpful in progressing engagement activities.
• The aims and objectives of engagement programmes need to be stated clearly from the outset.
• Consent from the child or young person and their parent or guardian is essential if names, quotes, drawings, or photos are used.
• Records of responses, consultation, and engagement should be treated as confidential and should be stored securely.
• Consider provision of training for children and young people, as it can provide them with transferable skills. Accreditation and recognition can assist in sustained engagement and participation.
• Use a broad range of communication strategies including social media/networking sites to advertise opportunities and to secure engagement and participation.
• Monitor and evaluate the effectiveness of engagement and the wider impact of child and youth participation.
• Put effective feedback mechanisms in place so that children and young people realize the impact of their contributions.
• Children and young people's representation is especially meaningful when they have a budget and the power to decide its allocation.
• Programmes should be frequent, child/youth led, and focused.

What to avoid

• Tokenism: organizations need to be committed to valuing input and acting on suggestions.
• Use of jargon or unnecessarily complex information.
• Exploiting children and young people and not giving credit for their contribution.

Key points
• Children and young people have a right to have their voices heard in healthcare.
• Children and young people want to and can be involved in making decisions about their healthcare services.
• Participation by children and young people needs to be valued and not tokenistic.
• Importantly, make it fun and have fun.

8 Observation of the well child

Figure 8.1 Assessment.

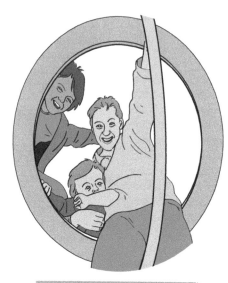

Airway

- Is the child talking or crying?
- Are there any abnormal noises?
- Is the child a normal colour?
- Is there any history of foreign body inhalation?
- Does the child have any history of known airway problems?
- Is the child drooling or unable to swallow their secretions?

Circulation

- Is the child a normal colour?
- Does the child have a normal heart rate?
- Is the child warm and well perfused?
- Is the child drinking sufficiently?
- Is the child passing urine sufficiently?
- Is the child vomiting?
- Does the child have diarrhoea?

Breathing

- Does the child have a rate within normal limits?
- Are there any added sounds?
- Is there any increased work of breathing?
- Is the child a normal colour?
- Is the child known to have any underlying breathing problems?
- Can they talk in sentences?
- Does the child appear breathless?

Disability

- Is the child alert?
- Is the child orientated?
- Does the child have normal tone?
- Is the child acting appropriately?

Exposure

- Does the child have a temperature within normal limits?
- Does the child have a rash?
- Is there any sign of trauma: bruising, bleeding, fracture, marks, burns?

If the parent is concerned, and the assessment shows the child is a well child, then reassurance may be all that is required. However, a parent knows their child best; if they are concerned, then ensure you have not missed something important. If you have assessed the child, and they appear to be a well child, but you still have a concern, then ensure they are reassessed by a senior colleague. Remember, a well child can rapidly become an unwell child. An unwell child can rapidly become a well child.

Children and Young People's Nursing at a Glance, Second Edition. Edited by Elizabeth Gormley-Fleming and Sheila Roberts.
© 2023 John Wiley & Sons Ltd. Published 2023 by John Wiley & Sons Ltd.

It is important for a children's nurse to be able, through observation and assessment (see Figure 8.1), to recognize a well child. Observing a child is generally considered a long-term activity that may occur in childcare settings to monitor the development of an individual. Children's nurses generally have a short snapshot opportunity to observe a child. Observation involves watching and listening to the individual child, noting their expressions, activity, and behaviour, and listening to them talk and interact with others – their peers or adults. Observations are often categorised into five areas:

- Cognition
- Social
- Emotional
- Physical
- Language

Children's nurses therefore need to be aware of the 'normal' development of children across the age span in order to make sense of their observations. However, involvement of the family is also key to understanding the child.

Example

A children's nurse observes a 3-year-old child quietly playing with bricks in the corner of an emergency room waiting area. The child builds a tower of three or four bricks before the tower topples over.

The children's nurse needs to have the knowledge that a 3-year-old should be able to build a tower of nine or ten bricks. Questions are required to ascertain if this is normal for this child – maybe they have never previously played with bricks – or whether this particular child has a visual or dexterity problem that means this is a difficult task for them. However, the nurse observes that the child can run up and down the stairs, one foot per step, a skill more often associated with a 4-year-old.

Stages of development or milestones are indicators of what may be expected; however, every child is unique, and the majority will develop at their own rate. Factors such as being unwell, tired, or anxious (such as being in a strange environment) will affect their activity, making the snapshot opportunity given to a children's nurse even more difficult to use as an indicator as to how well a child is. Factors such as previous experiences, position in a family (i.e. first or third child), and culture will all affect a child's development.

Key points

- Whether assessing or observing a child, the involvement of the family is paramount.
- Understanding the assessment process and the importance of observing and listening is a key skill for children's nurses.
- An apparently well child can quickly become an unwell child.

9 Observation of the sick child

Figure 9.1 Observation. AVPU, Alert, Voice, Pain, Unresponsive; GCS, Glasgow Coma Scale.

Use all your senses to observe what is happening and do not forget to communicate effectively to the child, young person, and family throughout. Do not forget that the vital sign normal range varies with the age of the child

Is the **airway** clear?
Can they talk/cry?
Look, listen, feel

Look at their colour: are they cyanosed?
Do they have mottled skin?
Are they flushed?

Count the **breathing** for a minute and record. Observe the pattern, effort, noise, movement

Listen for a stridor, which is a 'harsh sound coming from a narrowed upper airway, which can be heard on inspiration and/or expiration'. This is a sign of an airway obstruction

Listen for a wheeze, which is a 'high pitched sound heard on expiration in, e.g. children with asthma and bronchiolitis. It is caused by a narrowing of the airway, usually due to excess secretions (mucus)'

Oxygen saturation should not be measured alone; it needs to be combined with a respiratory assessment. Are they receiving oxygen?

Check **circulation**. Take the pulse and count beats for a minute. Observe the rate, rhythm, and volume

It is important to obtain an accurate temperature

Listen to parental concerns

Observe the child's behaviour, cry, position, how they interact with others, activity levels
Check their conscious level (AVPU, GCS)

Watch out for signs of respiratory distress:
• Respiratory rate/pattern/effort
• Nasal flaring
• Grunting
• Wheezing
• Stridor
• Dyspnoea
• Recession
• Use of accessory and intercostal muscles
• Change in chest shape
• Change in movement of chest
• Head bobbing in infants
• Tracheal tug
• Cyanosis
• Oxygen requirement

To measure capillary refill, press the skin firmly for 5 seconds with your finger take off, and count until the normal skin colouration returns
It may be measured centrally, by pressing on the sternum or the forehead, or peripherally, by pressing on the hands or feet. It may be worth measuring both peripherally and centrally. The peripheral capillary refill time will be affected first, but is also affected by factors such as ambient temperature
Normal children have a capillary refill of less than 2 seconds
Observe their urine output
What temperature is their skin?

Figure 9.2 Things to consider when a child or young person is in distress.

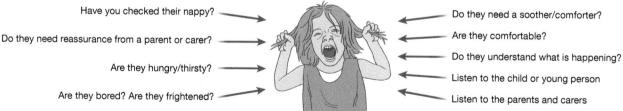

Are they in pain? Use a validated age-/development-appropriate tool to assess and document

Have you checked their nappy?

Do they need reassurance from a parent or carer?

Are they hungry/thirsty?

Are they bored? Are they frightened?

Do they need a soother/comforter?

Are they comfortable?

Do they understand what is happening?

Listen to the child or young person

Listen to the parents and carers

Information gained from the broader assessment of the infant, child, or young person should be recorded, e.g. crying, distress, laughing, playing
Observations and comments made by the child, young person, and parents/carers should be clearly recorded

Communicate effectively with the child or young person and family members to gain an understanding of what is happening

Children and Young People's Nursing at a Glance, Second Edition. Edited by Elizabeth Gormley-Fleming and Sheila Roberts.
© 2023 John Wiley & Sons Ltd. Published 2023 by John Wiley & Sons Ltd.

Introduction

This section will focus on observation of the sick child, in practical steps, and will work in conjunction with a recognized Paediatric Early Warning Score (PEWS), effective communication, and multiprofessional team working.

The importance of observation

At the point of registration, a nurse or nursing associate should be proficient in completing an accurate assessment and be able to accurately process the information gathered during that assessment in order to plan and implement evidence-based, child-centred care.

This needs to be a systematic process and the views of parents/carers must be included.

A baseline of vital signs (Figure 9.1), including temperature, heart/pulse rate, respiratory rate and effort, blood pressure, pain assessment, and level of consciousness of all infants, children, and young people is initially assessed, measured, and recorded on attending hospital and at varying frequencies from then on. Assessment needs to be a continuous process to be alert for changes. It is only through continual assessment that improvement or deterioration in the child or young person's condition can be identified. The healthcare practitioner should know the normal range for heart rate, respiratory rate, and blood pressure for the age of the child (Figure 9.2).

Respiratory rate

It is vital to measure, record, and monitor the respiratory rate, as a measure of either respiratory distress or more systemic problems such as septicaemia.

To measure the respiratory rate accurately, count each breath over a minute.

Crying or coughing can alter the rate considerably, so try to count when the child is calm.

The normal range varies with the age of the child, so check on your PEWS chart what the normal range is. As well as counting the breath rate, check for respiratory recessions, which are the indrawing of the respiratory muscles due to an increased effort of breathing.

Pulse oximetry

A pulse oximeter machine measures the amount of oxygen saturation in the blood using infrared light, giving the percentage of the haemoglobin that is saturated with oxygen.

In the child with no known cardiac or chronic lung disease, oxygen saturation of at least 96% in room air is considered to be within an acceptable normal range. Levels of less than 94% imply significant illness. Oxygen saturation levels below 90% are alarming and require immediate medical attention. Be cautious with monitoring, as movement, skin temperature, and probe placement can be factors affecting accuracy. Use your PEWS chart to record. Children whose normal oxygen saturations fall outside the normal acceptable limits should be documented, for example, a child with a cyanotic heart lesion

Pulse

The pulse is measured by lightly compressing the artery against firm tissue and counting the number of beats in a minute. The pulse varies with age so check your PEWS chart for the normal rate for your child/young person. To measure a peripheral pulse, palpate the radial pulse in an older child, while they are calmest if you can, or if a central pulse is needed use the carotid pulse.

In babies under 6 months old, the radial pulses can be difficult to measure, and the brachial or femoral pulse may be easier to feel. The brachial artery is located above the elbow on the inside of the arm and the femoral pulse is located in the groin. A stethoscope should be used to auscultate the apex heart rate of children less than 2 years of age. Electronic data should be cross-checked by auscultation or palpation of the heart/pulse rate. Electronic readings will not necessarily identify an irregular heart rate or pulse volume.

Capillary refill time

Capillary refill time is a measure of tissue perfusion, describing the time it takes for blood to re-enter capillaries after it has been squeezed out.

This indicates if a child has a compromised circulation, as you are observing whether their body has constricted the blood vessels to the arms and legs in order to preserve the more important central circulation, as would happen with serious bacterial sepsis or dehydration. This is a very useful measure of circulation in children, since blood pressure does not drop until the child is extremely ill, and tachycardia is not a 100% reliable sign. Normal capillary refill time is less than two seconds. The ambient temperature of the environment should be considered. Capillary refill time is normally measured by compressing the finger pulp on one of the fingers for five seconds. The hand should be held at heart height. Normal colour should return to the nail pulp within two seconds.

Blood pressure

Blood pressure can be difficult to measure in children because they can get upset when the cuff goes tight on their arm. The blood pressure is maintained until very late in the process of shock. This is because children have such good peripheral vasoconstriction to compensate. To measure the blood pressure, it is very important to use the right size of cuff. The cuff should measure two-thirds of the length of the upper arm.

Sucking, crying, and eating can influence blood pressure measurements and these should be noted.

Temperature

It is important to get an accurate temperature in children. A temperature should be recorded on all children who attend with an acute presentation of illness with the device applicable for their age.

Key recommendations from the National Institute for Health and Care Excellence (NICE) guideline on fever in children state that oral and rectal routes should not be routinely used to measure the body temperature of children aged 0–5 years. They recommend that 'in infants under the age of four weeks, body temperature should be measured with an electronic thermometer in the axilla' and 'in children aged four weeks to five years, healthcare professionals should measure body temperature by one of the following methods: electronic thermometer in the axilla, chemical dot thermometer in the axilla and infra-red tympanic thermometer'. Check your local Trust guidelines for which are used. Forehead chemical thermometers are unreliable and should not be used by healthcare professionals, but have become more widespread in their use recently.

Child-, young person-, and family-centred care

It is essential that all observations and assessments are carried out using effective communication appropriate for the age, development, and understanding of the child or young person, and with consideration of the family.

A full explanation of the procedure is needed when gaining consent.

Key points

- Vital signs should be documented on a PEWS chart.
- The correct site should be used for measuring heart rate.
- Communication is essential as gaining the cooperation and consent of the child is paramount.

10 Septic screening

Figure 10.1 Septic screening. AVPU, Alert, Voice, Pain, Unresponsive; IO, intraosseous; IV, intravenous.

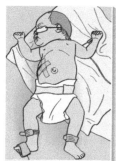

An ABCDE assessment should have been carried out before a septic screen proceeds:

Airway – patent. Apply 15 L oxygen through a non-rebreathe mask if required

Breathing – effective, check oxygen saturations, respiratory rate, and look for signs of respiratory distress

Circulation – is the infant stable enough to wait for IV access or is IO required? Check heart rate, blood pressure, colour, and capillary refill time

Disability – AVPU, or amended Glasgow Coma Score assessment completed, blood sugar sample obtained to rule out hypo-/hyperglycaemia, check pupil size

Exposure – assess for hypo-/hyperthermia. Check for any rashes (in particular petechiae). Look for injuries, bruises, marks, or burns

Stabilize the infant before considering septic screen and ensure reassessment is continuous while screening takes place

Septic screen consists of the following:
- Full blood count
- Blood culture lactate
- C-reactive protein
- Urine microscopy sensitivity and culture
- Stool sample
- Chest X-ray
- Cerebrospinal fluid (CSF) if not contraindicated
- Swabs of any wound sites
- Swab of throat, ears, nose, or eyes if indicated

Figure 10.2 Point-of-patient-care lactate measurement device.

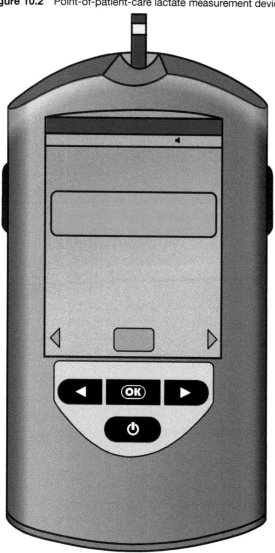

Figure 10.3 Heparanized syringe for arterial blood sample for lactate level.

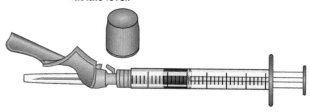

Box 10.1 Paediatric sepsis 6.

1. Give high-flow oxygen
2. Obtain intravenous (IV) or intraosseous (IO) access
3. Give IV or IO antibiotics
4. Fluid resuscitation
5. Get senior clinical colleagues
6. Consider inotropic support

Remember

1. Stabilize.
2. Assess ABCDE.
3. Obtain verbal consent if at all possible.
4. Consider pain management.
5. Document which tests have been carried out and when so results can be expected.

Children and Young People's Nursing at a Glance, Second Edition. Edited by Elizabeth Gormley-Fleming and Sheila Roberts.
© 2023 John Wiley & Sons Ltd. Published 2023 by John Wiley & Sons Ltd.

What is sepsis?

Sepsis is a whole-body inflammatory reaction to infection, usually pathogens in the blood and generally bacteria.

Clinical features include the following:

- Temperature less than 36°C or greater than 38.5°C (38°C if immunocompromised)
- Low blood pressure (late sign in children)
- Tachycardia
- Tachypnoea
- Limb pain
- Change in behaviour – sleepiness, irritability, lethargy, floppiness.
- Altered AVPU (Alert, Voice, Pain, Unresponsive)
- Prolonged capillary time >2 seconds
- Rash – non-blanching/mottled skin
- Cyanosis – SaO_2 <90%

Stabilization of the infant or child

Often, when procedures are carried out on sick children, medical professionals lose sight of the basics while they are concentrating on a task, for example taking blood. A shocked, septic, shut-down sick child requires stabilization and continuous assessment of their ABCDE (Airway, Breathing, Circulation, Disability, Exposure). The Paediatric Sepsis 6 should be commenced if there is a high suspicion that the child has sepsis (Box 10.1 and Figure 10.1).

It is dangerous to begin any procedure on an unstable child, as the procedure may exacerbate a problem and make the infant or child deteriorate further.

Sick infants do not like being handled. They are usually hypoxic, will become increasingly distressed, and their tachycardia and tachypnoea may advance. They may deteriorate further and become bradycardic and apnoeic.

Blood tests

Full blood count, lactate, C-reactive protein (CRP), blood glucose, and cultures can be taken from intravenous (IV) access or intraosseous (IO) access (although usually only enough bone marrow is obtained to carry out a blood sugar assessment). If bone marrow is sent to the laboratory, it is important to indicate that it is not venous blood, as it will look different under the microscope.

Serum lactate level is used as a marker to reflect systemic tissue hypoperfusion. It reflects the level of cellular dysfunction and is now included in the clinical criteria for septic shock. L-lactate is the end product of anaerobic glycolysis. Hyperlactatemia in sepsis is an important outcome indicator. It may originate from a deficit in oxygen delivery, impaired oxygen extraction, stress, peripheral shunting, or an increase in adrenergic stimulation. Lactate elevation primarily arises from tissue hypoxia that occurs from a deficit in the transport of oxygen. Normal lactate level is 0.5–2.2 mmol/L from arterial whole blood in all age groups. A lactate level of greater than 2.0 mmol/L indicates hyperlactatemia and requires urgent senior medical review of the child.

Lactate levels may be tested at the point of patient care. A heparinized blood gas syringe is required and the sample can be analysed on a blood gas analyser. Point-of-patient-care lactate measurement devices are now available and results can be made available quickly at the child's bedside (Figure 10.2).

If enough blood is obtained, a blood gas assessment is helpful to indicate how acidotic the infant or child is (Figure 10.3).

The blood test results should be available quite quickly, but the cultures take 48 hours to be processed.

Urine

A clean catch urine is recommended and this can cause some challenges, depending on the age and sex of the child. It may sometimes be necessary to obtain a catheter or a suprapubic sample from the infant or child.

Stool sample

This is easier to obtain from an infant's nappy, but if there are frequent abnormal stools, taking a sample is quite simple. Remember personal protective equipment at all times.

Chest X-ray

Ensure the infant or child is stable and has a parent and/or member of staff with them, and that the X-ray is carried out in a timely manner to help prevent hypothermia and possible deterioration from increased handling.

Results are available fairly quickly and help in the differential diagnosis of sepsis from pneumonia.

Lumbar puncture for cerebrospinal fluid sample

A lumbar puncture is often contraindicated in a child who is neurologically unstable, as it can have catastrophic consequences. It is unlikely that physicians will suggest a lumbar puncture when the patient is unstable, and it should always be questioned if considered.

If a lumbar puncture is required, ensure an ABCDE assessment is carried out before commencing the procedure, and ensure it is done in a safe environment with emergency equipment ready, including oxygen, bag valve mask, suction, and resuscitation trolley in case of further deterioration.

In an infant, observe the airway and breathing continuously, as the position of the infant has the potential to occlude the airway. It may be advisable to ask the parent to step outside the room while the procedure is being undertaken. In an older child, consider analgesia and provide reassurance, as it can be a frightening and painful procedure.

Specimens usually take 48 hours to be cultured.

Swabs

Swabs of wound sites, pegs, catheters, and discharging ears, noses, and throats can be useful in identifying the source of infection and are pain-free and quick. The results take 24–48 hours to culture.

Consent

Parental verbal consent should be obtained if at all possible and documented in the notes. A child that is Fraser competent may consent to a procedure, but also has the right to refuse. The involvement of parents, carers, and play specialists may be required.

Key points
- Know the red flag signs: hypotension, lactate >2 mmol/l, extreme tachycardia/tachypnoea, SaO_2 <90%, P or U on AVPU, immunocompromised, non-blanching rash, or mottled skin.
- If high suspicion of sepsis, get help, commence the Sepsis 6.

11 Advanced physical assessment

Figure 11.1 Rapid clinical assessment of a seriously ill child will identify any potential respiratory, cardiovascular, or neurological failures. Use the ABCDE approach for a systematic assessment of the child.

Airway and Breathing

- Is the child awake, talking? Do they sound breathless?
- Can you hear abnormal breath sounds?
- Is the child using accessory muscles to aid breathing?
- Are they breathing fast?
- Do they look pale or cyanosed?
- What position are they sat in?
- What are the O_2 saturations, do they reflect the child's actual condition?

Circulation

- Is the heart rate and BP normal for age range?
- Feel their hands and feet, are they warm or cold?
- Check the capillary refill time
- If they are in nappies, are they wet or dry?
- Are the lips dry and cracked?
- Check the fontanelle

Disability

- Is the child running and playing?
- Are they unsteady on their feet and falling over – do not presume this is normal
- Is the child meeting developmental milestones?
- If the child is crying, is it possible to console them?
- Check the blood sugar level as soon as possible if the child is having a fit or is unduly drowsy or irritable

Exposure

- Check the child's temperature
- Check from head to toe and back to front for the presence of any rashes, scars, bruises, or other injuries. Do not presume all injuries are accidental

If in doubt, discuss with a senior colleague and report in line with your local safeguarding policy

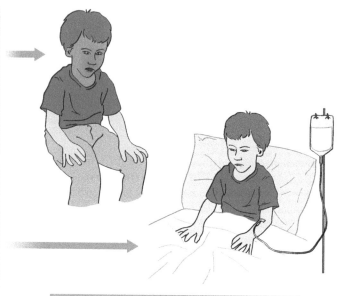

This chapter follows on from the section on observation of the sick child (Chapter 10), further developing these skills in the advanced physical assessment of children. Utilizing the ABCDE (Airway, Breathing, Circulation, Disability, Exposure) approach, this chapter will allow you to identify the deteriorating child and consider appropriate action.

While the majority of children who become unwell will recover with minimal intervention, the rapidity with which a child can deteriorate can lead to anxiety in even experienced practitioners. A rapid clinical assessment of a seriously ill child will identify any potential respiratory, cardiovascular, or neurological failures (Figure 11.1). Rapid assessment allows for initiation of appropriate treatment to prevent progression to respiratory or cardiac arrest

The ABCDE approach allows for a systematic assessment of the child to take place:
A – airway
B – breathing
C – circulation
D – disability
E – exposure

A baseline of vital signs includes temperature, heart/pulse rate, respiratory rate and effort, blood pressure, pain assessment, level of consciousness, and oxygen saturation. Physical assessment commences with observing the general appearance of the child and how the child interacts with the adults and others around them. Do they look well or unwell? Are they pale or flushed? Active or lethargic? Calm or agitated? Compliant or combative? What position are they in – sitting, lying, are they moving?

Airway

It is vital to establish that the airway is patent on immediate inspection and assessment of the child. Look for noises, secretions, coughing, and the presence of any artificial airways.

A crying, screaming, or talkative child indicates an airway that is patent at that time, whereas a child who appears floppy and quiet may require immediate airway support. If there are any concerns about a child's ability to maintain their airway, follow the Paediatric Life Support Algorithm. Look at the child: do they look cyanosed around the lips and nose? In children with darker skin it may not be immediately apparent, so check the tongue. If the child

Children and Young People's Nursing at a Glance, Second Edition. Edited by Elizabeth Gormley-Fleming and Sheila Roberts.
© 2023 John Wiley & Sons Ltd. Published 2023 by John Wiley & Sons Ltd.

seems to be drooling excessively, ask the parent or carer if this is normal. Difficulty in swallowing can be an indication of an airway problem. What sounds can you hear? A bark, seal-like cough, or noisy breathing on inspiration can indicate some narrowing of the upper airway, as in croup for example.

Breathing

Once a clear airway is established, breathing can be assessed. Remove the child's top with consent. Remember to maintain privacy, dignity, and warmth at all times. This assessment must take account of the work and effectiveness of breathing.

Look at the rate of breathing: is it within normal parameters for the child's age? Is the chest moving equally on inspiration? Auscultate the chest and listen for breath sounds. Bilateral air entry with the absence of adventitious noises and equal chest movement is the norm. If it is not, this may indicate a pneumothorax, infection, or inflammation.

Is there any drawing (recession) under the ribs (subcostal), between the ribs (intercostal), or in the sternal notch (tracheal)? While all infants 'tummy' breathe, if this is fast and drawing in excessively it can indicate a breathing problem.

Consider the child's general position. Are they in a relaxed position or playing? Children in respiratory distress will often adopt a tripod position. This is where they sit with their arms stretched out and pushing up against a table or their knees. They will stretch their head back and may possibly be blowing out when breathing in an attempt to improve ventilation.

Listen to the child talking. If they are only able to answer in short sentences or not at all, then these are signs of respiratory distress. Listen for any noises during breathing. Wheeze is the noise air makes as it is squeezed back out of the lungs. This is not necessarily a sign of respiratory distress in toddlers and infants if the other symptoms discussed are absent, but it can be a source of concern for parents.

Oxygen saturation levels, as discussed in other chapters, are a useful measure, but must be considered in the context of the child's overall condition.

As part of the ongoing physical assessment of the child, note oxygen requirements and delivery mode.

Circulation

Assessment of the child's state of hydration and circulation can take place once the respiratory system has been assessed. Checking the pulse is integral to assessing circulation. While palpating the pulse, consider not just the rate of the heart, but the volume and rhythm of the pulse. The location used should be noted. A thin, thready central pulse can indicate shock or severe dehydration. In infants and small children it is often easier to check the brachial pulse than the radial pulse, or consider using a stethoscope placed over the apex of the heart. For infants under 6 months of age, consider taking a femoral pulse when checking the nappy area. Remember, as with all procedures, to explain to the parent or carer what you are doing and why.

Look at the child's face and hands. Do they look pale or grey, are the lips dry and cracked? Look at the oral mucosa and nail-bed colour. Note any finger clubbing. Along with sunken eyes, this could indicate a child in shock or dehydrated. Skin turgor should be assessed and noted.

In infants with a patent fontanelle, ask the parents if it looks sunk in any way compared to its normal appearance. Capillary refill time is an important measure, but bear in mind that small infants and toddlers can be very sensitive to environmental changes and will have a sluggish capillary refill time due to a change in room temperature rather than shock. For this reason it is often better to check the capillary refill time on the forehead or chest. Consider urine output and ask the parent or carer how long the current nappy has been on if one is worn. If it is dry after being on for a few hours, consider the child's hydration status.

Disability

In the context of advanced assessment, when discussing disability it is not in relation to an existing condition, but rather to any acute changes in the child's level of consciousness. The use of the AVPU (Alert, Voice, Pain, Unresponsive) system allows for a rapid initial assessment of the child, and goes hand in hand with assessment of the airway. Is the child awake and responsive, or floppy and unconscious? The biggest risk to life in an unconscious child is an occluded airway. If the child is awake, ask the attending carers if the child is their usual self, or if anything has changed. Signs of a neurological problem are headaches, vomiting – especially on waking or after a head injury – dizzy spells, altered visual acuity, or a change in the appearance of the eyes. In infants, neurological signs can be more discreet, but a bulging fontanelle or inconsolable high-pitched crying is an indication of a problem.

A formal tool for assessing neurological status is the Glasgow Coma Scale, and an adapted paediatric version is available. This uses a scoring system to assess the level of neurological deficit and can provide an indication as to what treatment may need to be carried out. Infants have a poor ability to maintain their blood sugar level when unwell, so any signs of an altered level of consciousness in infants and small children should trigger checking of the blood glucose level. Identify any abnormal movement or gait. The use of mobility aids, prosthetics/orthotics, hearing aids, or glasses should be noted and recorded.

The growth and development of the infant and child should be noted. This will also include measurement of the head circumference, assessment of sensory function, and fine and gross motor skills.

Exposure

The final part of the advanced physical assessment is an overall review of the child. The skin should be assessed the colour, turgor, brushing wounds, lesions, rashes, and pressure injuries noted.

Infants and small children should be assessed from head to toe for the presence of any rashes, scars, bruises, or deformities. Remember to check the axilla, the nappy area, behind the ears, and around the nape of the neck. If you suspect there is a non-blanching rash, then have a high suspicion for sepsis until proven otherwise. While the majority of rashes seen will be normal, innocuous rashes associated with various common childhood conditions, they are often a source of anxiety for carers. If older children present acutely unwell, then check for the presence of rashes, but allow them the opportunity to undress in privacy before conducting the assessment. If the temperature has not been checked already then this should be done, but remember sepsis can present without fever, particularly in infants. Unusual marks or bruises must never be ignored and in the case of child protection concerns, reference should be made to local safeguarding procedures.

Gastrointestinal system

This will include inspection, light palpation, and auscultation of the abdomen. It will include the level of hydration and nutrition status of the infant or child, plus the normal feeding/dietary pattern, volume taken, and route (oral, nasogastric, gastrostomy, intravenous). A recognized nutrition screening tool should be used. Assessment of pain level, nausea, and vomiting is required, along with an assessment of their elimination pattern. Blood glucose should be considered as clinically indicated. The abdomen should be inspected for shape and symmetry, contours, distension, visible peristalsis, and any scars or stomas present. The umbilicus in neonates should be observed for redness, exudate, and the presence of a cord stump. Abdominal girth may be measured and auscultation will identify the presence of bowel sounds and bowel motility. Palpation will identify tenderness, pain, distention, and guarding. This must be performed with a light pressure.

Renal

Identify normal bladder and bowel routine. Note the pattern and hydration status of the infant/child. Any fluid restrictions should be noted. A urinalysis must be performed and blood is usually taken for biochemistry if indicated.

Musculoskeletal

Observation of the infant/child from a distance will be a good indication of musculoskeletal dysfunction. The inspection should include gait and ambulation, posture and body movement, and limbs and joints for swelling, redness, and any obvious deformity and the range of joint movements. Muscle strength, mass, and tone can be assessed by palpation.

Eyes

The infant/child will need to be fully compliant in order to competently assess their eyes. This will include noting that the eyes are bilateral in symmetry, shape, and placement in relation to the ears, size and shape of the pupil, and how the pupil reacts to light. The conjunctiva should be noted for inflammation, discharge, and colour, as should the sclera. The iris should be checked for up-slanting and down-slanting. Visual acuity should be checked if the child is old enough to comply. The presence of tears should be noted, particularly in the unconscious child, as they will need assistance to protect their cornea from drying out. Red-eye reflex should be assessed if indicated, as lesions of the retina are detected through visualization of the retina with an ophthalmoscope.

Ears/nose and throat

Upper respiratory infection, allergies, dental caries, trauma, and tonsilitis/pharyngitis are all common conditions in childhood. This involves inspection of the ears, nose, and mouth for symmetry, shape, patency, presence of blood or fluid or foreign objects, and odours.

Evaluation

All information from the assessment should be documented accurately. Abnormal findings will need to be actioned to the appropriate person and the care planned should be evidence based. Assessment is a continuous activity, as indicated by the clinical needs of the infant or child. Adaptation will be required depending on the age of the patient and the young person should have the HEADSSS tool (see Chapter 1) included in part of their physical assessment.

Key points

- Advanced physical assessment is a component of children's and young person's nursing practice.
- The children's and young person's nurse must be able to accurately process the information gathered during assessment to identify the care needs of the individual.
- The approach taken for physical assessment should be systematic, but there will be adaptations required for the various age groups.

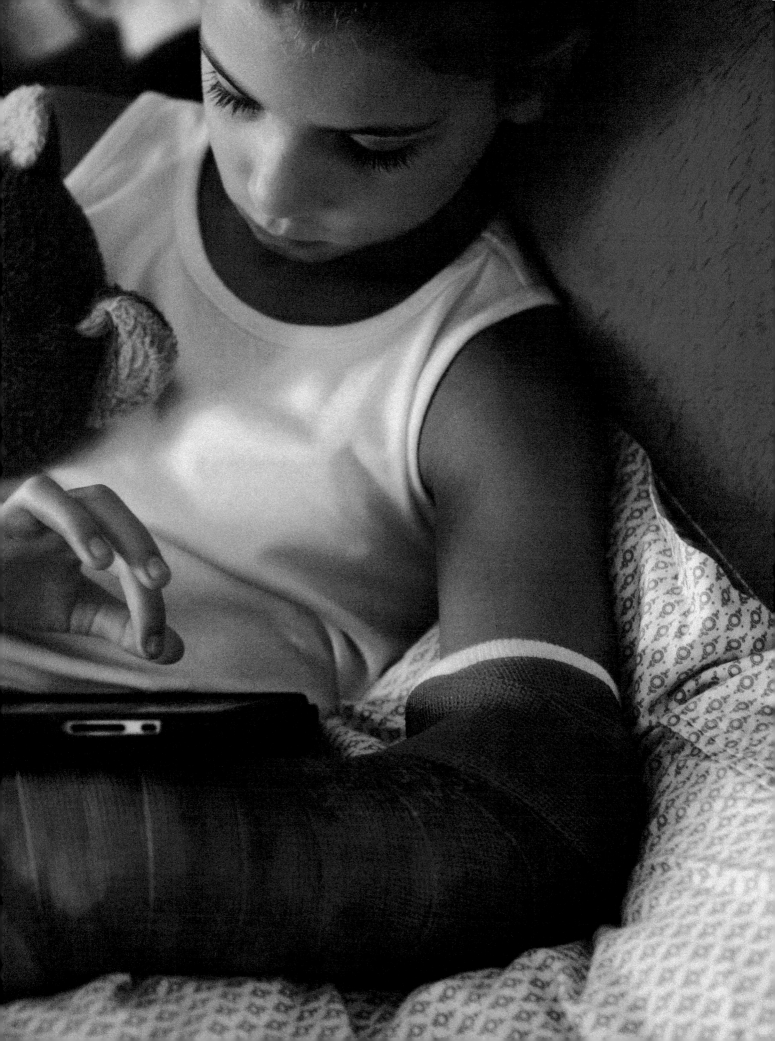

12 Developmental assessment

Figure 12.1 Developmental assessment.

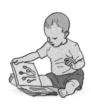

Birth to 2 years (sensorimotor stage)

Physical – rapid growth, key skills developed, gross/fine motor skills, milestones

Cognitive – learn and solve problems, perceptual development, reflexes, intelligence, speech and language development: pre-linguistic/linguistic stage, understand and use language

Personality – beginnings of self-concept, trust and mistrust, temperament, gender differences

Social – facial expressions (e.g. smiling), nature versus nurture, attachment/bonding, imitation, developing autonomy

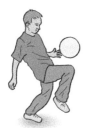

2–7 years (preoperational stage)

Physical – body shape, brain growth, sensory development, nutrition, safety, gross/fine motor skills development: skipping (gross motor skill); using a pencil to draw (fine motor skill)

Cognitive – egocentric, role of education, language development, cultural factors

Personality – self-concept, gender identity

Social – friendships, work of play, consideration of others, family life, moral development, behaviours

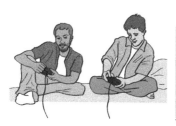

7–12 years (concrete operational stage)

Physical – slow steady growth, motor development, gross motor coordination; fine motor skills, draw detailed pictures

Cognitive – coherent, logical thought processes, appreciate others' perspectives, unable to consider abstract ideas

Personality – developing competence, appreciate own internal traits

Social – sensitive to the importance of friends, level of morality

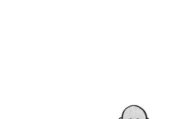

12 years to adulthood (formal operational stage)

Physical – primary and secondary sexual characteristics develop, puberty, growth spurts

Cognitive – abstract and hypothetical thoughts, consider consequences of actions, systematic problem solving, invulnerability

Personality – organized and accurate self-concept, identity formation, developmental self-esteem

Social – personal identity important, peer relationships, conformability, sexual experimentation, autonomy, parental/family conflicts

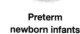

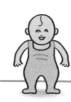
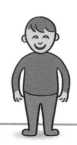
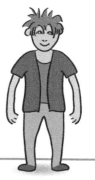
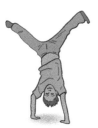

Preterm newborn infants

Term newborn infants (0–28 days)

Infants and toddlers (>28 days to 23 months)

Children (2–11 years)

Adolescents (12–18 years)

Children and Young People's Nursing at a Glance, Second Edition. Edited by Elizabeth Gormley-Fleming and Sheila Roberts.
© 2023 John Wiley & Sons Ltd. Published 2023 by John Wiley & Sons Ltd.

Development occurs throughout the life span and refers to changes that take place. These changes are complex and result in the individual developing capacity and capabilities towards achieving maturity.

Measuring and assessing development

Development is measured using recognized, validated scales and is divided into four main areas:

- Physical growth, hearing, vision, coordination, and locomotion
- Cognitive: language and understanding
- Psychosocial
- Emotional

The emphasis in the UK is on early detection and action, which is the philosophy of the Healthy Child Programme. Appropriate and timely referrals are subsequently made if action is required. Current practice advocates a full review at the age of 2.5 years.

Assessment is usually performed by a registered healthcare professional, such as a general practitioner, health visitor, or paediatrician. Children's and young people's nurses are required to have a comprehensive understanding of child development and be able to competently assess the child's level of development as part of the assessment process. Each child is assessed as an individual, considering their age, expected stage of development, and how this information relates to the various identified milestones. Birth and family history, alongside parental and professional observations of the infant's or child's movements, skills, awareness, and interactions, are important aspects of the assessment process. This process of assessment involves investigations, tests, and physical examination and should include the parent in supporting the child.

Genetics and nature versus nurture

Many debates on the nature of child development have centred on nature versus nurture. Genes are the blueprint of human development and cell function. These may manifest themselves in the inherited characteristics of the infant (e.g. eye and hair colouring). During the prenatal stages of development, natural mutations of the genes occur. These genetic factors can impact on the development of the foetus (e.g. Down's syndrome); this is referred to as the 'nature' side of development. The 'nurture' factors that impact on the child's development include the home, family, culture, school, social activities, and communities. Risks to any of these factors can affect the child's overall development (e.g. reading will develop a child's vocabulary; malnourishment may lead to poor brain development and suboptimal IQ). Cultural experiences can influence the child's social development as beliefs can guide and direct behaviours.

Developmental milestones

A developmental milestone is a skill that a child acquires in a specified period of time (Figure 12.1). For example, most children learn the skill of walking by the age of 9–15 months. If a child did not walk until they were 22 months, this would suggest a developmental delay, which must be closely observed and monitored by the parent and health professional.

Child development is very complex. Children develop along predicted progressive pathways within the main areas of development. The aspects of child development are linked, for example head control

must be achieved before the child can sit independently. This is referred to as cephalo-caudal development – head to toe via the spine.

The significant milestones are:

- Smiles – 5–8 weeks
- Laughs – 4 months
- Sits with support – 6 months
- Sits unsupported – 8–9 months
- Crawls – 8–9 months
- Stands/walks – 12 months
- Pincer grasp – 9 months
- Language – single syllables 6 months, one to three words by age of 1 year
- Walks backwards – 18 months

After each assessment a record is made and these developments are recorded within the child's personal health record – commonly referred to as the 'red book', which is now an electronic record. In order to assess developmental milestones, an underpinning knowledge of normal development must exist.

Developmental delay

Developmental delay is described as a recognized significant delay in the infant's achievement of predicted developmental milestones. This delay may affect only one aspect of development or include all aspects of development – generally referred to as global developmental delay. Natural or environmental factors may be linked to developmental delay and may be indicative of a more permanent setback or disability. Delays in development must be monitored and investigated by the healthcare professional, in order to give appropriate care and support to the child and family.

Implications for practice

Infants, children, and young people are changing every day in terms of their abilities and skills, learning new knowledge and simply growing. Children's nurses need to understand how children grow and develop in order to support both the child and their patients to understand their prospective development and how it may be disrupted or affected. Additionally, when children's nurses come into contact with an infant, child, or young person, they need to be able to plan and provide care that appreciates the patient's stage of development and understanding of what is happening to them and integrate this into care delivery. Children's nurses have a professional and ethical responsibility to preserve and safeguard the public and promote ethical practice in assessment and adherence to professional codes of practice. In performing developmental assessments, obtaining informed consent is considered a fundamental aspect of clinical practice for all healthcare professionals.

Key points

- It is important to know about normal child development so deviations from the expected are identified early and action taken.
- Development is sequential and skills are acquired in order to prepare the child for the next stage, e.g. head control before sitting
- The emphasis is on early detection and effective and appropriate referral to enable the child to achieve their full potential.

13 Paediatric early warning score

Figure 13.1 Paediatric Early Warning Scores (PEWS) are a systematic tool designed to detect early deterioration in children.

Benefits of PEWS

- A full set of vital signs are recorded and repeated as the child's condition dictates
- Aids early recognition of the sick child
- Empowers nursing and medical staff to escalate concerns
- Documents trends in the child's condition – improvement or deterioration
- Reduces risk of cardiorespiratory arrest
- Reduces number of unexpected paediatric intensive care admissions

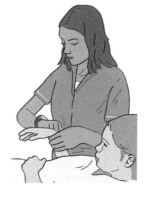

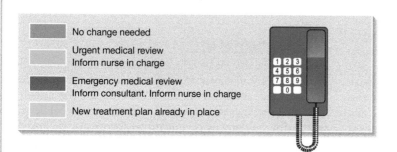

No change needed

Urgent medical review
Inform nurse in charge

Emergency medical review
Inform consultant. Inform nurse in charge

New treatment plan already in place

Once the vital signs have been recorded and scored, the treatment algorithm should be consulted, actioned, and documented. The Situation, Background, Assessment, and Recommendation tool should be used to communicate findings when escalating concerns

The vital signs that must be recorded are heart rate, respiratory rate, and blood pressure. Oxygen saturation should also be recorded.

However, there are many variations of early warning scores in use that may require measurement of other physical signs.

Age-appropriate parameters

Age (years)	Respiratory rate	Heart rate (beats/min)	Systolic BP (mmHg)
<1	30–40	110–160	80–90°
1–2	25–35	100–150	85–95°
2–5	25–30	95–140	85–100°
5–12	20–25	80–120	90–110°
>12	15–20	60–100	100–120°

Children and Young People's Nursing at a Glance, Second Edition. Edited by Elizabeth Gormley-Fleming and Sheila Roberts.
© 2023 John Wiley & Sons Ltd. Published 2023 by John Wiley & Sons Ltd.

The Paediatric Early Warning Score (PEWS) is a systematic clinical tool (Figure 13.1) used to facilitate and detect the signs of clinical deterioration in the patient. Initially, early warning systems were devised as a method of early identification and prediction of which children are likely to deteriorate and necessitate high dependency or intensive care, as it is known that children who die or require intensive care have exhibited signs of deterioration prior to collapse. Regular recording of vital signs will also indicate the child's response to treatment. This combined method of observations and recording makes healthcare staff situationally aware of the child's condition. They are now an integral part of the care of the majority of acutely ill children in hospital. They may have some use as a triage tool in the A&E department. PEWS is a risk management tool and may also be referred to as 'track and trigger'. PEWS tools should be used in conjunction with the National Institute for Health and Care Excellence (NICE) Traffic Light System.

Calculating the paediatric early warning score

The score is calculated by adding the numerical values together that have been assigned to the routine observations that are undertaken on infants and children. Once the score is calculated, the nursing and/or medical staff refer to the algorithm on the chart, which will indicate the action required. If using triggers from one parameter and there is an increase in PEWS above 0 or there is concern about the child's condition, all parameters should be measured to give a holistic clinical picture of the child's condition. Age-appropriate charts must be used (Box 13.1).

This multiparameter scoring system includes routine observations:

- heart rate
- respiratory rate
- blood pressure
- oxygen saturation level
- temperature
- conscious level

Observations may also include assessing a more detailed level of consciousness and capillary refill time. Both of these require clinical judgement. The other measure that is recorded on the PEWS chart is the amount of oxygen the child is receiving. Other observations and treatments may also be considered, but these will not be part of the scoring system.

Each parameter is allocated a score, which are then added together to give an overall score. The greater the deviation from normal for the physical sign being measured, the higher the score. Generally, if the child's clinical condition is deteriorating the score is high, thus alerting the nursing and medical team that early intervention is required in anticipation of preventing adverse outcomes. Early intervention may prevent the need for transferring the child to a higher level of care. It may also indicate the need for more frequent observation of the child and a revision of their treatment plan. Escalation guidelines must be followed in accordance with local protocol.

Box 13.1 The age ranges of PEWS scoring systems.

0–11 months
12–23 months
2–4 years
5–11 years
12 years+

How often should a PEWS be undertaken?

The frequency with which a PEWS is undertaken will be determined by the clinical condition of the child, and the type of treatment they are receiving. For example, high-risk treatment such as chemotherapy, blood transfusion, or specific disease pathways may indicate the need for frequent assessment of the child's vital signs. Other situations may include:

- On admission and thereafter with frequency indicated by the child's condition during the acute phase of their hospitalization.
- Where there is concern of serious illness and risk of deterioration.
- Postoperatively, to reflect the clinical needs of the child.
- Chemotherapy.
- Blood transfusion.
- Decreased level of consciousness.
- Any increase in PEWS.
- Clinical judgement.
- Parental concerns.

PEWS provides nursing and medical staff with a framework to escalate their concerns about a child to a more senior team member. Abnormal observations recorded by healthcare support workers and students should be verified as per local policy. PEWS is a tool and not a replacement for clinical judgement. Medical help should be sought if the child is deteriorating irrespective of their PEWS (Box 13.2).

Education on how to use the PEWS tool effectively should be considered.

Limitations

There is currently limited research into the trigger points for scoring and escalating concerns. Inconsistency in the use of PEWS and scoring systems make it difficult to validate its effectiveness.

There are a variety of scoring systems in existence, but with limited methodological assessment to identify their reliability or validity. Work has commenced on developing a national PEWS system for England following the success of the development and rollout of the adult National Early Warning Score 2.

Box 13.2 Escalation if PEWS >0 or concern.

If child is deteriorating suddenly – call resuscitation team 2222
If PEWS is >0 then:

Child should be reviewed as per escalation guide.
New plan of care should be agreed and documented. This may include investigations
and interventions.
Identify when the child will be next reviewed and document in their care records.

Key points

- PEWS has become increasingly used to prevent unexpected intensive care admissions.
- Always escalate if you have concerns about the child's condition irrespective of the PEWS.
- PEWS enables healthcare professionals to intervene early and prevent deterioration of the child's condition.
- PEWS provides healthcare professionals with a framework to escalate their concerns.
- There are many scoring systems in use, some of which have limited methodological assessment.

14 Paediatric critical care

Figure 14.1 Intensive care transport team.

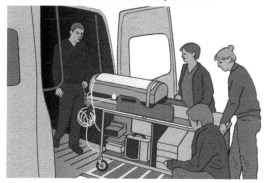

Figure 14.2 Monitoring of vital signs.

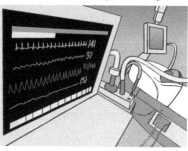

141
91
8 1/44
(5)

Figure 14.3 Non-rebreather mask.

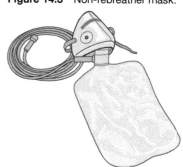

Figure 14.4 Oropharyngeal airways.

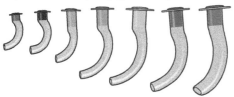

Figure 14.5 Self-inflating (Ambu) bag.

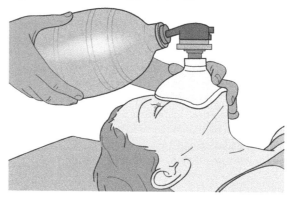

Figure 14.6 Insertion of endotracheal tube.

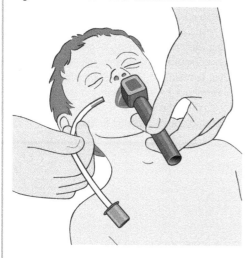

Figure 14.7 Capnography.

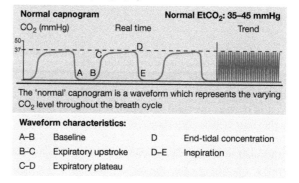

Normal capnogram   **Normal EtCO$_2$: 35–45 mmHg**

CO$_2$ (mmHg)   Real time   Trend

The 'normal' capnogram is a waveform which represents the varying CO$_2$ level throughout the breath cycle

Waveform characteristics:

A–B	Baseline	D	End-tidal concentration
B–C	Expiratory upstroke	D–E	Inspiration
C–D	Expiratory plateau		

Figure 14.8 Syringe pump for drug administration.

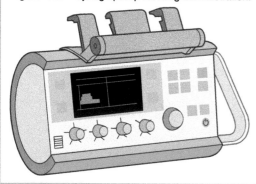

Figure 14.9 Insertion of intraosseous needle. IV, intravenous.

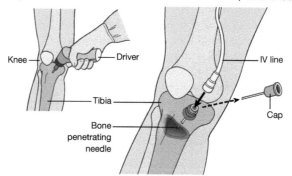

Knee — Driver
— IV line
Tibia
Bone penetrating needle
Cap

Children and Young People's Nursing at a Glance, Second Edition. Edited by Elizabeth Gormley-Fleming and Sheila Roberts.
© 2023 John Wiley & Sons Ltd. Published 2023 by John Wiley & Sons Ltd.

Paediatric critical care describes an enhanced level of care when children require observation, monitoring, and interventions that cannot be delivered in another setting. Children require intensive care for a variety of reasons: for example, respiratory difficulty due to an airway infection, a mechanical obstruction in the airway, septicaemia, seizures, or following a serious traumatic incident or major surgery.

There are three levels of paediatric critical care identified:
Level 1: Basic-level critical care
Level 2: Intermediate-level critical care
Level 3: Advanced-level critical care

Levels 1 and 2 are aligned to high-dependency care, so may be delivered in secondary care settings, whereas level 3 is defined as intensive care, therefore requiring specialist paediatric services.

Most children present to their local hospital and receive immediate care delivered by the emergency department, and paediatric and anaesthetic staff. If the child is assessed to be seriously ill they will require specialist intensive care advice and treatment in a tertiary children's hospital. A transfer will usually be required. This could involve travelling long distances, especially if the child lives in a rural location.

The centralization of intensive care services for children has seen the development of standards that address the needs of critically ill children and their families from the time of arrival at secondary care centres to the quality of care they receive in a tertiary paediatric intensive care unit. This includes the requirement for tertiary centres to provide transport for children requiring intensive care. Transport requirements include specially equipped land ambulances and air transport. Results from numerous studies have demonstrated decreased morbidity and a lower critical incident rate (e.g. endotracheal tube dislodgement) during transfer by a specialist team.

Each geographical region of the UK has provision to mobilize a specialist paediatric intensive care transport team (Figure 14.1). This could be a standalone team or a team based in one of the 31 paediatric intensive care units. The Paediatric Intensive Care Society (PICS) has produced standards of practice for the transportation of the critically ill child. This outlines areas such as staffing, education, communication, and a recommended equipment list. These services also provide advice and support for staff caring for the seriously ill child while the transport team is mobilizing and travelling to the hospital.

Recognition and management of the seriously ill child

The assessment of the vital signs (heart rate, blood pressure, respiratory rate, temperature, capillary refill time) by age is essential to recognize the seriously ill child. The Paediatric Early Warning Score (PEWS) assessment tool should be used (see Chapter 13). This enables early recognition of the deteriorating child through changes in their observations (Figure 14.2). A senior team needs to be alerted to ensure that treatment is administered quickly.

If the child is breathing spontaneously, a non-rebreather mask (Hudson type) is recommended (Figure 14.3). Oxygen administration is essential and should be available via a flow meter that can deliver 15 L per minute.

There are two commonly used airway adjuncts that can be utilized until a definitive airway is achieved. Oropharyngeal airways (Guedel) are available in a variety of sizes (Figure 14.4) and are used to provide a clear passage along the tongue and posterior pharyngeal wall. A nasopharyngeal airway tube is inserted via the nasal passage and is often better tolerated as it is less likely to cause laryngospasm. Insertion of these airway adjuncts should only be undertaken by a trained member of staff.

If the child's breathing requires support, this can be achieved by using a self-inflating bag (Ambu® bag, Ambu, Ballerup, Denmark; Figure 14.5) or an Ayres T-piece or Mapleson T-piece.

Definitive airway support is achieved when a tube is passed via the mouth or nose into the trachea (windpipe; Figure 14.6). This requires the expertise of a senior anaesthetist. In order to place the tube, anaesthetic induction agents will be required via intravenous drugs or the inhaled route. Endotracheal tubes range from 2 to 8 mm (internal diameter) and require tape to secure to the child's cheeks.

To ensure that the tube is inserted to the correct length, a chest X-ray should be requested when tracheal intubation has been established. Accidental extubation is always a potential risk. Exhaled gases from the lungs contain carbon dioxide. Sampling the exhaled gas can be carried out to alert the team if the tube is dislodged from the trachea (Figure 14.7). Ventilation can be maintained after intubation by a mechanical ventilator that is suitable for a child.

The child will require a gastric tube to ensure that the stomach can be emptied. Air can be forced into the stomach during bag valve mask ventilation. This air, if not removed, can splint the diaphragm and cause difficulties in establishing mechanical ventilation.

Intravenous access is essential to facilitate drug administration (Figure 14.8). Peripheral cannulation can be difficult to achieve in the seriously ill child. The insertion of an intraosseous needle allows rapid delivery of drugs and fluids (Figure 14.9).

Intravenous drugs are required to ensure that the child remains asleep and able to tolerate the endotracheal tube. An infusion of an opiate such as morphine, combined with a sedative (e.g. midazolam), is frequently used. A paralyzing agent is also administered to control the child's breathing rate.

Accurate measurement of the child's urine output can be very useful to determine renal efficiency and intravascular fluid volume. A Foley catheter may be required to record urine output hourly.

Blood sampling and analysis form an important diagnostic tool. The results are relied upon to interpret the efficacy of the treatment provided. Blood glucose levels should be frequently checked, as all children, especially infants, can become hypoglycaemic when seriously ill.

Neurological assessment using the AVPU scale (Alert, Voice, Pain, Unresponsive) is a system by which a healthcare professional can measure and record the child's responsiveness. Pupil reaction to light should be recorded regularly, as changes in the response of the pupil could indicate a serious brain disorder or injury.

Communication with the child and parents or carers should never be ignored. Explanation and information will allay fears in most situations, so it is important to explain things as clearly and simply as possible.

Key points

- Early recognition of the seriously ill or deteriorating child is crucial.
- Alert senior medical personnel and request they attend the child's bedside.
- Prompt treatment and resuscitation as appropriate (children can deteriorate quickly).
- Utilize telephone advice provided by the paediatric intensive care services.
- A structured approach to managing a seriously ill child can focus the care delivered.
- Effective communication with the child and family is essential.

15 Understanding investigations

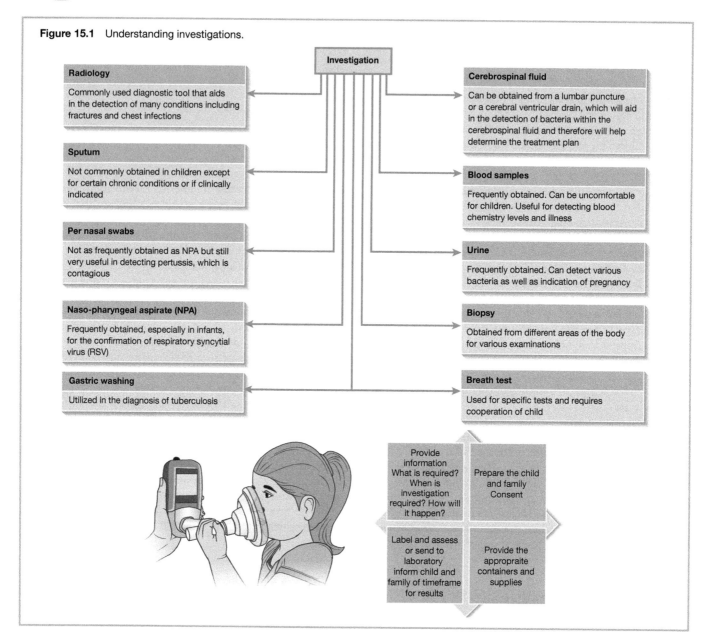

Figure 15.1 Understanding investigations.

Investigation

Radiology
Commonly used diagnostic tool that aids in the detection of many conditions including fractures and chest infections

Sputum
Not commonly obtained in children except for certain chronic conditions or if clinically indicated

Per nasal swabs
Not as frequently obtained as NPA but still very useful in detecting pertussis, which is contagious

Naso-pharyngeal aspirate (NPA)
Frequently obtained, especially in infants, for the confirmation of respiratory syncytial virus (RSV)

Gastric washing
Utilized in the diagnosis of tuberculosis

Cerebrospinal fluid
Can be obtained from a lumbar puncture or a cerebral ventricular drain, which will aid in the detection of bacteria within the cerebrospinal fluid and therefore will help determine the treatment plan

Blood samples
Frequently obtained. Can be uncomfortable for children. Useful for detecting blood chemistry levels and illness

Urine
Frequently obtained. Can detect various bacteria as well as indication of pregnancy

Biopsy
Obtained from different areas of the body for various examinations

Breath test
Used for specific tests and requires cooperation of child

Provide information
What is required? When is investigation required? How will it happen?

Prepare the child and family
Consent

Label and assess or send to laboratory inform child and family of timeframe for results

Provide the appropraite containers and supplies

Investigations are carried out to determine the cause of illness and require consent from the child and family (Figure 15.1). A large number of investigations come under the umbrella of radiology.

Radiology

Radiology includes *plain static X-rays*, which can be used to look at bone or soft tissue in any area of the body, chest infections, or the position of an endotracheal tube in an intensive care unit patient. It is the most common imaging investigation in hospital. Plain X-rays can be obtained in the radiology department or, if the child is too unwell to be transferred, they can be obtained via a portable machine.

Fluoroscopy uses pulsed X-rays that create a real-time image and is utilized for procedures such as a barium swallow to examine the gastrointestinal tract, micturating cystourethrogram to examine the bladder and urethra, and intravenous urography to examine the urinary tract.

Ultrasound uses sound waves and is very useful in examining areas of soft tissue within the body or structures that contain fluid. It is not as useful at examining structures that contain gas because the ultrasound waves pass straight through the gas, so there is poor image quality.

Children and Young People's Nursing at a Glance, Second Edition. Edited by Elizabeth Gormley-Fleming and Sheila Roberts.
© 2023 John Wiley & Sons Ltd. Published 2023 by John Wiley & Sons Ltd.

Computerized tomography (CT) is a very useful addition to diagnostic medicine. It uses multiple X-ray images and, with the assistance of a computer, creates a cross-sectional image of various parts of the body. It is not only used to distinguish between normal and abnormal structures within the body, but can also assist in procedures where instruments need to be placed with accuracy.

In *nuclear medicine* a radioisotope is injected into the child or young person via a cannula or butterfly needle. The radioisotope emits gamma rays, which are then recorded by a gamma camera. It is a very useful tool in diagnostic medicine.

Magnetic resonance imaging (MRI) is a way of looking inside the body and producing two- and three-dimensional images without using X-rays. The images are gained by using radiowaves, a magnet, and a computer. Metal objects cannot enter the same room as the magnet. Occasionally, a small amount of contrast is injected into the child or young person so that a clearer picture can be obtained.

Sampling of cerebrospinal fluid

A sample of cerebrospinal fluid (CSF) may be obtained from a lumbar puncture examination (the insertion of a needle into the back) to determine the diagnosis of conditions such as meningitis or encephalitis.

Blood samples

Blood samples are used to determine the different haematological, biochemical, immunological, and microbiological components of blood to aid in the diagnosis of illness. They can also be used to determine certain antibiotic and drug levels, which dictate the dose required for the child. Blood cultures can be obtained if a child's clinical condition is deteriorating as they can detect bacteria in the bloodstream.

Blood samples are obtained frequently, as they can be used to determine levels of blood chemistry as well as detect illness. Children generally do not like blood being taken as it can be uncomfortable or painful unless managed well using local anaesthetics and distraction. Point-of-patient-care testing is now more frequently used to provide immediate information that will enable accurate and timely treatment to be planned and implemented, such as serum lactate levels. At the point of registration, the children's and young person's nurse is required to undertake venepuncture and cannulation and blood sampling. They need to be able to interpret normal and common abnormal blood profiles and venous blood gases.

Sputum samples

Sputum samples are obtained for the microbiological diagnosis of respiratory tract infections. They are routinely obtained in children with cystic fibrosis.

Breath test

Breath testing may be used to test for lactose intolerance. The hydrogen breath test is a non-invasive means of determining if a child is lactose intolerant. The child is required to blow into a balloon-like bag. The breath sample is tested to identify the amount of hydrogen present, measured in parts per million. The child is then given a drink of a lactose solution and the breath test is repeated every 15 minutes for a few hours. If the breath contains hydrogen levels greater than 20 parts per million, it is likely that a diagnosis of lactose intolerance will be confirmed.

Heliobacter pylori may be detected from urea breath testing. Breath testing in young children is possible, but local guidelines should be followed.

Gastric washings

Gastric washings can be obtained when children do not produce enough sputum to detect the presence of *Mycobacterium tuberculosis*.

Nasopharyngeal aspirate

A nasopharyngeal aspirate (NPA) sample is mainly obtained for the diagnosis of viral infections such as respiratory syncytial virus (RSV), influenza, and parainfluenza.

Pernasal swabs

These are used to help diagnose pertussis. Pertussis, commonly known as whooping cough, is a highly contagious bacterial infection that causes episodes of violent coughing and respiratory obstruction.

Urine samples

Urine samples can be collected in various ways, but the most reliable way is via a midstream specimen or a clean catch. This is difficult to obtain in a very young child, so it is important to ensure that the nappy area and genitalia are as clean as possible prior to obtaining a urine specimen. Urine samples can be used to detect various bacteria within the urine if sent to the microbiology laboratory for analysis. However, bedside urine tests can detect the presence of blood, protein, and other constituents in the urine, which in turn will dictate whether further laboratory tests on the urine need to be considered.

Stool samples

The most frequent reason for a stool sample is to identify pathogenic bacteria or parasites. Yeast infection and malignancies can also be detected in faecal matter. Results from a stool sample will report as 'isolated' if a pathogen has been identified. Some pathogens in the stools are notifiable to the public health authority, as it may be necessary to identify the source of infection, for instance salmonella infection from contaminated food.

Biopsy

Biopsies can be obtained from different areas of the body to determine the diagnosis of specific conditions. Specimens are sent to a relevant laboratory so that a histopathological and microbiological examination can occur.

There are too many investigations to cover them all in this chapter; however, it has provided you with some useful information about the most common ones. It is important to consider the needs of the child and family and to explain why such procedures are being undertaken and, importantly, when the results will be obtained.

Key points
- Children and their families must be adequately prepared prior to any investigations being undertaken.
- Preparation for the procedure/investigation is key and all essential equipment and specimen containers should be available, with spare containers accessible.
- The child and family should be informed of when results can be expected and how they will receive this information.

16 Understanding blood gas analysis

Figure 16.1 Blood gas analysis.

A disturbance in acid–base balance occurs as a result of either respiratory or metabolic disorders. Alteration in the acid–alkali balance in the body is a common problem in sick children that requires urgent intervention. Measurement of these substrates through blood gas analysis is an important part of the assessment of the sick child.

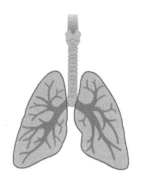

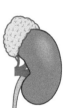

Common causes of acidosis or alkalosis

Metabolic acidosis pH 7.35	• Severe gastroenteritis • Diabetic ketoacidosis (DKA) • Shock: hypovolemic, cardiogenic • Birth asphyxia
Metabolic alkalosis pH >7.45	• Pyloric stenosis • Diuretics • Excessive nasogastric tube losses
Respiratory acidosis	• Respiratory failure due to illness or any other cause, e.g. asthma, inadequate mechanical ventilation, central nervous system depression
Respiratory alkalosis	• Hyperventilation • Excessive mechanical ventilation

Analysis of arterial blood gas (ABG)

In order to interpret the ABG of a child correctly, the clinical history, treatment given, findings from examination, and previous laboratory investigations need to be considered

A systematic approach such as the five-step method may be utilized:

• How is the child?
• What is the pH?
• What is the $PaCO_2$?
• What is the base excess?

Normal range for acid–base and blood gas measurements

Arterial pH	7.36–7.42
Arterial $PaCO_2$	4.7–5.5 kPa
Arterial PaO_2	1–14 kPa (8–10 kPa in neonates)
Arterial or venous bicarbonate	17–27 mmol/L
Base excess	>0–2 mmol/L

Measured (37.0 °C)		Derived Parameters	
pH	7.21	HCO_3^-	33.2 mmol/L
pCO_2	11.1 kPa	HCO_3std	27.3 mmol/L
pO_2	6.3 kPa	TCO_2	35.7 mmol/L
Na^+	133 mmol/L	BE(B)	3.6 mmol/L
K^+	5.6 mmol/L		
Ca^{++}	1.37 mmol/L		
Glu	5.2 mmol/L		
Lac	2.3 mmol/L		
Hct	30%		

Changes in the blood gas and acid–base values depending on type of acidosis or alkalosis

*Compensated state	Metabolic acidosis	Metabolic alkalosis	Respiratory acidosis	Respiratory alkalosis
pH	Low	High	Low	High
PO_2	Normal	Normal	Normal or low	Normal or high
PCO_2	Normal or low*	Normal or high*	High	Low
Bicarbonate	Low	High	Normal or high*	Normal or low*

Indication for measuring blood gas

• Respiratory distress
• Management of mechanical ventilation
• Altered level of consciousness
• Shocked child: sepsis, cardiogenic
• Trauma
• Ingestion of poison
• Metabolic disorders, inborn and DKA
• Ongoing evaluation of resuscitation treatments

Interpreting the result from blood gas analysis is a skill the children's and young person's nurse is required to have. The value of a blood gas is its ability to provide an immediate reflection of the physiology of the sick infant, child, or young person, which will then direct the type of treatment they require. A blood gas may be taken to assess the effectiveness of ventilation, circulation, and perfusion and to assess metabolic and renal function (Figure 16.1).

A blood gas measures three main components:
• pH of the sample
• Oxygen level
• Carbon dioxide level

Children and Young People's Nursing at a Glance, Second Edition. Edited by Elizabeth Gormley-Fleming and Sheila Roberts.
© 2023 John Wiley & Sons Ltd. Published 2023 by John Wiley & Sons Ltd.

pH

pH is the term used to describe the acidity or alkalinity of a solution. The pH scale is based on the number of hydrogen ions and is expressed in mmol/L. If a solution has a pH of 7, then it is considered to be a neutral solution such as water, where the hydrogen (H+) ions are present in equal concentration with the hydroxyl ions OH+.

A pH below 7 is an acid solution. This dissociates into H+ ions and OH+ ions, with more H+ ions than OH+ ions.

A pH greater than 7 is an alkaline solution. This dissociates into OH+ ions and H+ ions, with more OH+ ions than H+ ions. In the human body there needs to be a balance between intake and removal of H+ if normal body function is to be maintained. Three systems regulate the acid–base balance:

- Buffers – metabolic
- Lungs – respiratory
- Kidney – metabolic

In the event of abnormalities, these three systems function together in an attempt to compensate.

Buffers

The function of the buffers is to counteract changes to the pH by either increased absorption or release of H+. The carbonic acid–bicarbonate is the most important buffer system. Carbonic acid (H_2CO_3) is the weaker acid and sodium bicarbonate ($NaHCO_3$) is the weak base. In solution, dissociation occurs:

$$H_2CO_3 \leftrightarrow H + + HCO_3$$
$$NaHCO_3 \leftrightarrow Na + + HCO_3$$

When the blood becomes acidic, the sodium bicarbonate disassociates to buffer the acid; this increases the concentration of carbonic acid and decreases the sodium bicarbonate, resulting in an increase in the pH as the carbonic acid is weak.

If the blood is alkaline (strong base), then the concentration of sodium bicarbonate increases and carbonic acid will be utilized as the buffer.

The protein buffer system is activated in the body cells and plasma. The haemoglobin–oxyhaemoglobin buffer system buffers carbonic acid in the blood. The phosphate buffer system works in red blood cells and renal tubular fluids.

Respiration

The level of carbon dioxide (CO_2) is regulated by respiration. The respiratory system balances the pH by offsetting the production of H+ ions by clearing the CO_2 through ventilation. This CO_2 dissolves in water, forming carbonic acid, which is weak and unstable. If there is an elevation in H+, the respiratory system will increase the rate and depth of the child's breathing in an attempt to remove more CO_2, which inhibits the formation of carbonic acid. This is called respiratory acidosis; the PCO_2 is high and this occurs rapidly. The reverse of this process is called respiratory alkalosis and the PCO_2 will be low.

Base deficit

This indicates the level of base in the blood. Base deficit is the amount of base that needs to be added to return the pH to normal. The base excess is the amount of base that needs to be removed to return the pH to normal. Thus, a high base excess above +3 suggests metabolic alkalosis and if it is less than −3 then metabolic acidosis may be present.

Renal tubular secretion

Renal tubular secretion assists with the control of the pH level of the blood by continuous filtration of bicarbonate ions. If the pH is acidic, then the secretion of H+ is increased and sodium Na+ is displaced, which combines with bicarbonate to form sodium bicarbonate, which is absorbed into the bloodstream. H+ is lost from the body and the pH becomes less acidic.

Anion gap

The anion gap is calculated to identify the cause of the metabolic acidosis if it is not known. The anion gap is the sum of:

$$\begin{pmatrix}\text{plasama sodium} + \text{plasam potassium}\end{pmatrix}$$
$$- \begin{pmatrix}\text{bicarbonate} + \text{chloride}\end{pmatrix}.$$

The normal value is 5–12 mmol/L.

Sampling

Blood is taken from the following:
- Artery – usually the radial or femoral.
- Arterial cannula.
- Capillary prick of heel or ear lobe – this is less accurate as venous and arterial blood is mixed.

This is a painful procedure in the non-ventilated child, so careful consideration is given prior to drawing a sample. The Allen test needs to be undertaken prior to arterial puncture from the radial artery. Direct pressure must be applied to the puncture site for 3–5 minutes after sampling has occurred. Capillary refill time should be monitored post procedure.

A pre-heparinized syringe or a capillary tube is required. Avoid dead space and bubbles in the tube blood, as this will alter the results.

Minimize metabolism in the sample by placing the specimen on ice if there is likely to be any delay in analysis (i.e. >15 minutes).

The blood is then analysed immediately and a printed result is generated. Fraction of inspired oxygen (FiO) and temperature need to be noted when analysing the sample.

Three steps to consider when analysing blood gas:
- What is the pH? If it is raised, it is alkalosis; if it is low, then it is acidosis. This is the overall status of the child.
- What is the $PaCO_2$? Does the CO_2 agree with the pH? If there is low pH and a high CO_2 (acidosis) or a high pH and a low CO_2 (alkalosis), then the child is in either respiratory acidosis or alkalosis, respectively. If the CO_2 disagrees with the pH, it is compensating for a metabolic abnormality.
- What is the base excess? This will confirm your findings. If the base excess agrees with the pH – that is, a low pH with a negative base excess means acidosis and a high pH with a positive base excess means alkalosis – then the overall picture is one of metabolic acidosis or alkalosis. If the base excess disagrees with the pH, then the child is compensating for a respiratory abnormality.

Interpreting blood gas can be challenging. The results should be correlated with other clinical data in order to give an accurate picture of the child's condition. Understanding each element and what it means will help with comprehending the impact on the child's physiological status.

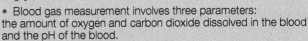

Key points
- Blood gas measurement involves three parameters: the amount of oxygen and carbon dioxide dissolved in the blood and the pH of the blood.
- Blood gas can be taken as an arterial, venous, or capillary sample and this is important to note.
- Blood gas provides clinical useful information that will determine the course of treatment for the child. The children's nurse is expected to understand normal values for blood gas levels.

17 Understanding blood chemistry

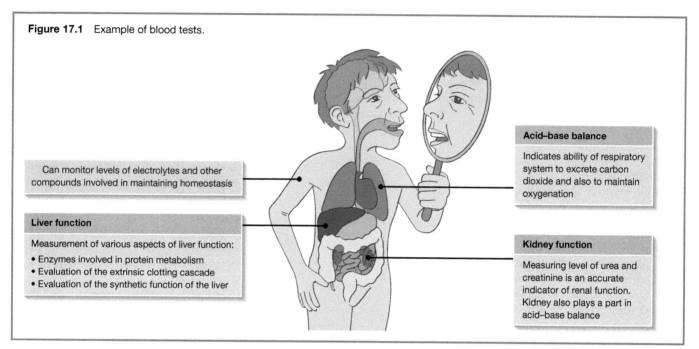

Figure 17.1 Example of blood tests.

Acid–base balance

Indicates ability of respiratory system to excrete carbon dioxide and also to maintain oxygenation

Can monitor levels of electrolytes and other compounds involved in maintaining homeostasis

Liver function

Measurement of various aspects of liver function:
- Enzymes involved in protein metabolism
- Evaluation of the extrinsic clotting cascade
- Evaluation of the synthetic function of the liver

Kidney function

Measuring level of urea and creatinine is an accurate indicator of renal function. Kidney also plays a part in acid–base balance

Introduction

Children and young people will have blood tested and interpreted to identify their current health status. Blood is tested for screening, disease management, and prognosis and for risk assessment. It will also be tested prior to treatment being initiated and to monitor the effectiveness of treatment. All newborns will be screened for genetic and metabolic diseases. Children may have blood screened for iron deficiency anaemia, type 2 diabetes, or immunodeficiencies.

Children's and young people's nurses will often perform venepuncture on the child or young person, so should be conversant with the normal reference intervals for the relevant biochemistry tests. At the point of registration, the children's and young person's nurse is required to undertake venepuncture and cannulation and blood sampling. They need to be able to interpret normal and common abnormal blood profiles and venous blood gases. Clinical diagnosis and treatment are informed by blood chemistry (Figure 17.1). The children's and young person's nurse should notify the relevant member of the multidisciplinary team once results are known.

Routine biochemistry testing

- *Potassium*: normal range 3.5–5.0 mmol/L. Important in neuromuscular function. Low level, usually below 3.0 (hypokalaemia), can lead to cardiac arrhythmias. High level, usually above 5.5 (hyperkalaemia), slows heart rate and can cause cardiac arrest.

- *Calcium*: total calcium 2.23–2.57 mmol/L, ionized calcium 1.15–1.27 mmol/L. Allows cardiac muscle to work without becoming tired. Ionized calcium (available for body to use). Low level can lead to decreased muscle contractility.
- *Sodium*: normal range 135–145 mmol/L. Most of body's sodium is in the extracellular fluid. Controls water distribution as well as extracellular volume. Hyponatraemia (usually below 135 mmol/L) = water into cells. Hypernatraemia (usually above 150 mmol/L) = water out of cells.
- *Phosphate*: normal range 0.81–1.45 mmol/L. Intracellular. Critical component of adenosine triphosphate, which the body uses as fuel. Also important in muscle function, red blood cells, and nervous system. Hypophosphataemia: muscle weakness and reduced cardiac contractility. Hyperphosphataemia: reduced calcium levels, tingling of fingers. Precipitation of calcium phosphate in the kidney.
- *Magnesium*: normal range 0.65–1.05 mmol/L. Intracellular: involved in enzyme reactions. Extracellular: neuromuscular transmission, neuronal control, cardiovascular tone. Low levels (usually below 0.6 mmol/L): muscle weakness, cardiac arrhythmias. High levels (usually above 1.1 mmol/L): bradycardia, reduced skeletal muscle function.
- *Glucose*: normal range 2.5–6.0 mmol/L. Energy source for the body. Hypoglycaemia (usually below 3 mmol/l): confusion, anxiety, weakness, hunger, dizziness, shaking, coma. Hyperglycaemia: increased urine output, excessive thirst, damage to major organs, reduced resistance to opportunistic infections.

Children and Young People's Nursing at a Glance, Second Edition. Edited by Elizabeth Gormley-Fleming and Sheila Roberts.
© 2023 John Wiley & Sons Ltd. Published 2023 by John Wiley & Sons Ltd.

- *Lactate*: normal range 0.6–1.7 mmol/L. Produced as an end result of energy production. Level rises in anaerobic respiration and contributes to acidosis. Increased in inherited metabolic disorders and also bacterial and fungal infections.
- *Chloride*: normal range 97–110 mmol/L. Needed to maintain normal cellular and organ function. Also fluid levels. Diarrhoea, nausea and vomiting, and increased sweating can decrease chloride levels.
- *C-reactive protein* (CRP): increased in bacterial infection as it is an acute-phase reactant. Normal range <5 mg/L.
- *Ferritin*: to detect iron deficiency and iron overload. Normal range: males 22–322 ng/mL; females 20–290 ng/mL.
- *Haemoglobin A1C*: monitoring of glycaemic control in diabetes mellitus only. Normal reference range 20–42 mmol/L.

Kidney function

- *Urea*: normal range 2.9–8.9 mmol/L. Waste product produced from protein metabolism.
- *Creatinine*: normal range, neonate 2–90 µmol/L; infant <1 year 11–34 µmol/L; child <14 years 21–65 µmol/L; >14 years 49–104, µmol/L; >18 years 53–133 µmol/L. Breakdown product of creatine phosphate in muscle. Affected by muscle mass, muscle breakdown, protein intake, and glomerular function.

Liver function

- *Ammonia*: sick/premature <150 µmol/L; neonate <150 µmol/L; child <16 years <50 µmol/l. Deamination of amino acids during protein metabolism. Increased levels = reduced synthetic liver function. Can cross the blood–brain barrier and lead to hepatic encephalopathy.
- *Albumin*: 0–5 days 26–36 g/L; 6 days–3 years 34–42 g/L; 4–6 years 35–50 g/L; >7 years 30–50 g/L. Plasma protein responsible for maintaining plasma oncotic pressure. Low levels maty reflect kidney or gastrointestinal losses, infection, malnutrition, haemodilution, or redistribution.
- *Prothrombin time*: 10–14 seconds. International normalized ratio (INR) 0.8–1.2. Clinical evaluation of extrinsic clotting cascade. If longer than normal then could have clotting problems. INR altered if on anticoagulant therapy such as warfarin or heparin.
- *Alanine aminotransferase* (ALT): 0–3 years 50 units/L; 4–10 years 40 units/L. Catalyst for protein metabolism.
- *Aspartate aminotransferase* (AST): 1–5 days 35–140 units/L; 6 days–3 years 20–60 units/L; 4–15 years 15–40 units/L. Involved in protein metabolism.

- If levels of ALT or AST altered, then the ability to break down protein will be affected.
- *Alkaline phosphatase* (ALP): 0–1 years 110–320 units/L; 1–9 years 145–420 units/L; 10–15 years male 130–525 units/L; 10–15 years female 70–230 units/L. Phosphate metabolism.
- *Alpha fetoprotein* (AFP): produced by the foetal liver and yolk sac during gestation and up to 1 year of age. Used alongside other tests to diagnose and monitor hepatoblastoma. >1 year <7k U/L. Under 1 year of age will need to be discussed with biochemist.
- *Bilirubin*: may be raised with hepatocellular dysfunction, breast milk jaundice, or with haemolysis. 14 days–16 years: <21 mmol/L.
- *Bilirubin split* (conjugated and unconjugated): differential diagnosis of jaundice. Unconjugated bilirubin predominates in haemolytic or 'breast milk' jaundice. Conjugated bilirubinaemia indicates other possible causes such as infection, biliary atresia. Direct bilirubin >33% of the total is generally considered conjugated in hyperbilirubinaemia.

Acid–base balance

- *pH*: 7.35–7.45. Measurement of the concentration of hydrogen ions in body fluids. Important in maintaining homeostasis (hydrogen ions: 35–45 mmol/L).
- *PCO_2*: 4.7–6.0 kPa. Measurement of amount of CO_2 present in blood. If respiratory rate low, then level will be raised, and if respiratory rate high, then level will be low.
- *Standard bicarbonate*: 21–26 mmol/L. Measurement of level of sodium bicarbonate in the blood. Important in maintaining homeostasis.
- *Base excess*: –2 to +2. Measurement of how many extra basic chemicals are present in blood or amount of acid that would have to be added to blood to bring pH back to normal.
- *PO_2*: 9–13 kPa. Measurement of amount of oxygen in arterial blood.

Key points
- Age- and sex-appropriate thresholds may be required for some biochemistry analysis.
- Children under 1 year of age and those in puberty can have altered biochemistry due to their dynamic physiology.
- Different clinical laboratories may have different thresholds to identify abnormal results, so be aware of this.

18 Understanding pathology specimen collection

Figure 18.1 Principles of pathology specimen collection.

Urine sample

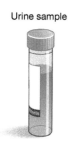

Stool sample

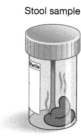

Some additives to blood bottles
- Gel
- EDTA
- Sodium
- Trisodium citrate
- Lithium heparin
- Sodium heparin

Safe transportation

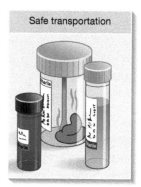

Figure 18.2 Blood collection tubes. ACTH, adrenocorticotropic hormone – from the pituitary gland; APTT, activated partial thromboplastin time – to check function of clotting factors; DAT, direct antiglobulin test – to establish if antibodies are present on red blood cells; EDTA, ethylenediaminetetraacetic acid – to assess kidney function; ESR, erythrocyte sedimentation rate; HBA1c, haemoglobin A1c –average blood sugar over preceding 2–3 months; INR, international normalized ratio – to check blood clotting time; PT, prothrombin time – also clotting time.

Sample tube/Chemical/Test	Tube
Red/brown top: Plain gel. Biochemistry	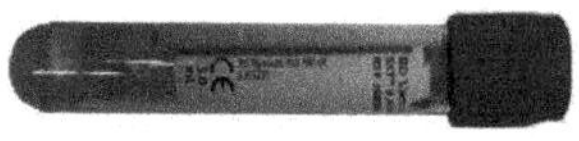
Purple top: EDTA. Full blood count and ESR. HBA1c ACTH	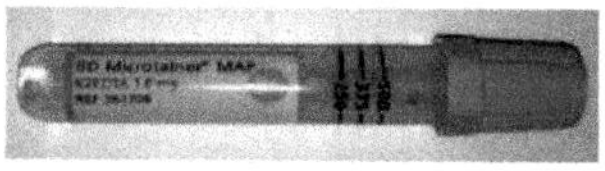
Green top: Heparin. Chromosomes, troponin, amino acids	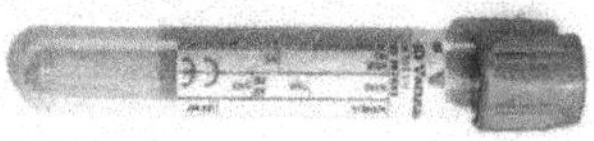
Grey top: Sodium fluoride. Glucose	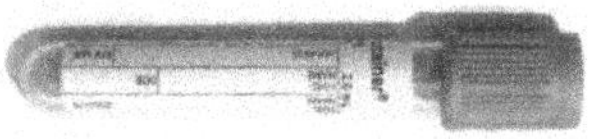
Blue top: Sodium citrate. Coagulation testing, INR, APTT, PT	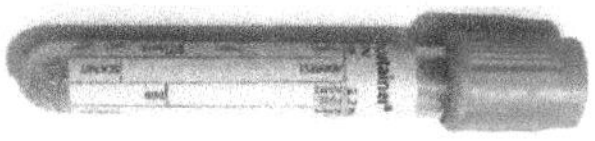
Gold top: Clot activator. Immunology	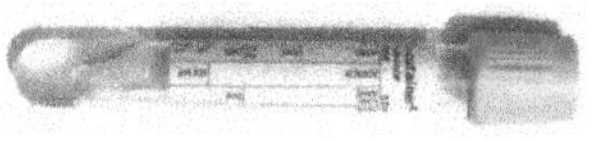
Pink top: EDTA. Transfusion samples (Group & Save, Crossmatch, Direct Coombs Test [DAT]	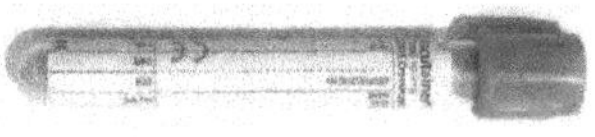
Paediatric microvette. No additive. Antibiotic levels.	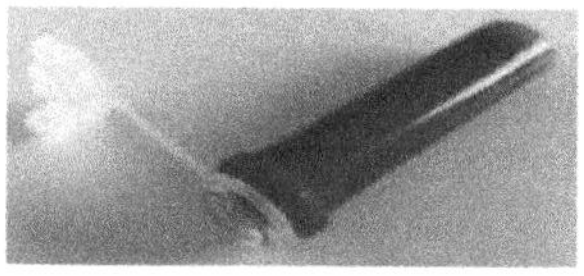
Blood cultures	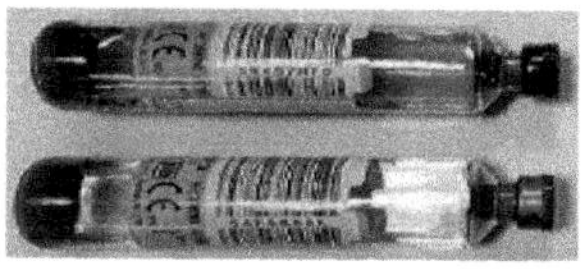

Children and Young People's Nursing at a Glance, Second Edition. Edited by Elizabeth Gormley-Fleming and Sheila Roberts.
© 2023 John Wiley & Sons Ltd. Published 2023 by John Wiley & Sons Ltd.

Important principles when collecting specimens

It is crucial that the following are adhered to when collecting specimens:
- Required investigations are confirmed with reference to medical records.
- Checks are made to ensure it is the correct child and that name, date of birth, and hospital number match.
- Any labels used must match the child's details.
- The child's name must match their hospital record, as they may be known to their family/nurse by a shortened version, for example Ed, when their full name is Edward if handwriting is used on sample tubes.
- The correct tubes or bottles are selected prior to sampling (Figure 18.1).
- Correct laboratory request forms are used and labelled.
- Expiry dates on the tubes or bottles must be checked.
- Tubes and bottles must be intact and not damaged.
- Any materials should be prepared before the procedure.
- It is the responsibility of the person undertaking the intervention to ensure it is the correct child, tests, tubes, and labels.
- Any specimens must be stored correctly and transported following local policy and procedures.

Obtaining blood samples

Blood samples can be obtained through a variety of methods:
- *Heel prick*: mainly used on neonates, where small samples of blood are preferred so as not to reduce their blood volume.
- *Fingerprick*: often used for measuring blood glucose levels in children with diabetes or in those who have drunk alcohol.
- *Peripheral venepuncture*: this method involves the insertion of a butterfly cannula or a standard needle to obtain samples for a variety of investigations. This is the most common method utilized.
- *Large vessel venepuncture*: in some cases it is not possible to obtain blood samples from smaller veins and so larger vessels are utilized.
- *Arterial blood sampling*: mainly used for ascertaining blood gas levels and involves taking a sample directly from an artery (often the radial or femoral arteries) or from an arterial line. The former is a distressing procedure and so preparation and analgesia are crucial.
- *Intraosseous sampling*: in emergency situations when venous access is not available. The laboratory needs to be informed that this is bone marrow and not blood, so blood collection tubes need to clearly identify this.

Staff required to obtain blood samples must be trained in the intervention, deemed competent, and maintain their competence. At the point of registration, the children's and young person's nurse is required to undertake venepuncture and cannulation and blood sampling. They need to be able to interpret normal and common abnormal blood profiles and venous blood gases. All staff must prepare the child ensure local anaesthetic is applied, and monitor their response to the intervention. If unable to perform the technique (e.g. difficult venepuncture), the staff member must seek help from a more experienced colleague. Repeated attempts by inexperienced staff should not occur, but in circumstances where this does happen the nurse must advocate on behalf of the child, thus ensuring their safety and wellbeing.

The recommended order to obtain blood samples is:
1 Blood cultures.
2 Coagulation tubes.
3 Tubes with other additives (this will avoid contamination of the other samples).

Blood samples are collected either by venepuncture with a standard needle and syringe and then transferred to a tube, or a vacutainer system is used. The vacutainer is a tube already attached to a needle or is attached on venepuncture, and then the vacuum draws out the blood sample, so a syringe is not necessary.

Once the blood sample has been obtained, it is important to ensure that each of the tubes is inverted, which allows for mixing of the blood with the chemical inside the bottle. If the blood is not mixed, then it may lead to inaccurate results. The total amount of times that the tube should be inverted is detailed on the side of the blood bottle or tube.

There are various departments that blood samples can be sent to depending on the investigation required:
- Biochemistry
- Haemotology
- Microbiology

The blood bottles (Figure 18.2) have various additives that aid in the accuracy of the test. The correct bottle must be used.

Urine collection

Depending on the investigation required, different urine collection methods are utilized including clean catch, catheter, early morning, midstream urine, or 24-hour collection.

Early-morning sampling is normally collected immediately when the child wakes. It is important to collect as much as possible of the morning's first urine into the supplied container.

The collection of midstream urine is particularly useful when testing for a bacterial culture. The child or young person must void the first portion of urine into the toilet. Next they must pass the midportion of urine into an appropriate container to fill it to the mark on the container, while not contaminating the inside of the container with the hand. This can be especially difficult for young children as it requires control of the bladder. Some departments perform an in–out catheterization procedure; this depends on the age and compliance of the child and the parent's wishes.

Stool specimens

Stool samples are useful in diagnosing bacteria in the gastrointestinal tract. Many children do not like to provide stool samples as they feel embarrassed, so it is important to maintain their privacy and dignity. When obtaining a stool sample, it is vital to inform the child that they must ensure that the sample avoids contact with urine. It is therefore easier if they pass the stool directly into a bedpan. Should be transferred into to specimen pot. The bottle should be sealed and labelled with the child's details, and the date and time of collection.

Transporting specimens

All specimens must be handled according to local procedures and policies. The primary container for all specimens must be leakproof. Ensure that lids of containers are secure. Each specimen must be placed inside a secondary container for transport. The secondary container is a securely sealed plastic bag labelled with the patient's information and a biohazard symbol if necessary.

All specimen bottles must be individually labelled. Using patient labels is acceptable practice, as they have a barcode and the label must be applied to the sample correctly.

This chapter provides a brief overview of pathology specimen collection and transportation. Practitioners involved in the collection and transportation of specimens must refer to local guidelines and procedures to ensure safe and effective practice.

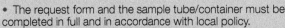

Key points
- The request form and the sample tube/container must be completed in full and in accordance with local policy.
- The child should be prepared, and consent obtained prior to collecting the sample, unless it is an emergency.

19 Understanding X-rays

Figure 19.1 How an X-ray is performed.

To take a good X-ray you need:
- A radiation source – to provide the X-rays
- Image receptor – like photographic film for a camera
- Cooperation – from both the child and the parent
- Help – from the parent to keep the child still
- A radiographer – to take the X-ray
- A radiologist – to interpret the images
- Protection – for everyone present not being X-rayed
- Communication – to work well together as a team

Image receptor
- This is a square hard box that goes next to the body part of interest
- It houses the technology that holds the image of the patient after the X-ray is taken until it has been processed and converted into an X-ray image (like a photograph before it is processed)
- As X-ray plates can be hard or uncomfortable for distressed patients who may have to lie on them, the radiographer knows that speed and comfort are key!

X-ray images
- The X-rays pass through some body structures easier than others, which is why an X-ray image has different shades of grey and white areas
- X-rays pass through air most easily, and so these parts appear black
- X-rays cannot pass through dense bones, and so these parts appear white
- Body tissues between these two extremes appear grey, such as fat, muscle and blood vessels

Radiation protection
- General radiation protection when taking X-rays is achieved by wearing a protective lead rubber apron
- Any person holding a patient or by standing behind a protective screen in the room must be suitably protected
- On the ward a safe standing distance if not wearing a lead rubber apron is no less than 2 metres away from the patient
- It is important that the lead rubber apron fits correctly, X-ray departments usually have a range of sizes available

Radiation source
- This is what generates radiation (X-rays)
- X-rays are then channelled as an 'X-ray beam' at the body part being imaged
- Light rays are used to indicate exactly where the X-rays are being channelled, like a torch
- An 'X-ray' is used to refer to both the radiation beam that passes through the patient, and the image that is generated from an X-ray machine

Advantages of X-ray
- Imaging that can be performed quickly
- As it is so quick and flexible (think about how an X-ray is taken) it accounts for the vast majority of imaging undertaken
- It offers a detailed image of each body part at a time

Disadvantages of X-ray
- Uses radiation to take images
- Children do not like having to lie still
- Several body parts being imaged may need a larger dose of radiation or lots of separate X-ray images
- X-rays cannot always be used during pregnancy

Figure 19.2 Types of X-ray.

X-rays can be used to image several body parts, examples of which are given below. All of these techniques use X-rays in different ways. X-rays can be used in conjunction with dense contrast material to make tubes and lines appear dark on an X-ray image, such as in studies of vessels or the gut

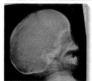
A skull X-ray in a child

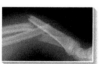
A fractured bone in a child's arm

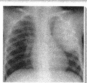
White parts of an X-ray can show abnormalities, such as infection

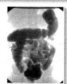
Adding a dense material such as barium helps to show the inside of the bowel, or dense contrast to show blood vessels of the hand

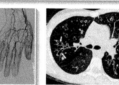
Applying several X-rays at the same time can help create a 3D image of the body (here showing the lungs) using computerized tomography

Table 19.1 Procedures and X-ray doses

	Effective dose (mSv)	Equivalence to how many chest X-rays?	Equivalence to NBR (2.6mSv/yr)		Effective dose (mSv)	Equivalence to how many chest X-rays?	Equivalence to NBR (2.6mSv/yr)
Chest X-ray	0.04	1	6 days	CT head	2.0	50	9 months
Abdominal X-ray	0.4	10	2 months	CT chest	2.5	62.5	11.3 months
Ultrasound exam	0	0	0	CT abdomen/pelvis	5.0	125	22.6 months
Bladder fluoroscopy test	1.5	37.5	6.8 months	MRI exam	0	0	0
Swallow fluoroscopy test	1.0	25	6.8 months	Nuclear medicine test, e.g. kidneys	0.7	17.5	3.4 months

CT, computerized tomography; MRI, magnetic resonance imaging; NBR, normal background radiation.

Children and Young People's Nursing at a Glance, Second Edition. Edited by Elizabeth Gormley-Fleming and Sheila Roberts.
© 2023 John Wiley & Sons Ltd. Published 2023 by John Wiley & Sons Ltd.

How do X-rays work?

Patients and their families often have questions about the risks and benefits of having an X-ray taken. Understanding X-rays is key to answering these questions.

The X-ray tube points directly at the body region of interest, which lies in contact with the image receptor, a digital detector. X-rays then travel from the tube through the patient and onto the image receptor. Some structures block the X-rays due to their density and appear white (bone), while air-filled structures allow the radiation to pass through and appear black (lungs). The various shades of grey in between will vary depending on the density of the structures in the image. These X-rays are extremely useful in high patient-throughput areas (chest X-ray imaging) or when a speedy answer is needed to an urgent clinical question (e.g. fracture?).

What is radiation?

X-rays use ionizing radiation, which, although fairly safe in small doses, is associated with a very small increased risk of certain cancers later in life. Having a single higher dose, or repeated X-rays over time, can increase this risk. Different procedures use a different dose of X-rays, so it is important to understand the relative differences between these (Table 19.1). Radiographers need to be able to 'justify' any X-ray request as a legal requirement, to ensure that it is the best way to address the medical needs of the patient.

The importance of staying still

X-rays are taken like photographs, a snapshot in time. So a moving patient appears as a blur on an X-ray image, just like a photo. For this reason, the radiographer will try to keep the patient as still as possible when they are taking the image, with the help of parents or guardians.

Children often need additional help to stay still. This can include foam pads held by a parent to keep a wriggling child's head still, or a chest chair (as in Figure 19.1) can be used to hold both the cassette and the patient in an upright position when they would struggle to keep upright by themselves. Other immobilization devices may also be used in addition to the help of a holder.

Other types of imaging

Depending on what the doctor's concern is about the patient, they might request different types of imaging technique (Figure 19.2).

Ultrasound uses high-frequency sound waves rather than radiation to build an image of an organ or tissue. A probe is placed over the body part of interest and the sound waves that bounce back from body structures produce an image. This is particularly useful for fluid-filled structures, such as the bladder or imaging an unborn baby during pregnancy, but cannot take pictures of air-filled structures like the lungs, or dense structures like bone.

Fluoroscopy is a method of using a steady stream of X-rays to produce a real-time video image on a monitor screen of what is going on inside a patient. Usually, an extra substance is given to the patient to make certain structures appear dense on the X-ray, such as barium or iodine. This is most useful when moving structures need to be imaged, such as in the gut, where contrast can be given by mouth (barium swallow), or during imaging of blood vessels (angiography). Fluoroscopy can also be useful to take pictures rapidly elsewhere in the hospital, such as in theatres where a broken limb is being repaired. Using these techniques means that doctors can see the effects of their surgery immediately or treat problems such as using catheters in blood vessels.

Computed tomography (CT) is a way of using several X-rays simultaneously to produce a detailed 3D image of a body part with computer software. A CT machine resembles a ring doughnut with the patient table lying in the centre. Within the CT machine are two main parts: an X-ray source and a series of detectors to capture the image. By spinning both of these around the patient, lots of images are taken, which resemble cross-sections of anatomy and so are sometimes referred to as 'slices'. The advantage of CT is that it is fast and gives very detailed high-quality images. The downside is the high radiation dose to the patient. For this reason, CT should never be undertaken unless clinically justified and a close eye should be kept on the number and frequency of CTs requested on any patient. Often, injections of contrast agents are used to highlight and differentiate structures on a CT scan.

Magnetic resonance imaging (MRI) machines resemble a long tube with a bed inside, which a patient must pass into in order for their imaging to be undertaken. It uses no X-rays at all to produce an image, but instead strong magnetic fields image tiny changes in the body's water molecules, and reconstruct these into images by computer. MRI is excellent for detecting very subtle anatomical changes, especially in soft tissues such as the brain. While ionizing radiation is not used, MRI scans can take a long time in a noisy cramped space, and this can be frightening for children. For this reason many children will be medicated to make them sleepy, or be given an anaesthetic.

Nuclear medicine tests use tiny amounts of radioactive material to look at how certain parts of the body work, like blood flow and activity within certain organs. This requires an injection and then the radioactivity is collected using a gamma camera, which can take a long time. For this reason, it is used only for particular tests in children, such as how the kidney functions, among others.

Key points
- There are a range of different radiological investigations that a child/young person may need. It is important that the children's nurse understands what these are.
- Preparation for the child/young person and parent is key to ensuring that a safe procedure can take place, specifically the importance of keeping still.

20 Pulse oximetry

Figure 20.1 Pulse oximetry.

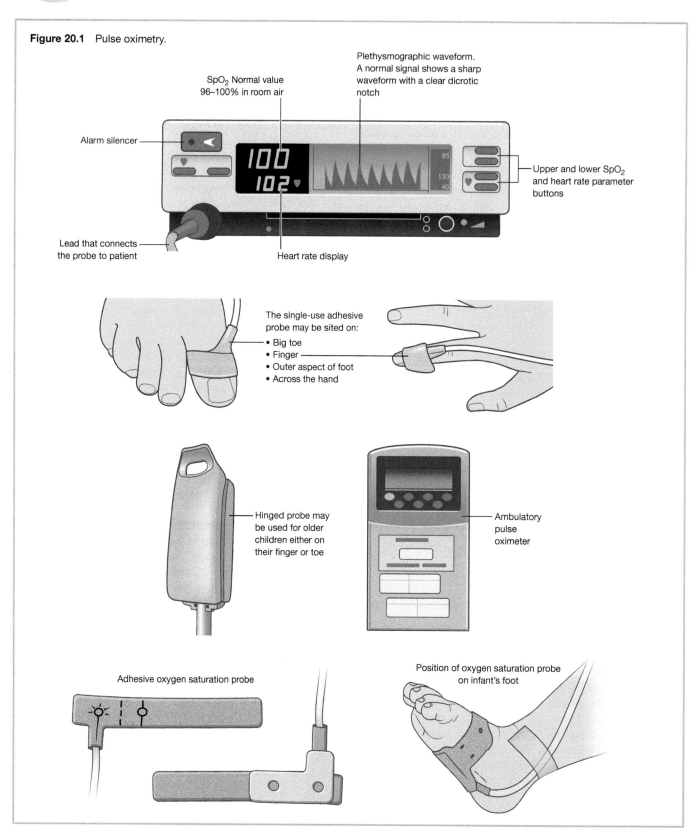

SpO$_2$ Normal value 96–100% in room air

Plethysmographic waveform. A normal signal shows a sharp waveform with a clear dicrotic notch

Alarm silencer

Upper and lower SpO$_2$ and heart rate parameter buttons

Lead that connects the probe to patient

Heart rate display

The single-use adhesive probe may be sited on:
- Big toe
- Finger
- Outer aspect of foot
- Across the hand

Hinged probe may be used for older children either on their finger or toe

Ambulatory pulse oximeter

Adhesive oxygen saturation probe

Position of oxygen saturation probe on infant's foot

Children and Young People's Nursing at a Glance, Second Edition. Edited by Elizabeth Gormley-Fleming and Sheila Roberts.
© 2023 John Wiley & Sons Ltd. Published 2023 by John Wiley & Sons Ltd.

Pulse oximetry is used in both the acute care environment and the community. It is routinely used as part of the assessment of the respiratory status of infants and children by measuring the oxygen saturation of the arterial blood flow through their extremities. The oxygen saturation level is expressed in SpO_2. Advantages of using pulse oximetry are that it is non-invasive, can be used for continuous monitoring and intermittent monitoring, and is accurate if the SaO_2 is >70%.

The pulse oximeter

Pulse oximetry consists of a pulse oximeter monitor that is connected to the patient by a probe. The pulse oximeter display shows the oxygen saturation of the patient, a plethysmographic waveform that indicates the pulsatile nature of the blood flow through the patient's extremities, and the heart rate. The heart rate displayed is an average recorded over 5–20 seconds. There is also an audible signal that varies in pitch depending on the saturation level and heart rate level. The pulse oximeter displays a motion indicator that indicates the signal quality, thus identifying the accuracy of the saturation level and heart rate.

Pulse oximetry is based on two physical principles: the presence of a pulsatile signal generated by arterial blood, which is reasonably independent of non-pulsatile arterial blood; and oxygenated and deoxygenated blood have different absorption spectra. The two light-emitting diodes emit red and infrared wavelengths through the tissues to a photo detector and work together. The detector measures the colour difference between the oxygenated and deoxygenated haemoglobin during each cardiac cycle, so the probe requires a constant supply of arterial blood. The absorption of light by the haemoglobin is dependent on the level of oxygenation. This information is then analysed in the calibration algorithm of the microprocessor of the pulse oximeter and the estimated arterial saturation level is displayed. This is displayed as a percentage and a plethysmographic waveform. A normal signal shows a sharp waveform with a clear dicrotic notch. Movement artefact and decreased perfusion will distort the waveform.

The pulse oximeter probe

The probe is available in two types: a hinged clip-on type for the older child or an adhesive single-use only type for the neonate, infant, and young child. Some probes are weight specific.

The probe consists of two parts: light-emitting diodes and a photo detector. This needs to be placed where a pulse can be detected. In the infant, this will be on the big toe or the lateral aspect of the foot. For the child, the adhesive probe may be sited on the finger or big toe over the nail-bed area or across the hand. With the older child, a finger-clip probe may be used on the thumb or big toe (see Figure 20.1). The orientation of the nail bed is identified on the probe by the manufacturer. The probe position should be changed on a regular basis and only secured as indicated by the manufacturer's instructions.

Indications for use and clinical application

Pulse oximetry is used for monitoring and as a screening tool in infants and children in the following circumstances:
- Potential for respiratory failure.
- Respiratory illness.
- Oxygen therapy is being received.
- Haemodynamic instability.
- Sedation or anaesthesia is required.

- Complex surgical procedures have been undertaken.
- In infants who are post surgery.
- During the administration of continuous respiratory depressant medication (e.g. patient-controlled analgesia).
- During transportation of infants and children between departments or hospitals, if they are at risk of respiratory compromise or are already receiving oxygen therapy.

Limitations of pulse oximetry

Pulse oximetry has a number of limitations that the user needs to be aware of, as these may lead to inaccurate readings:
- Inadequate positioning of the probe. Excessive light entering straight through the photo detector may give a false high reading.
- When the child has low cardiac output, hypothermia, or vasoconstriction, peripheral perfusion may be impaired and as oximetry relies on detecting a pulse, it may be difficult for the sensor to detect a true signal.
- When the SpO_2 is <70%. The presence of carboxyhaemoglobin that the two wavelengths of light cannot distinguish make pulse oximetry unreliable.
- Elevated methaemoglobin caused by either structural changes of iron in the haemoglobin or drug induced as with local anaesthesia may lead to tissue hypoxia as oxygen binding to haemoglobin is inhibited.
- Smoke inhalation and carbon monoxide poisoning. The pulse oximeter cannot distinguish between haemoglobin saturated with oxygen and that saturated with carbon monoxide.
- Motion artefact accounts for a significant number of errors and false alarms, thus shivering can cause problems with detecting saturation level and give a false high pulse.
- Use of intravenous dyes such as methylene blue can give false low readings, so nurses need to know which dye has been used and its half-life.
- Presence of oedema will lead to inaccurate measurement of saturation level.
- High bilirubin levels will affect the accuracy of readings.
- Inaccurate readings will also occur in the presence of nail varnish and acrylic nails.
- Dried blood and dirt on the skin can affect the accuracy of readings and need to be removed.
- Bright overhead lighting and external light may cause overestimation of saturation level.

Pulse oximetry at home

Pulse oximeters are now affordable and their use in the home has become more widespread, particularly since the arrival of the Covid-19 pandemic. Parents need to know that the pulse oximeter is a rapid diagnostic tool and also be aware of the appropriate action to take when a drop in saturations occurs.

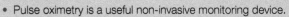

Key points
- Pulse oximetry is a useful non-invasive monitoring device.
- The correct-sized probe needs to be used and it needs to be sited correctly.
- It may be used continuously or intermittently.
- Users need to be aware of the limitations of saturation monitoring.

21 Central venous access devices

Figure 21.1 Advantages and disadvantages of central venous access devices (CVADs).

Advantages

- Easy to access
- Reduced anxiety, distress, and trauma associated with treatment as less frequent venous access required
- A safer route of administration for vesicant drugs and fluids that are unsuitable for peripheral cannula infusion
- Provides long-term venous access

Disadvantages

- Permanent indwelling catheter can impact on activities and body image
- Greater risk of infection
- Care and maintenance required to maintain
- Port – needle access required

Figure 21.3 Tunnelled device

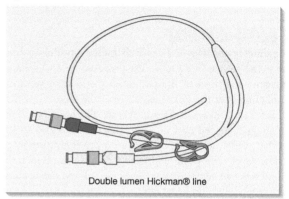

Double lumen Hickman® line

Figure 21.2 Advantages and disadvantages of each central venous access device (CVAD).

	Non-tunnelled	Peripherally inserted central catheter (PICC)	Tunnelled device	Port
Insertion under general anaesthetic	No	No	Yes	Yes
How long will it last?	Days–weeks	Weeks–months	Months–years	Years
Needle access	No	No	No	Yes
Dressing	Yes, changed weekly	Yes, changed weekly	No	No (only when in use)
Participation in sport	No	Some with caution	Some with caution	Most
Able to go swimming	No	No	No	Yes

Figure 21.4 Implantable ports.

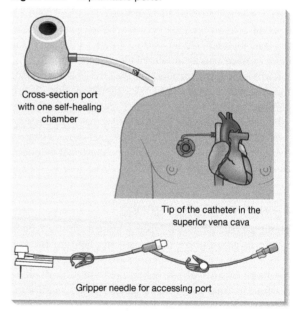

Cross-section port with one self-healing chamber

Tip of the catheter in the superior vena cava

Gripper needle for accessing port

Indications for use – choice

- **Non-tunnelled** – more than three peripheral cannulae required; <7 days irritant solutions being administered, blood samples required, inpatient
- **PICC** – treatment therapy >3 weeks; irritant solutions being administered; patient can be discharged home between infusions or home therapy
- **Tunnelled device** – treatment therapy >1 month–years; blood samples required, irritant solution therapy, inpatient or home therapy
- **Port** – treatment therapy >1 month–lifelong; blood samples required, irritant solution therapy, inpatient or home therapy

Indications for use – treatment

- Drug administration, specifically vesicant drug therapy
- Administration of fluids/electrolytes/inotropes
- Long-term total parenteral nutrition (TPN) administration
- Blood sampling
- Blood or blood product transfusion
- Monitoring – haemodynamic status
- Haemodialysis/haemoflitration

Children and Young People's Nursing at a Glance, Second Edition. Edited by Elizabeth Gormley-Fleming and Sheila Roberts.
© 2023 John Wiley & Sons Ltd. Published 2023 by John Wiley & Sons Ltd.

A central venous access device (CVAD) is an intravenous device that is inserted into the central circulation, reducing the need for frequent venepuncture or intravenous cannulation. It may be used for both short- and long-term care. CVADs are most commonly used for fluid or drug administration and blood sampling. It a crucial role in the administration of treatment to children within various care settings and the home environment.

The type of device selected for use will vary according to:
- Age of the child or young person
- Type of treatment required
- Frequency of use
- Length of time treatment is required:
  - Short term – <7 days/weeks
  - Intermediate – weeks/months
  - Long term – a month or longer/years/indefinite

Types of CVAD

There are four main types of CVAD:
- Non-tunnelled devices
- Peripherally inserted central catheters (PICCs)
- Tunnelled devices (Hickman line)
- Implantable ports

All CVADs have advantages and disadvantages (Figures 21.1 and 21.2), which may influence the child's, parent's, or clinician's choice of device (if appropriate).

Non-tunnelled devices

A non-tunnelled device is a short-term venous access device, most commonly used within high-dependency and intensive care settings within the hospital environment. There are three main insertion sites:
- Internal jugular vein
- Subclavian vein
- Femoral vein

Such catheters vary in size – length and gauge – and number of lumens. The line is usually secured in place with skin sutures at the entry point, covered with a sterile semipermeable transparent dressing.

Peripherally inserted central catheters

For intermediate use, the catheter length is measured prior to insertion, and then inserted peripherally under antiseptic non-touch technique (ANTT) conditions. The catheter is advanced through the vein to the required length, until the catheter tip position is located in the superior vena cava (SVC); the position is confirmed with imaging. The line is secured in place, usually with wound closure strips, and then covered with a sterile semipermeable transparent dressing. On occasion it may be sutured to the skin and sutures must be removed prior to line removal.

Tunnelled devices

For long-term use a skin-tunnelled catheter, known as a Hickman® or Broviac® line (Bard Access Systems, Murray Hill, NJ, USA; Figure 21.3), is inserted under general anaesthetic. The catheter is tunnelled under the skin for 10–15 cm before the catheter enters the vein. The skin entry site and the vein entry point are therefore a distance apart; the catheter tip's final position is in the SVC. Fibrosis initiated by a Dacron cuff within the device anchors the line in the subcutaneous skin tissues. Lines are most commonly single or double lumen, but can be triple, depending on the clinical requirements of the patient, with an external clamp.

Regular dressings are not required once the catheter is secured in place.

Implantable ports

For long-term use, a Port-a-Cath® (ICU Medical, San Clemente, CA, USA; Figure 21.4) can be used. This is a form of tunnelled catheter attached to a reservoir. The entire device is surgically implanted under general anaesthetic under the patient's skin. The port (chamber) is secured to the underlying tissues with sutures. Ports vary in size and are single or double chamber, depending on the physical size of the patient and clinical requirement of use. Ports are accessed with a non-coring needle – Gripper or Huber needle – which pushes through the skin and silicone septum of the port into the chamber. A semipermeable transparent dressing is applied when the needle is *in situ*.

Accessing CVADs

All personnel who use CVADs must have knowledge, be trained, and undergo competency assessment in the use and care of these devices. The child and family members can be taught and competency assessed as appropriate in accessing CVADs and managing treatment, allowing independence for long-term treatment delivery. Before accessing any line, it is important to observe the skin-line entry site, checking for any signs of damage to the line or any attachments and, during access and administration, to observe for signs of leakage of blood or fluids, documenting findings within nursing notes as standard practice. CVADs have a needleless valved access device on the end of the lumen.

Care of CVADs

Catheter-related blood stream infection (CRBSI) is a common complication and is associated with both insertion of the device and with maintenance. CRBSIs remain a significant risk to the child and family, as infection will increase the length of hospitalization. Guidelines must be followed in all aspects of CVAD care and use, before, during, and after procedure(s).

General principles

- *Prevention of infection*: thorough handwashing, decontamination of the hub or needleless device prior to accessing CVAD, and maintaining principles of asepsis with all equipment and throughout the procedure. The principles of ANTT must be followed.
- *Maintenance of a patent catheter*: adequate flushing, pulsating flushing, heparin flush to fill lumen between use, routine flushing, ensure line is clamped under pressure. Heparin flushing maintains patency of lines when they are 'locked' and will not be used for 24 hours. If the line is being used frequently, then it may be flushed with 0.9% sodium chloride using a positive pressure technique.
- *Preventing damage to catheter*: 10 mL syringes or larger will need to be used when first accessing any CVAD. Smaller syringes produce greater pressure and can result in fracture if the line is blocked, so *must not* be used.

Nurses have a key role in the care of these lines. In addition to performing the practical procedures, they are responsible for the education of the child or young person and family on their CVAD.

Line may fracture and repair kits must be available, only to be used by trained and competent staff.

Key points
- The choice of device to be inserted will be determined by clinical need.
- ANTT practices must be adhered to when accessing the device.
- CRBSI is a significant risk to the child or young person and every step should be taken to avoid this.

22 Tracheostomy care

Box 22.1 Tracheostomy care

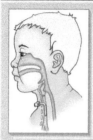

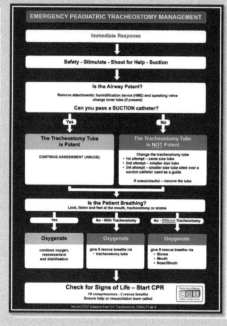

EMERGENCY PEADIATRIC TRACHEOSTOMY MANAGEMENT

Immediate Response

Safety - Stimulate - Shout for Help - Suction

Is the Airway Patent?
Remove attachments: humidification device (HME) and speaking valve
change inner tube (if present)

Can you pass a SUCTION catheter?

Yes — No

The Tracheostomy Tube is Patent

CONTINUE ASSESSMENT (ABCDE)

The Tracheostomy Tube is NOT Patent
- Change the tracheostomy tube
- 1st attempt – same size tube
- 2nd attempt – smaller size tube
- 3rd attempt – smaller size tube sited over a suction catheter used as a guide

If unsuccessful – remove the tube

Is the Patient Breathing?
Look, listen and feel at the mouth, tracheostomy or stoma

Yes — No - With Tracheostomy — No - Without Tracheostomy

Oxygenate
continue oxygen, reassessment and stabilisation

Oxygenate
give 5 rescue breaths via
- tracheostomy tube

Oxygenate
give 5 rescue breaths via
- Stoma
- Mouth
- Nose/Mouth

Check for Signs of Life – Start CPR
15 compressions : 2 rescue breaths
Ensure help or resuscitation team called

Issued 2022 Adapted from UK Tracheostomy Safety Project

- Suction apparatus and appropriate-size suction catheter.
- Spare tracheostomy tubes; one the same size and one a size smaller.
- Double round-ended scissors, water-soluble lubricant
- Spare set of tracheostomy tapes and dressing.
- Normal saline ampoules and gauze.
- A suction catheter to act as a guide over which the new tracheostomy tube is placed in the event that the smaller-size tube is unable to be passed.
- +/– Oxygen connection tubing for a tracheostomy.
- +/– Spare inner cannula.
- +/– Syringe to deflate the cuff.
- +/– One-way resuscitation valve, bag–valve mask (Ambu bag)

Paediatric tracheostomy emergency resources

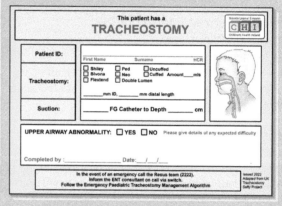

This patient has a
TRACHEOSTOMY

CHI Children's Health Ireland

Patient ID:		
Tracheostomy:	First Name Surname HCR	
	☐ Shiley ☐ Ped ☐ Uncuffed	
	☐ Bivona ☐ Neo ☐ Cuffed Amount____mls	
	☐ Flextend ☐ Double Lumen	
	_____ mm ID, _____ mm distal length	
Suction:	_____ FG Catheter to Depth _____ cm	

UPPER AIRWAY ABNORMALITY: ☐ YES ☐ NO   Please give details of any expected difficulty

Completed by : _____   Date:___/___/___

In the event of an emergency call the Resus team (2222).
Inform the ENT consultant on call via switch.
Follow the Emergency Paediatric Tracheostomy Management Algorithm

Issued 2022 Adapted from UK Tracheostomy Safety Project

- Bedhead signs communicate a child's specific airway, the tracheostomy tube, and suction details.
- Algorithms guide staff through tracheostomy emergency management.
- These resources are freely available from the National Tracheostomy Safety Project website, www.tracheostomy.org. They can be adapted to suit your organization's practice and needs.

Indications
- Upper airway obstruction including:
  - Pierre Robin sequence
  - Subglottic stenosis
  - Bilateral vocal cord palsy
  - Tumours, cystic hygroma
- Ventilation insufficiency including:
  - Prolonged ventilation
  - Tracheomalacia/bronchomalacia
  - Neurological disease
  - Pulmonary disease
- Protection of the tracheobronchial tree
  - Aspiration risk

Emergency equipment
Essential equipment should accompany the child at all times and is checked each shift.

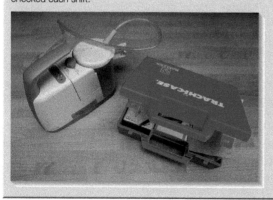

Children and Young People's Nursing at a Glance, Second Edition. Edited by Elizabeth Gormley-Fleming and Sheila Roberts.
© 2023 John Wiley & Sons Ltd. Published 2023 by John Wiley & Sons Ltd.

The term 'tracheostomy' refers to a surgically created opening in the anterior wall of the trachea, into which a tube is placed to provide an artificial airway (Box 22.1). In paediatrics, a tracheostomy is performed in theatre under a general anaesthetic. Children with a newly formed tracheostomy are nursed in a paediatric intensive care or high-dependency unit where staff are skilled in tracheostomy care and management. This ensures that the child is continuously observed and monitored and early potential life-threatening events such as tube obstruction or accidental dislodgement are avoided. During surgery, the otolaryngologist will have placed 'stay sutures' at either side of the incision in the trachea; these are secured on to the chest wall and clearly labelled. The purpose of the stay sutures is to assist with an early or difficult tube change. Once the first tube change has occurred, and the child is deemed as having a safe tract by the otolaryngologist, the stay sutures are removed, after which the child may transfer to a ward.

Most children who require a tracheostomy are under 4 years of age. The tracheostomy tube can be removed once the underlying pathology has been surgically corrected or has improved with growth. This often occurs by the age of 18 months–2 years.

The approach to care is multidisciplinary. The nurse acts as a resource for the child, parents, and staff for education, training, advocacy, consultancy, and emotional and social support. Children who have a tracheostomy will also have input from a speech and language therapist, physiotherapist, and psychologist for a holistic approach to care. Parental education is completed during hospitalization and parents must demonstrate competence in caring for their child's tracheostomy before discharge home.

Stoma and skin care

Stoma care and the care of the skin under the tapes are attended to daily, on alternate days or as needed in an older child; the areas are checked for any alteration to skin integrity.

Mucus or exudate lying on the skin can contribute to skin breakdown. The stoma is cleaned using gauze squares that have been dampened with normal saline. A tracheostomy keyhole dressing can be inserted under the flanges of the tube, which absorbs mucus and exudate and also provides padding. The skin under the tapes is washed with warm water and a pH-neutral wash; it is then rinsed and dried thoroughly. Avoid products that contain small fibres, powders, creams, and cotton wool, which could accidently enter the stoma.

Suctioning

Suctioning is performed when clinically indicated. Staff wear the appropriate personal protective equipment (PPE) during the procedure. Prior to the procedure the following information needs to be established:
• *Catheter size*: the diameter of the catheter should be half the internal diameter of the tracheostomy tube.
• *Depth of insertion*: the catheter is advanced to 0.5 cm past the end of the tracheostomy tube.
• *Suction pressure*: between 80 and 100–120 mmHg, depending on the child's age.
• *Duration of suctioning*: 5–10 seconds is recommended.

Humidification

After a tracheostomy has been formed, inspired air bypasses the upper airway, contributing to a loss of filtering, warming, and humidification. Lack of humidification can lead to thicker secretions and increased risk of mucus plugging, which can cause the tracheostomy tube to block. In the initial postoperative period, humidification is replaced by the use of a heated humidity system. Children progress to the use of heat and moisture exchangers (HMEs); these are changed once they become contaminated with secretions. Normal saline nebulisers are administered to liquefy and loosen secretions.

Tube CHANGES

The frequency of tracheostomy tube changes varies from weekly to monthly depending on the material of which the tube is made. The tracheostomy tube is held in position by the use of a tracheostomy tube holder. Two competent caregivers perform routine tube changes. A blockage or dislodgement of the tube is a life-threatening emergency that necessitates the tube being changed immediately. If a second person is not available, one person will perform the tube change. Signs of a blocked tube include failure to pass a suction catheter, increasing respiratory distress, pallor, and cyanosis; all of which may lead to eventual respiratory arrest if not recognized and acted upon promptly by staff or parents.

Safety

While a child with a tracheostomy is encouraged to live as normal and active a life as possible, some precautions are necessary. Care must be taken to avoid water going into the tracheostomy tube or into the trachea via the stoma during bathing and hair washing. Swimming is not allowed. Care must also be taken with sand. Clothing that does not cover the tracheostomy or shed fibres should be selected. Avoidance of inhaled irritants such as cigarette smoke, pet hair, powder, and aerosol sprays is advised.

Communication

As the majority of airflow bypasses the upper airway, children with a tracheostomy may have an altered ability to vocalize. Early involvement of the speech and language therapist allows the use of aids appropriate to the child's needs and abilities to promote communication. Check with the otolaryngologist if the child has a patent upper airway and is suitable for the placement of a speaking valve.

Feeding

The presence of a tracheostomy tube does not preclude oral feeding. An assessment of the child's swallow is performed by the speech and language therapist before oral feeding is commenced. As the majority of airflow bypasses the upper airway, children with a tracheostomy have a reduced sense of smell and taste.

Complications

Early complications include tube obstruction, accidental tube dislodgement, haemorrhage, pneumothorax, and false passage formation.

Late complications include tube obstruction, accidental tube dislodgement, chest infections, suprastomal collapse, granulation tissue, and laryngotracheal stenosis.

Key points
• Children are at a greater risk of tube obstruction than adults because their airways are smaller and paediatric tracheostomy tubes generally have a single lumen.
• A blocked or dislodged tube is life-threatening and requires immediate action.
• Paediatric tracheostomy care must be implemented by competent personnel.

23 Infant resuscitation

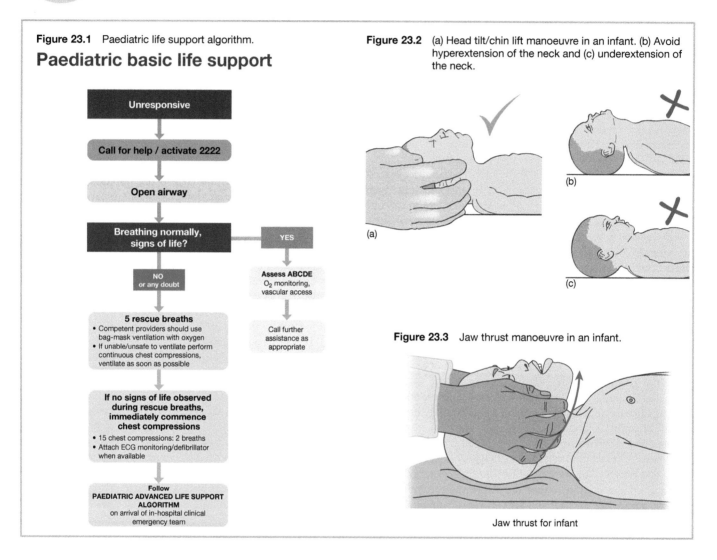

Figure 23.1 Paediatric life support algorithm.

Paediatric basic life support

Unresponsive

Call for help / activate 2222

Open airway

Breathing normally, signs of life? → **YES** → **Assess ABCDE** O₂ monitoring, vascular access → **Call further assistance as appropriate**

NO or any doubt

5 rescue breaths
- Competent providers should use bag-mask ventilation with oxygen
- If unable/unsafe to ventilate perform continuous chest compressions, ventilate as soon as possible

If no signs of life observed during rescue breaths, immediately commence chest compressions
- 15 chest compressions: 2 breaths
- Attach ECG monitoring/defibrillator when available

Follow PAEDIATRIC ADVANCED LIFE SUPPORT ALGORITHM on arrival of in-hospital clinical emergency team

Figure 23.2 (a) Head tilt/chin lift manoeuvre in an infant. (b) Avoid hyperextension of the neck and (c) underextension of the neck.

Figure 23.3 Jaw thrust manoeuvre in an infant.

Jaw thrust for infant

Cardiorespiratory arrest is an uncommon event for most children's and young people's nurses, but the ability to perform the procedure effectively and efficiently is paramount. Competence is required for professional practice. Most paediatric cardiac arrests occur due to decompensated respiratory or circulatory failure. Early intervention and recognition of the sick infant are essential, as outcomes for cardiorespiratory arrest are poor. This chapter deals specifically with infant resuscitation (i.e. any child less than 1 year of age but not a newborn baby). This is a concise version of the full procedure offered by the Resuscitation Council (UK) and all readers are strongly advised to read this guidance to ensure up-to-date practice while performing this procedure (Figure 23.1). The Paediatric Basic Life Support guidance does not include advice for the layperson and covers the actions of healthcare professionals with a duty of care (for the full guidance visit www.resus.org.uk). Systematic assessment is required to ascertain physiological alterations and direct focused interventions.

Covid-19 guidance published by the Resuscitation Council 2021 advised on the use of full aerosol-generating procedure (AGP) personal protective equipment (PPE) for staff attending cardiac arrests. Airway management must only be performed by competent individuals. The risk of Covid-19 should be stated when the cardiac arrest call is made, and personnel should be restricted in the resuscitation area. Equipment must be disposed of in accordance with local infection control guidelines.

Unresponsive – shout for help!
- Gently stimulate the infant by loudly asking 'Are you all right?' or calling the infant's name.
- If this infant is responsive, leave them in the position you found them unless they are in immediate danger or the airway is at risk.
- If there is no response, shout for help.
- If there is more than one responder, get them to call 999 (outside hospital), or if in a National Health Service hospital call 2222.

Children and Young People's Nursing at a Glance, Second Edition. Edited by Elizabeth Gormley-Fleming and Sheila Roberts.
© 2023 John Wiley & Sons Ltd. Published 2023 by John Wiley & Sons Ltd.

Open airway

- Turn infant on their back on a firm surface where you are able to be directly above them.
- Head tilt should be used initially by placing your hand on the forehead to gently tilt the head. While placing your fingertips onto the bony prominence of the child's jaw, lift the chin into a neutral position. Do not put any pressure on the soft tissues under the chin, as this may cause airway occlusion.
- If there is difficulty opening the airway or you are concerned about cervical injury, perform a jaw thrust. There should be a low threshold for using a jaw thrust if a neck injury is suspected.
- Place fingers either side of the infant's mandible (jawbone) and push the jaw forward.
- Once the airway is open, position the side of your face close to the infant's face.
- LOOK for chest movement.
- LISTEN for breath sounds.
- FEEL air movement on your cheek.
- Be able to differentiate between normal breathing and noisy gasps. The infant may continue to make infrequent attempts at breathing immediately after going into cardiac arrest.
- This should take no more than 10 seconds. If in doubt, assume breathing rate is abnormal and take action.
- While assessing breathing, you should be looking for other signs of life. These include coughing, movement, and normal breathing rather than gasps.

   If the infant is breathing normally:
- Place them in a recovery position or maintain the current position with their airway opened.
- Seek help, ideally while remining with the infant. The infant should only be left if there is no means of getting help.
- Continue to observe the infant.

Rescue breaths

If breathing is not normal or is absent, clear the airway of any secretion or airway obstructions (do not use finger sweeps to remove obstructions) and give five rescue breaths.

   With the head in the neutral position (Figure 23.2):
- Take a breath and cover the nose and mouth with your mouth.
- A good seal can be obtained by not overly opening your mouth and keeping your lips soft.
- Blow steadily over one second until the chest visibly moves.
- Maintain the neutral position while removing your mouth to watch the chest fall before applying the next breath.

   If you are unable to get a good seal around the nose and mouth in the older infant you may:
- Attempt to just seal the nose or the mouth with the rescuer's mouth.
- If using the nose, be sure to close the mouth while securing the airway to ensure air is not lost.

   In the hospital setting, a bag-mask device is likely to be available and therefore should be used by trained staff as soon as one is accessible at the cot side.

Difficulty in achieving effective breaths

If there is difficulty in achieving effective breaths, airway obstructions should be considered.
- Open the infant's mouth and carefully remove any visible obstructions. Do not perform a blind finger sweep.
- Try to reposition the head to open the airway, making sure there is adequate head tilt/chin lift.
- If this is unsuccessful, use the jaw thrust method (Figure 23.3).
- Attempt to give five effective breaths. If this is unsuccessful, move to chest compressions.

Following rescue breaths if there are signs of life

If you are confident that you can detect signs of life, then:
- Continue rescue breaths, if necessary, until the infant starts breathing on their own.
- If the infant is unconscious, not in cardiac arrest but breathing normally, keep their airway opened either by head tilt/chin lift or jaw thrust. If there is a risk of vomiting, place the infant into the recovery position.
- Reassess the infant frequently.

After rescue breaths if there are no signs of life

There are two methods of performing chest compression in an infant, the two-finger technique and the two-thumb encircling technique. The two-thumb encircling technique is preferable, but a lone rescuer may prefer to use the two-finger technique. Palpating for a pulse has been determined as an unreliable method to establish if there is effective or inadequate circulation. Palpation of a pulse is not the determinant for the need for chest compressions either. The two-finger technique is outlined below:
- The tips of two fingers to be placed on the sternum just below the nipples. This equates to one finger breath up from the end of the sternum (xiphisternum).
- Depress the sternum by at least one-third the depth of the chest –approximately 4 cm for an infant (do not be afraid to push too hard).
- Release the pressure to allow the chest to recoil, and avoid leaning on the chest at the end of each compression. Allow time for the chest to recoil. Around 50% of the whole cycle should be the relaxation phase, from the start of one compression to the next.
- The aim is to achieve a rate of 100–120 chest compressions per minute.
- The compression to breath rate should be 15 : 2.
- Reassess after one minute, looking for signs of life.
   The encircling technique requires:
- The two thumbs on the lower half of the sternum.
- Thumbs should be pointing towards the infant's head.
   You must continue resuscitation until:
- The infant shows signs of life.
- Further qualified help arrives.
- You become exhausted.
   Get help as quickly as possible:
- If there are two rescuers, one begins cardiopulmonary resuscitation (CPR) while the second person call for emergency medical assistance.
- If only one rescuer is present, undertake resuscitation for one minute before going for assistance.
- If there is one rescuer with a mobile phone, call for help with the speaker function on immediately after giving rescue breaths.
- With an infant it may be possible to carry them to further assistance to minimize interruptions.
- There is one exception to performing one minute of CPR before seeking help and that is the witnessed, sudden collapse of an infant when the rescuer has no phone, is alone, and primary cardiac arrest is suspected. The infant may need defibrillation for a shockable rhythm, so help should be sought immediately.

Key points
- This chapter reproduces the basic life support guidance published on the Resuscitation Council's website.
- Children's and young people's nurses must always keep up to date with life support training.
- Regularly visit the website to ensure you have the most up-to-date information for your practice (www.resus.org.uk).

24 Child and young person resuscitation

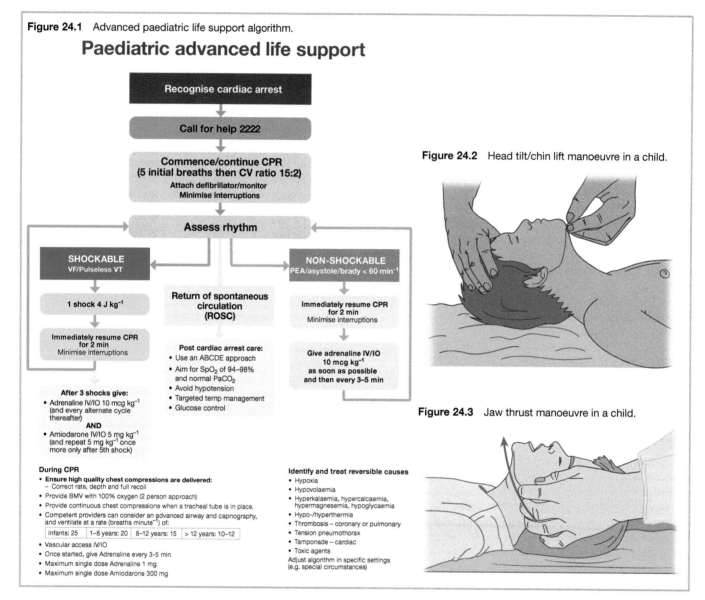

Figure 24.1 Advanced paediatric life support algorithm.

Paediatric advanced life support

Recognise cardiac arrest

Call for help 2222

Commence/continue CPR
(5 initial breaths then CV ratio 15:2)
Attach defibrillator/monitor
Minimise interruptions

Assess rhythm

SHOCKABLE
VF/Pulseless VT

NON-SHOCKABLE
PEA/asystole/brady < 60 min⁻¹

1 shock 4 J kg⁻¹

Return of spontaneous
circulation
(ROSC)

Immediately resume CPR
for 2 min
Minimise interruptions

Immediately resume CPR
for 2 min
Minimise interruptions

Give adrenaline IV/IO
10 mcg kg⁻¹
as soon as possible
and then every 3–5 min

Post cardiac arrest care:
- Use an ABCDE approach
- Aim for SpO₂ of 94–98% and normal PaCO₂
- Avoid hypotension
- Targeted temp management
- Glucose control

After 3 shocks give:
- Adrenaline IV/IO 10 mcg kg⁻¹ (and every alternate cycle thereafter)
  AND
- Amiodarone IV/IO 5 mg kg⁻¹ (and repeat 5 mg kg⁻¹ once more only after 5th shock)

During CPR
- **Ensure high quality chest compressions are delivered:**
  – Correct rate, depth and full recoil
- Provide BMV with 100% oxygen (2 person approach)
- Provide continuous chest compressions when a tracheal tube is in place.
- Competent providers can consider an advanced airway and capnography, and ventilate at a rate (breaths minute⁻¹) of:

| Infants: 25 | 1–8 years: 20 | 8–12 years: 15 | > 12 years: 10–12 |

- Vascular access IV/IO
- Once started, give Adrenaline every 3-5 min
- Maximum single dose Adrenaline 1 mg
- Maximum single dose Amiodarone 300 mg

Identify and treat reversible causes
- Hypoxia
- Hypovolaemia
- Hyperkalaemia, hypercalcaemia, hypermagnesemia, hypoglycaemia
- Hypo-/hyperthermia
- Thrombosis – coronary or pulmonary
- Tension pneumothorax
- Tamponade – cardiac
- Toxic agents
Adjust algorithm in specific settings
(e.g. special circumstances)

Figure 24.2 Head tilt/chin lift manoeuvre in a child.

Figure 24.3 Jaw thrust manoeuvre in a child.

When involved in resuscitation, it must be noted that there are differences to the resuscitation algorithm that are dependent on whether the patient is an infant (under 1 year of age), a child or young person (between 1 and 18 years of age), or an adult. For the purposes of this chapter, resuscitation is focused on a child or young person who is between 1 and 18 years of age. The variation in child and adult resuscitation guidelines is based on their different aetiology. The rescuer should work within the guidelines (Figure 24.1) that they believe best reflect the age group of the patient if unsure of the age group.

Covid-19 guidance published by the Resuscitation Council 2021 advised on the use of full aerosol-generating procedure (AGP) personal protective equipment (PPE) for staff attending cardiac arrests. Airway management must only be performed by competent individuals. The risk of Covid-19 should be stated when the cardiac arrest call is made, and personnel should be restricted in the resuscitation area. Equipment must be disposed of in accordance with local infection control guidelines.

Safe to approach

Always ensure that it is safe to approach the patient and that there are no obvious hazards.

Stimulate

Try to gain a response from the patient. This can be by calling their name or stroking their forehead or ears. If they respond, keep them comfortable and call for help. If they are unresponsive, continue with the young person resuscitation algorithm.

Children and Young People's Nursing at a Glance, Second Edition. Edited by Elizabeth Gormley-Fleming and Sheila Roberts.
© 2023 John Wiley & Sons Ltd. Published 2023 by John Wiley & Sons Ltd.

Shout

Shout for help and ensure that someone contacts the paediatric arrest team so that further assistance is provided. In a National Health Service setting, call 2222 as this is the cardiac arrest emergency number. The caller should state clearly where they are: location Ward X, Room Y.

Airway

Ensure that the mouth is clear from obstruction and then place the head into a 'head tilt/chin lift' (Figure 24.2) until the head is extended into a sniffing position. This will enable the airway to be fully opened. If there are concerns that the young person has been involved in a trauma, then a jaw thrust (Figure 24.3) should be performed to ensure that the head remains in a neutral position and is in alignment with the cervical spine. To open the child/young person's airway using jaw thrust, place the first two fingers of each hand behind each side of the mandible and push the jaw forward. Have a low threshold for suspecting neck injury and if any suspicion is present then the jaw thrust movement should be utilized.

Once the airway has been opened it is important to look, listen, and feel for breathing for 10 seconds:

- LOOK to see the rise and fall of the chest.
- LISTEN for any breath sounds.
- FEEL for breath being expelled from the mouth and/or nose.

While assessing breathing, you should be looking for other signs of life. This includes coughing, movement, and normal breathing rather than gasps.

Breathing

If there is no breathing or ineffective breathing, then five effective rescue breaths must be given:

- Pinch the soft part of the nose closed with the index finger and thumb of the hand, tilting the child's forehead.
- Take a breath and place your lips around the child's mouth, making sure there is a good seal.
- Blow steadily into their mouth over one second. The chest should rise.
- Maintain the airway opening position and remove your mouth while watching the chest wall fall as air is expelled.
- Take another breath and repeat this sequence four times while continuing to watch the chest rise and fall with each breath given.

If any of the breaths are not effective, then reassess the airway. Open the child/young person's mouth and if there are any visible obstructions, they should be carefully removed. Do not perform a blind finger sweep.

- Reposition the head and ensure there is adequate head tilt/chin lift. Do not overextend the neck.
- If this does not work satisfactorily, use the jaw thrust opening method.
- Make five attempts to give effective breaths and if still unsuccessful move to chest compressions without delay.

In the hospital setting a bag-mask valve set will be available and should be used with haste by those competent in its use.

If there are signs of life following rescue breaths

If you are confident that you can detect signs of life, then:

- Continue rescue breaths, if necessary, until the child/young person starts breathing on their own.
- If the child/young person is unconscious, not in cardiac arrest but breathing normally, keep their airway opened either by head tilt/chin lift or jaw thrust. If there is a risk of vomiting, place the child/young person into the recovery position.
- Reassess the child/young person frequently.

If there are no signs of life following rescue breaths or you are uncertain

- Commence chest compressions if there are no signs of life or if you are uncertain whether there are.
- The landmark for chest compressions is one finger breadth above the xiphisternum; using the heel of the hand or both hands interlocked, deliver the chest compressions depressing the lower half of the sternum by at least one-third of the anterior–posterior dimension, which is approximately 5 cm.
- Lift the fingers off the chest when performing chest compressions.
- The best position for the rescuer delivering chest compressions is to be vertically over the child/young person's chest with arms straight.
- Allow the chest to return to a resting position between each compression. Approximately 50% of the cycle should be in the relaxation phase. Continue in a ratio of 15:2 compressions:ventilations.
- While cardiopulmonary resuscitation (CPR) is being carried out it is vital that a monitor is attached to the young person to determine what rhythm their heart is in and therefore if it is a shockable or unshockable rhythm.
  - *Shockable rhythms*: pulseless ventricular tachycardia and ventricular fibrillation.
  - *Unshockable rhythms*: pulseless electrical activity (PEA) and asystole.
- If the young person requires defibrillating, the amount of energy that should be used is 4 J per kg.
- If the young person is in cardiac arrest, the pulse and heart rhythm must be rechecked every two minutes and the appropriate course of action taken.

Definitive care

It is important to note that while not all young people have a spontaneous return of circulation, some do make a very good recovery from a cardiac arrest. If a young person responds to the treatment, then plans should be made for them to be admitted to either an intensive care unit on site or to another hospital that has the expertise and facilities to care for them.

If the young person does not survive the cardiac arrest, it is imperative that support services are put in place for the family to offer comfort during their bereavement, and also that a debrief is carried out for all staff who were involved in the resuscitation to allow them an opportunity to discuss their feelings and the situation.

Key points

- The primary cause of cardiopulmonary arrest in young people is hypoxia. For this reason, if a young person is found unresponsive and not breathing, the first action to be taken is for the rescuer to deliver five rescue breaths before seeking further help.
- Early recognition of the sick child/young person is desired in order to prevent deterioration.
- Effective ventilation and oxygenation may prevent a cardiac arrest from occurring in young people.

25 Emergency care of children

Figure 25.1 Common presentations of the unwell baby.

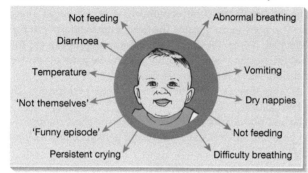

Not feeding
Diarrhoea
Temperature
'Not themselves'
'Funny episode'
Persistent crying

Abnormal breathing
Vomiting
Dry nappies
Not feeding
Difficulty breathing

Box 25.1 Common presentations of the preschool child.

- Foreign body to ear, nose, or swallowed
- Toddler's fracture
- Clavicle fracture
- Finger-tip injury
- Head injury
- Minor wounds to head
- Pulled elbow
- Torus fracture to distal radius
- Supracondylar fracture
- Burn
- Accidental ingestion
- Fever
- Otitis media
- Otitis externa
- Viral illness/rash
- Asthma
- Febrile convulsion

Box 25.2 Common presentations of school-age children.

- Head injury
- Clavicle fracture
- Torus fracture to distal radius
- Long bone fracture
- Metacarpal and phalangeal fracture
- Ankle injury (soft tissue and bony injury)
- Wound
- Foreign body in wound
- Animal bite
- Transient synovitis
- Septic arthritis/osteomyelitis
- Legg–Calve–Perthes disease

Box 25.3 Common presentations of adolescents.

- Muscular skeletal injury
- Head injury
- Assault
- Alcohol intoxication
- Illicit drug use
- Fever
- Rash
- Abdominal pain
- Headache
- Mental health problems including deliberate self-harm and overdose
- Sexual health – including emergency contraception
- Concealed pregnancy
- Gynaecological problems
- Osteoarthritis or septic arthritis
- Slipped femoral epiphysis

Box 25.4 Safeguarding red flags.

- Inappropriate delay in presentations
- Injury and mechanism of injury mismatch
- Immobile children with long bone fracture
- Head injury on children under 1 year old
- High frequency of attendances
- Domestic abuse, alcohol, substance misuse, or mental illness in the household
- Other concerns: home safety, supervision, bullying, parent–child interactions

Children and Young People's Nursing at a Glance, Second Edition. Edited by Elizabeth Gormley-Fleming and Sheila Roberts.
© 2023 John Wiley & Sons Ltd. Published 2023 by John Wiley & Sons Ltd.

Introduction

A child or young person attending an Emergency Department may be frightened and overwhelmed, as can their parents/carers. An attendance at an Emergency Department is unplanned and usually because of sudden injury or illness. Children or young people often present in pain or acute illness and can at times attend initially without their parent or carer (teacher, sports coach, youth leader). The emergency children's nurse faces a unique, challenging, rewarding, and privileged aspect of practice. In emergency care the children's nurse develops refined skills, from meeting a patient to promptly assessing, managing, and recognizing critical illness, crisis, or vulnerability in a short period with no prior medical or social history on the patient. Developing trusting therapeutic relationships with the patient and accompanying parent/carer is core to working in this speciality.

There is an enhanced understanding of the importance of pre-hospital care and why children and young people attend hospital for emergency care. New models of care delivery provide different levels of care, with an ambition of achieving cost-effective and efficient care for the child/young person and their families. The National Health Service (NHS) offers a range of emergency care centres ranging from minor injury units, to walk-in centres, to major trauma centres. A network approach to care is now well established in the NHS.

Children's emergency care is a relatively new speciality. Facing the Future, Standards for Children, from the Royal College of Paediatrics and Child Health, provides 70 standards for emergency care. These standards reflect the significant changes and complexity of needs for emergency care for children and young people. They advocate an integrated approach, ensuring that children are seen in the right place and by the appropriate, competent clinicians.

The emergency children's nurse requires knowledge of other specialities covered in other chapters in this book, such as fever, asthma, fractures, plaster care, resuscitation, Paediatric Early Warning Score (PEWS), physical assessment, safeguarding, head injury, and coma management. Nurses working in emergency settings are delivering care at the starting point of the breadth of speciality pathways. A governance framework must be in place with speciality teams to ensure that pathways are safe, risks are assessed, and updated practice is shared. This chapter provides a snapshot of common presenting complaints to an Emergency Department in relation to the developmental stages of childhood.

The unwell baby

The unwell baby is a common presentation to an Emergency Department (Figure 25.1). Babies present a different challenge to the emergency nurse, which can range from a worried parent and a minor viral illness to a severely sick baby requiring critical care or resuscitative management. Essential skills of listening to the history of illness, and understanding infant physiology, feeding regimes, response to illness, and safeguarding are required in these presentations. The children's nurse is crucial during the assessment of these babies, with the assistance of a PEWS to identify severe illness and prompt escalation to the appropriate senior clinician.

Parents are very aware of the careful balance between breathing, feeding, and production of wet nappies. A change in one of these will lead to the baby being brought to an Emergency Department. These concerns can also be accompanied by a fever, rash, or history of a 'strange episode'. There is no way of predicting at what stage in the baby's illness they will present. Bronchiolitis, viral-induced wheeze, gastroenteritis, febrile convulsion, and oesophageal reflux are commonly diagnosed.

Common presentations in preschool children

The preschool child has endless adventures seeking out their environment during a time of rapid physical and intellectual development (Box 25.1). Socializing with other children both aids their development and can lead to injury. Their immunity is developed by the daily sharing of minor infections. There is a predictable pattern of illness and injury of preschool children.

Common presentations in school-age children

The school-age child is more aware of their personal safety and that of others around them (Box 25.2). They develop more responsibility for themselves and have some independence in their activities away from their parents. It is a stage when regular physical activity becomes embedded into their daily lives, which does influence their pattern of injury.

Common presentations in adolescents

It can be a challenge to meet the needs of the adolescent in healthcare (Box 25.3). This time of their development includes increasing risk-taking behaviours as well as mental health presentations. The Covid-19 pandemic has exacerbated already existing pressures on services caring for children and young people presenting with mental ill health.

Safeguarding

Safeguarding children and young people in an Emergency Department is core to all nursing practice (Box 25.4). Nursing children and families who are not previously known, in a short period of time, requires a thorough and rapid assessment for 'red flags' to identify any safeguarding risks relating to their presentation.

Key points
- Receive a child to your department with compassion, allowing for play and distraction.
- Listen to what the child or young person is telling you.
- Eyes and ears are your best assessment tools (use the physical assessment skills you have been trained in).
- Listen to the history given by the parents, and clarify what their biggest concern is – they know the child better than anyone.
- Consider safeguarding risks for all children and young people.

26 Resuscitation drugs

Figure 26.1 Use and doses of resuscitation drugs.

Adrenaline

Uses: cardiorespiratory arrest, bradycardia of <60 beats per minute after initial steps to improve oxygenation have been taken and anaphylaxis with hypotension

Dose: 10 µg/kg (0.1 mL/kg of 1 : 10 000 solution) This can be repeated every 3–5 minutes as needed

If anaphylaxis: intramuscular adrenaline should be given (1 : 1000 solution)
    <6 years 150 µg (0.15 mL)
    6–12 years 300 µg (0.3 mL)
    >12 years 500 µg (0.5 mL)

Atropine

Uses: bradycardia as a result of vagal stimulation

Dose: 20 µg/kg (minimum dose 100 µg)

Oxygen

15 L via bag-valve mask if not breathing or ineffective breathing or via non-rebreather mask if breathing not compromised

0.9% Sodium chloride

Uses: children in cardiac arrest or circulatory failure, or with hypovolaemia causing a circulation compromise must be given fluid resuscitation

Dose: 20 mL/kg

Glucose

Uses: hypoglycaemia

Dose: 2 mL/kg of 10% glucose followed by an infusion to prevent rebound hypoglycaemia once child has been successfully resuscitated

Amiodarone

Uses: refractory ventricular fibrillation (VF) or pulseless ventricular tachycardia (VT). If VF or pulseless VT remains after the third defibrillation shock, amiodarone should be given with adrenaline. This should then be given again after the fifth shock if defibrillation is unsuccessful

Dose: 5 mg/kg

If defibrillation was successful but VT or VF recurs, the amiodarone can be repeated and a continuous infusion commenced

Adenosine

Uses: supraventricular tachycardia (SVT). It is safe because it has a short half-life (10 seconds). This should be administered intravenously via upper limb or central veins to minimize the time taken to reach the heart. Give adenosine rapidly, followed by a flush of 3–5 mL normal saline

Dose: 100 µg/kg (maximum dose 6 mg) for first bolus. Second bolus can be doubled up to a maximum of 12 mg

Figure 26.2 (a) Intraosseous access line and needles. (b) Intraosseous access to medial surface of the anterior tibia. (c) Landmarks for intraosseous access.

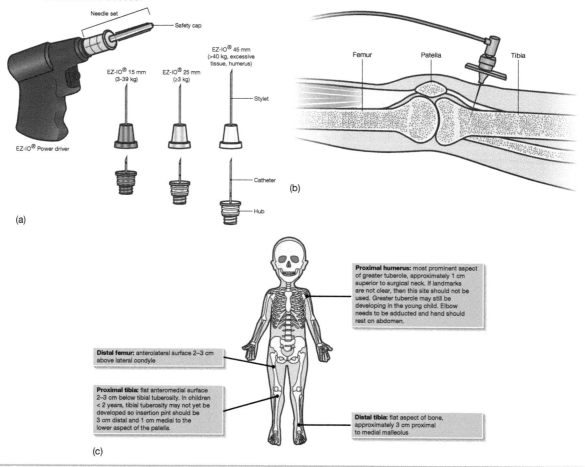

Children and Young People's Nursing at a Glance, Second Edition. Edited by Elizabeth Gormley-Fleming and Sheila Roberts.
© 2023 John Wiley & Sons Ltd. Published 2023 by John Wiley & Sons Ltd.

Effective drug administration is an imperative in the resuscitation of all infants and children. The primary cause of cardio-respiratory arrest in children is hypoxia, therefore effective ventilation is also essential and oxygen is a vital drug in the management of infants and children who require resuscitation. Access to emergency drugs is crucial and sufficient amounts must be readily available so as not to delay treatment of the critically ill child. Familiarity with the medication used during resuscitation is all-important for patient safety (Figure 26.1).

Drug calculation in an emergency situation

Body weight estimation is frequently required in emergency situations to calculate drug dosages and fluid volume in the absence of knowing the infant's or child's actual body weight. Body weight may be estimated using a body length tape (the Paediatric Advanced Weight Resuscitation Emergency Tape, PAWPER, or Broselow tape). The PAWPER tape relates to the child's height and provides the medication doses as well as other key information (e.g. voltage). Broselow is a colour-coded tape measure. It relates to the child's height as a measure of their weight, which then provides drug doses, size of equipment, and the amount of voltage that may be used. The child needs to be in a supine position and the red end of the tape is placed at their head; the colour zone at the child's heels provides their approximate weight and their colour zone. Caution in its use is required. Some departments have adopted this methodology for their resuscitation trolley layout.

An age-based weight calculation formula is commonly used for children up to the age of 10 years.

If the child is obese, their ideal body weight should be used to calculate drugs. If their actual body weight is used it may cause drug toxicity.

A paediatric emergency drug chart must be available in the resuscitation room as this will provide accurate dosage information.

The maximum adult doses of drugs should not be exceeded in young people.

WETFLAG is an emergency calculation tool that is frequently used in advance of the arrival of the child in the Emergency Department in order to prepare drugs and fluid volumes (Box 26.1). This tool relies on the age of the child as the basis for estimation of their weight.

Oxygen administration

Oxygen is an essential drug for all resuscitations. Oxygen should be administered via a bag-mask ventilation (BMV) using a high concentration of 100% immediately. If BMV is not successful, then the child may need to be intubated. Once positive-pressure ventilation has been achieved, ventilation can be continued via BMV or the child can be placed on a mechanical ventilator. where the fraction of inspired oxygen can be titrated to maintain oxygen saturations of 94–98%.

Route of drug administration during resuscitation

Vascular access must be established early, as it is essential to enable drugs and fluids to be given during resuscitation. However, this can be difficult to establish during resuscitation of an infant or child, particularly if they are hypovolaemic.

Intravenous (IV) and intraosseous (IO) routes are both acceptable. IV access is preferable, but if this cannot be obtained within one minute then IO access should be attempted. The preferred site is the antecubital fossa.

Some medication, for example adrenaline, may be administered via endotracheal tube if required and other access routes are not available.

If IV access is not available, then the IO route should be used. IO access is obtained using an EZ IO™ (Teleflex, Morrisville, NC, USA; Figure 26.2a). Securing the access route is vitally important and should be achieve in accordance with local guidelines and policy. The preferred site is the medial surface of the anterior tibia (Figure 26.2b), but if this is not accessible other landmarks may be used (Figure 26.2c). A sample of bone marrow taken from the IO site can be sent to the laboratory for analysis. It is important to note on the sample that this is bone marrow and not blood.

Scalp veins should not be used during resuscitation as the risk of extravasation injury is increased.

Resuscitation and other emergency drugs

Adrenaline

Adrenaline should be administered within three minutes in the presence of a non-shockable rhythm. In the presence of a shockable rhythm, adrenaline should be administered immediately after the third and then alternate shocks (fifth, seventh, etc.). Additional doses can be administered every three to five minutes.

Amiodarone

Amiodarone should be infused slowly >20 minutes in children who have a perfusing rhythm: ventricular tachycardia with a pulse or supraventricular tachycardia. This should prevent bradycardia and cardiac arrest.

In the presence of a shockable rhythm, an IV bolus can be administered immediately after the third shock.

Known to cause thrombophlebitis, amiodarone should be administered into a central vein if possible. If this is not possible then it must be adequately flushed with 0.9% sodium chloride or glucose 5%.

Atropine

Atropine is used in resuscitation to treat symptomatic bradycardia and atrioventricular (AV) block. It blocks the effects of the vagus nerve on the sino-atrial node. This increases sinus automaticity and therefore the heart rate increases. It may be used as an antidote following overdose or poisoning of angiotensin-converting enzyme (ACE) inhibitors or muscarinic mushrooms.

Box 26.1 WETFLAG calculation tool

W – Weight kg <1 year of age: 0.5 × age in months + 4
    1–5 years: (2 × age) + 8
    >5 years: (3 × age) + 7
E – Energy 4 J/kg
T – Tube diameter: (age/4) + 4. Oral tube length: (Age/2) + 12. Nasal tube length: (Age/2 + 15)
F – Fluid
L – Lorazepam 0.1 mg/kg
A – Adrenaline (intravenous) 0.1 mL/kg of 1 : 10 000
G – Glucose/dextrose 10% 2 mL/kg

Adenosine

A naturally occurring nucleoside, adenosine slows conduction through the AV node by opening the acetylcholine-sensitive potassium channels and block calcium influx in the nerve cells. This leads to hyperpolarization. Conduction time is decreased, and this leads to an antiarrhythmic effect. Vascular smooth muscle is relaxed, and this leads to an increase in blood flow through the coronary arteries. Adenosine has a short half-life and is best administered in a vein close to the heart, such as the antecubital fossa.

Lidocaine

Lidocaine blocks sodium channels, which results in a shortening of the cardiac action and a decrease in the rate of cardiac contractions. The initial dose is administered by IV injection and this is followed immediately by IV infusion. It may be used for shock-resistant ventricular fibrillation or pulseless ventricular tachycardia.

Magnesium

Magnesium is a major intracellular cation. It is a cofactor in many enzymatic reactions. Its use is well documented in children with hypomagnesium and polymorphic ventricular tachycardia.

Calcium

Calcium is essential for the cellular mechanisms responsible for myocardial contractability. It should only be administered in a cardiac arrest when specifically indicated (hyperkalaemia, hypocalcaemia, hypermagnesium, and in overdoses of calcium-channel blocking medication). It must be administered over 5–10 minutes.

High plasma concentration post administration has been known to cause ischaemia to the myocardium and to impair cerebral recovery.

Glucose

Glucose is essential for normal cell function. It provides the energy required by all cellular function. Low glucose levels mean that the contractility of the heart muscle can be decreased, which in turn reduces cardiac output.

Fluids in CPR

Hypovolaemia is a reversable cause of cardiac arrest. If the child is volume depleted, then fluids should be administered IV or IO rapidly in boluses. A mix of crystalloids or 0.9% saline should be used for initial volume resuscitation. Blood or blood products may be indicated for trauma patients. Dextrose-based solutions must not be used for volume replacement. These will cause rapid redistribution of fluid away from the intravascular spaces, leading to hyponatraemia and hyperglycaemia and altering neurological status.

Key points

- A sufficient amount of emergency drugs and fluids should be available.
- All drugs administered should be recorded and signed for with date and time noted by an identifiable member of staff.
- Additional drugs required post resuscitation should be available.
- Emergency drugs should be checked for expiry dates in accordance with local protocols.

Part 2

27 Partnership

Figure 27.1 Effective partnership. MDT, multidisciplinary team.

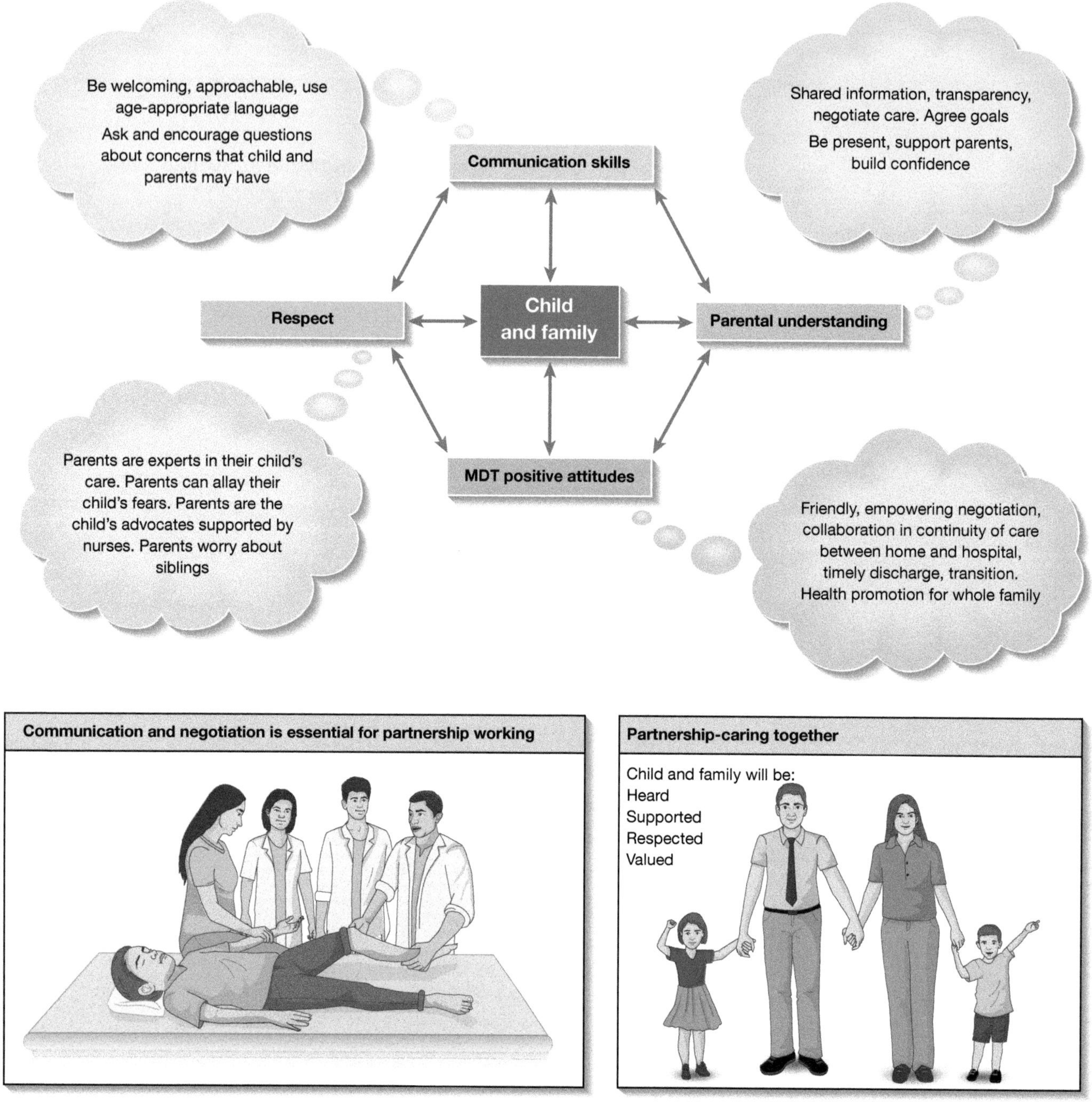

Be welcoming, approachable, use age-appropriate language

Ask and encourage questions about concerns that child and parents may have

Shared information, transparency, negotiate care. Agree goals

Be present, support parents, build confidence

Communication skills

Respect

Child and family

Parental understanding

MDT positive attitudes

Parents are experts in their child's care. Parents can allay their child's fears. Parents are the child's advocates supported by nurses. Parents worry about siblings

Friendly, empowering negotiation, collaboration in continuity of care between home and hospital, timely discharge, transition. Health promotion for whole family

Communication and negotiation is essential for partnership working

Partnership-caring together

Child and family will be:
Heard
Supported
Respected
Valued

Children and Young People's Nursing at a Glance, Second Edition. Edited by Elizabeth Gormley-Fleming and Sheila Roberts.
© 2023 John Wiley & Sons Ltd. Published 2023 by John Wiley & Sons Ltd.

Working in partnership with the child and family is well established in the practice of children's nursing. International health policy advocates that patient-centred care is embedded into care delivery and that professionals and patients/carers work in collaboration. It is vital that nurses and the multidisciplinary team (MDT) realize that parents are the experts with regard to their child and that valuable knowledge and skills can be gained from parents regarding their child's routines. Parents want to contribute to discussion and decisions about their child, but may not always be invited to or consider that their contribution is of value.

The partnership model of care recognizes that the family are expert carers with regard to their child.

Care of the child needs to be negotiated with the child, family members, and the nurse. The nurse's role is supporting, teaching, and assisting the family to make informed decisions about their child's care. Parents are the child's advocate and nurses provide support to ensure that the child's wishes and feelings are taken into account.

A plan of care is discussed and agreed. Direct care is carried out as planned. The nurse shares information, provides support, monitors progress, and, with the family's consent, coordinates care with other professionals. Parents will be concerned about the effects that hospital admission will have on the child and their siblings.

Effective partnership

For partnership care to be effective, nurses must have a positive attitude, respect for the family, good communication skills, and an understanding of the complexity of the parents' role. This requires the following:

- Building of trust.
- Listening to concerns.
- Valuing the parents' knowledge and incorporating it into clinical care.
- Respecting and being sensitive to the family's context.
- Mutual exchange of information.
- Supporting the parents in their role.

Partnership and the multidisciplinary team

Nurses and members of the MDT (Figure 27.1) have to be non-judgemental and work together with the family to discuss options, and participate in negotiation and decision making. It has been found that negative staff attitudes could result in the delayed discharge of children with complex care needs. Carers may feel that their parenting skills are on public display and that staff might disapprove of their family set-up, cultural differences, or parenting styles.

Parental stress and partnership

Nurses need to recognize that parents will have additional stressors when their child is admitted to hospital. These may be financial, personal, or time pressures. Information is shared with parents to make them aware that there may be financial support available, and this knowledge can reduce some anxieties. Parents of children with long-term conditions may have unique challenges around hospitalization as they are more likely to require frequent healthcare appointments and lengthy stays, which can have significant impacts on many aspects of family life.

Parents will engage in a collaborative partnership with the MDT to ensure continuity between hospital and care at home. This provides an opportunity for parents to share their concerns about how the admission of a child will affect their siblings. Parents' fears can be allayed by the nurse, ensuring that the child is involved in decision making regarding their care. Nurses can also work in partnership with the family to ensure a timely discharge for the child as well as initiating health promotion for the family. When a child is admitted to hospital, parents can feel lonely and unsupported. Nurses need to provide emotional support before parents reach crisis point.

Parental needs

Effective partnership may be hindered by the lack of recognition of parental needs. Staff need to respect the family's social, religious, and cultural beliefs and this can reduce negative interpretations. The child and parents may need to be prepared and supported to engage in partnership care prior to admission. This must be done without making the parents feel as though they are being forced to take part in the child's care. Nurses must realize that partnership is not always easy. Working in partnership means that care does not have to be shared equally between the family and the nurse. It is important that nurses are aware that the amount of family participation will vary and that this must be negotiated between the family and the children's nurse responsible for care planning

Communication

Excellent communication with the child and family is vital for partnership in care to be successful. When communicating with children, professionals need to communicate in a manner that is age appropriate and suitable for the child's intellectual ability. Parents need to be part of the decision-making process, which keeps the child at the centre of care. The MDT needs to ensure that the child and family are listened to and that they participate in the negotiation of care. Sharing information, reviewing the care plan with the family, and maintaining a presence help achieve this.

The partnership model of care continues to evolve and when effective partnership care is achieved, the child, family, and nurse express satisfaction with the care that has been received.

Key points
- The partnership model of care recognizes the expertise of the parents, and that this must be valued.
- Certain conditions are needed to enable true partnership and this requires collaboration, negotiation, and support.
- Recognizing that parents must be involved in decisions that affect their child can sometime be challenging to the healthcare professional.

28 Family-centred care

Figure 28.1 Principles of family-centred care.

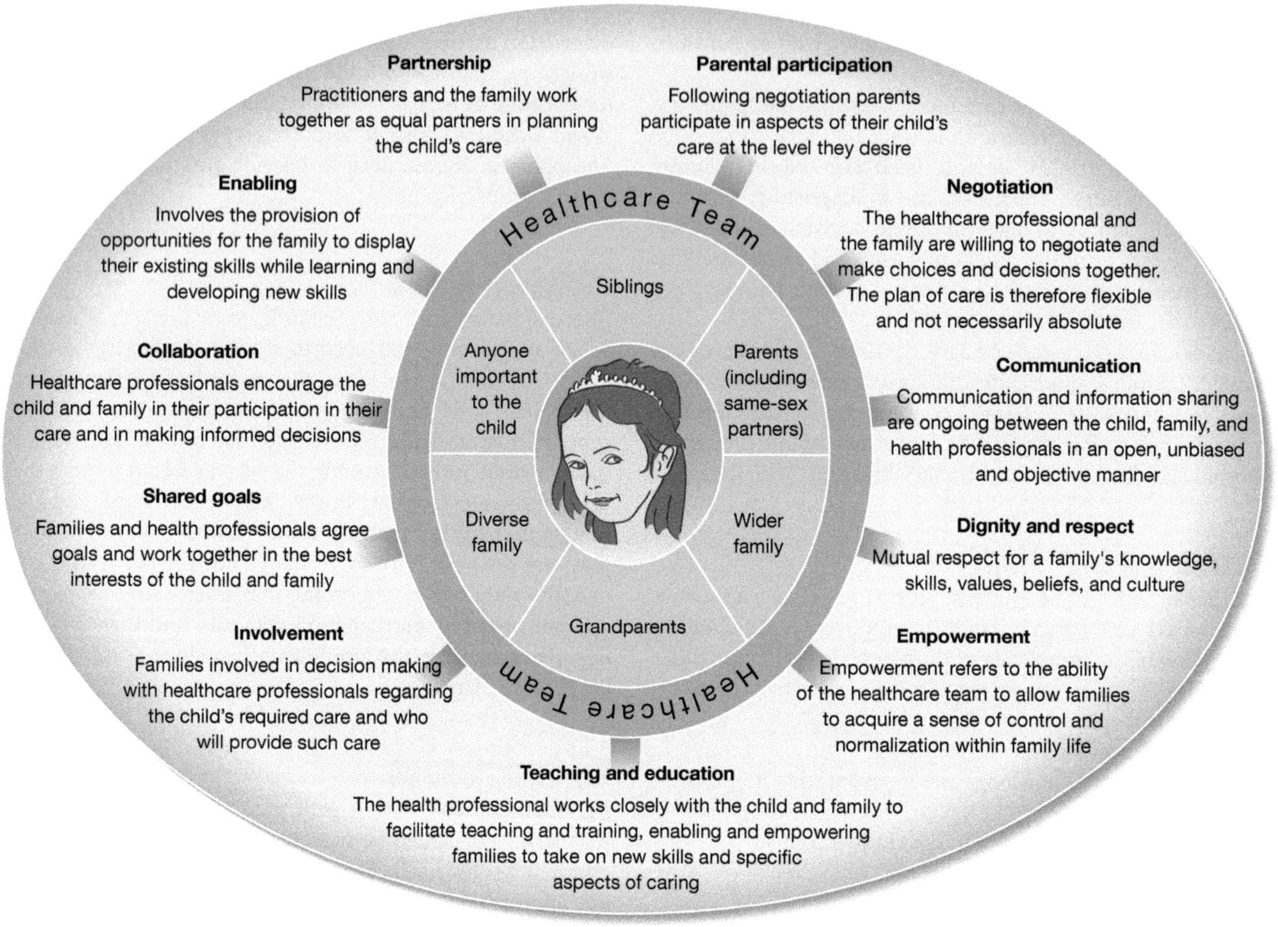

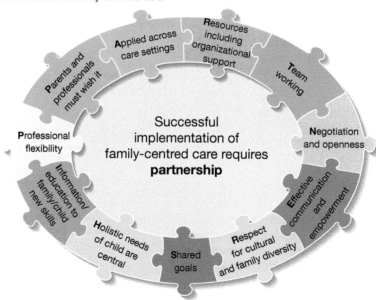

Partnership
Practitioners and the family work together as equal partners in planning the child's care
Parental participation
Following negotiation parents participate in aspects of their child's care at the level they desire
Enabling
Involves the provision of opportunities for the family to display their existing skills while learning and developing new skills
Negotiation
The healthcare professional and the family are willing to negotiate and make choices and decisions together. The plan of care is therefore flexible and not necessarily absolute
Collaboration
Healthcare professionals encourage the child and family in their participation in their care and in making informed decisions
Communication
Communication and information sharing are ongoing between the child, family, and health professionals in an open, unbiased and objective manner
Shared goals
Families and health professionals agree goals and work together in the best interests of the child and family
Dignity and respect
Mutual respect for a family's knowledge, skills, values, beliefs, and culture
Involvement
Families involved in decision making with healthcare professionals regarding the child's required care and who will provide such care
Empowerment
Empowerment refers to the ability of the healthcare team to allow families to acquire a sense of control and normalization within family life
Teaching and education
The health professional works closely with the child and family to facilitate teaching and training, enabling and empowering families to take on new skills and specific aspects of caring
Healthcare Team
Siblings
Parents (including same-sex partners)
Wider family
Grandparents
Diverse family
Anyone important to the child
Healthcare Team

Figure 28.2 Successful implementation of family-centred care.

Successful implementation of family-centred care requires **partnership**
Parents and professionals must wish it
Applied across care settings
Resources including organizational support
Team working
Negotiation and openness
Effective communication and empowerment
Respect for cultural and family diversity
Shared goals
Holistic needs of child are central
Information/ education to family/child new skills
Professional flexibility

Children and Young People's Nursing at a Glance, Second Edition. Edited by Elizabeth Gormley-Fleming and Sheila Roberts.

Family-centred care (FCC) has become firmly established as a cornerstone of children's nursing practice, and is frequently referred to as a philosophy of care. Concern exists regarding FCC due to misunderstandings about what FCC is and how it can be implemented. Children's nurses use FCC to advocate for child-friendly environments, parental involvement in care, and securing children's nursing as a distinct field of practice.

As a philosophy of caring for children in partnership with their families, FCC ensures that care is planned around the unique and individual needs of the whole family. A family-centred approach recognizes the family as central in a child's life and that it should also be central in the child's plan of care. Within children's nursing, therefore, not only the child is viewed as a recipient of care, but also other family members.

While FCC embraces diversity in family structures, cultural backgrounds, choices, strengths, and needs, acknowledgement exists that no single approach is right for all families.

Families and the healthcare team need to collaborate and work as partners in planning the child's care. Policies and organizational structures also need to be in place to successfully implement a true family-centred approach. Families should be involved in decision making about who will provide the required care and negotiation over whether they want to participate in care and if so at what level. Figure 28.1 shows the various components of FCC, illustrating how the healthcare team works in partnership with families around the child. The key prerequisites to success are summarized in Figure 28.2.

What is family?

At the core of FCC is the understanding that the child's family offers a primary source of support and strength, while upholding the child's best interests at all times. Family can be viewed as anyone who is important to the child and the concept must recognize the ever-changing structure of families in society. Families can be big, small, extended, or multigenerational. They can include parents, siblings, grandparents, extended families, foster families, stepfamilies, and same-sex parents.

The casey model to facilitate a family-centred approach to care

Casey developed the partnership model of care, which was based on the assumption that 'The care of the children, well or sick, is best carried out by their families, with varying degrees of assistance from members of a suitably qualified health care team whenever necessary.' Care is planned in negotiation with the families, who are considered as equal partners in their child's care. The model has five components: child, family, health, environment, and the nurse.

Advantages of family-centred care

Advantages for the child
- Can improve clinical outcomes.
- Reduces child's anxiety.
- Promotes familiarity in an unfamiliar environment.
- Reduces impact of separation in short and long term.
- Supports the child in learning about and participating in their care and decision making.
- Promotes an individual and developmental approach.
- Supports transition to adulthood.

Advantages for the family
- Acknowledges that the family is the constant in the child's life.
- Supports and empowers the family to work in partnership and make decision in relation to their child's care.
- Reduces feelings of anxiety and guilt.
- Increases confidence and control.
- Honours cultural diversity and family traditions.
- Encourages family-to-family and peer support.
- Builds on family strengths and resources.
- Recognizes different methods of coping.
- Promotes holistic care.

Advantages for professionals and organizations
- Greater job satisfaction.
- Parental insight can help in planning individualized care.
- Reduced inpatient stay and associated costs.
- Potential for fairer allocation of resources.
- Recognizes the importance of community-based services.
- Assurance that the design of the healthcare delivery system is flexible, accessible, and responsive to family need.

Challenges of family-centred care

One of the significant challenges to FCC is the lack of evidence demonstrating that it is anything more than concept espoused by children's nurses. Organizational structures have been developed to promote and engender FCC such as visiting times, but challenges still persist. Some of these are:
- Individual attitudes/anxieties, knowledge, and understanding.
- Staff shortages/skill mix.
- Surrounding environment.
- Communication issues.
- Lack of understanding and/or practical guidance.
- Situations when family intention is not focused on the best interests of the child (e.g. issues relating to safeguarding).
- Limited support from organizations/policies to support FCC.

Key points
- FCC has inherent advantages for the child, the family, and healthcare professionals. Implementing successful FCC in practice requires partnership.
- Despite the challenges around FCC, it remains a central concept in children's nursing practice.

29 Family health promotion

Figure 29.1 Family health promotion.

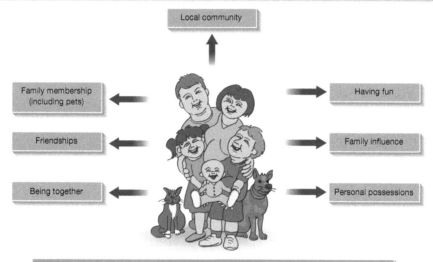

Scenario: Sue, a community children's nurse, visits Anika, a 7-year-old girl who is recovering from recent elective surgery. During the visit, Sue realizes that all the family members appear to be overweight and do very little physical activity. She therefore decides to consider how their health could be promoted. The family comprises mum, dad, three children (aged 6 months, 7, and 9 years), and their pet cat and dog. The children's maternal grandparents live approximately 2 miles away. Initially, Sue considers the positive aspects of the family's life and the things they enjoy (these are identified in the figure and discussed further in the text).

Local community

Family membership (including pets)

Having fun

Friendships

Family influence

Being together

Personal possessions

Next Sue considers the tools and approaches that she will utilize to promote the family's health

Tools for promoting family health

- Leaflets
- Posters
- Games, toys
- School, work presentations
- Magazines, comic books, newspapers
- Radio, television
- Bulletin boards
- Internet, including government and social media sites

Sue decides to visit her local health promotion unit to collect some games that the family can play together to help to promote health messages about diet and exercise

Being positive

- Encouraging family participation
- Making achievable suggestions that are engaging and fun for everyone, such as:
  - The identification of parks where the family can go together to play and walk the dog
  - Identification of low-cost activities such as family swim sessions
  - The use of computer games that have a physical activity component
  - Cooking together and learning new recipes
  - Doing activities with other family members and friends

Benefits of a family approach

- The opportunity for the family to spend more time together
- The family works together to enhance everyone's health and wellbeing
- Positive reinforcement for all family members
- A healthier environment is created for the whole family, not just the person who is at risk

It is recognized that the family unit is both a resource and a priority group requiring both preventative and curative health services and support across the life span. Family-orientated health promotion (Figure 29.1) is an important public health strategy, as the family unit may support and nurture one another in maintaining good health and in disease prevention. Families form a basic societal unit and therefore can be the producers of individual and community good health. Most families want to be proactive in terms of enhancing health and wellbeing; therefore, for children's nurses, health promotion is about working with children, young people, and their families to achieve this aim.

While the structure of the family continues to evolve and reform in the twenty-first century, the diverse and complex nature of the family needs to be considered. Children continue to be strongly influenced by the people they have close relationships with.

Health promotion has focused upon specific poor health behaviours in the past – particularly areas that have the potential to be resource intensive in the long term, such as obesity and lack of physical activity. There has been a tendency to be reactive rather than working towards the general enhancement of health and wellbeing. Contemporary health-promoting family models can

Children and Young People's Nursing at a Glance, Second Edition. Edited by Elizabeth Gormley-Fleming and Sheila Roberts.
© 2023 John Wiley & Sons Ltd. Published 2023 by John Wiley & Sons Ltd.

Table 29.1 Characteristics of the family as a health-promoting setting.

Characteristic	Description
Maternal characteristics	Education, age, marital status, mental health, engagement with child, ideologies about parenting and women's roles, economic independence, maternal affection
Paternal characteristics	Presence in child's life, behaviour and characteristics, employment status, health
Child characteristics	Attachment and emotional security, self efficacy, regulation of behaviour, resilience, competence, health, parental influence
Family characteristics	Shared values, supportive relationships, communication, attitudes and flexibility, sense of identity, health status, family routines, family composition and structure, family emotional climate, boundaries, social support, family coping, family cohesion
Family composition	Single parents, divorce, step-family, teenage parents, size of family, extended family involvement, number of siblings.
Potential stressors	Ill health, family break-up, unpredictable events, teenage years, children with a disability or a parents with a disability, loss of economic status

provide scaffolds that will shape the health behaviours required for a healthy lifestyle.

There are a number of health-promoting settings that the child and young person may be familiar with, including health-promoting schools, outdoor environments, and workplaces. Within these settings there is a well-articulated context where public health, education, and environment all interlink to form a partnership with the aim of health promotion.

Promoting family health not only provides the opportunity for a more holistic approach, but offers the opportunity to enhance the health and wellbeing of all family members.

What is important to the family?

There are a number of key issues that need to be considered when promoting family health; these can be termed as 'assets', as they are positive factors within family life. This suggests that health assets are resources that people have that can be used to promote health and protect against ill health – that is why it is crucial to spend time identifying the areas that are particularly important to people. Following are some core examples.

Family membership

Family membership relates to the structure of the family and includes both blood relatives and step-family members. This can mean that the family is large and complex, but it is important to identify the close relationships so that the relevant family members can work together to promote each other's health, with professional support – for example, children often have very close relationships with grandparents. In addition, family members may extend beyond the human element to embrace pets.

Being together

Families enjoy undertaking activities together, so if these can be identified it will help to facilitate family engagement in health-promoting activities. It is important to note that family health promotion is concerned with overall quality-of-life enhancement, so opportunities for families to eat meals together can be enormously beneficial from a psychological as well as a physiological perspective.

Family influence

Parents positively influence children in relation to a range of activities. This sometimes results from their own personal interest (perhaps, for example, a mother or father has always been an avid football supporter), motivating the parent to identify suitable sports or activity venues, pay for the child's lessons or training, and take the child to and from the relevant classes. In addition, parents can influence their children's activities through the purchase of

play equipment, toys, and games consoles. Understanding both parental and the child's interests is therefore an important consideration in terms of promoting family health. Evidence exists to show that parents' characteristics such as employment status, education, and health are all influencing factors on how they promote health within their family. Table 29.1 summarizes key aspects of the family that could be considered when promoting health.

Lifestyle

Family life is busy and this needs to be considered if realistic suggestions are to be made (and achieved) in terms of the enhancement of family health. School, work, and personal commitments all have an impact upon the family. However, a busy life has the potential to be positive, as it means that there is often a clear routine, it fosters a family teamwork approach, and can mean that parental work responsibilities generate more material resources, such as holidays and personal possessions – these can then promote emotional as well as physical health and wellbeing in the long term.

Local community

The local community has been recognized as influential in terms of health and wellbeing. The proximity of other family members and friends, as well as physical resources (such as parks, swimming pools, clubs), means that children develop a knowledge of their community.

Friendships

Children tend to form friendships easily, and these are highly valued across the age spectrum. Friends can be particularly influential in terms of activities undertaken, common interests can be developed, and children, and their families, are able to share them. Friendships can also facilitate independence, as children and young people are more likely to be allowed freedom if in the company of their peers. Positive relationships through friendships will enhance confidence and overall wellbeing.

Personal possessions

Our lives are undoubtedly influenced by the availability of physical resources and possessions, many of which can enhance our physical and emotional health. Identifying the possessions that families have access to will naturally influence the health promotion advice provided.

Having fun

Having fun is important to all of us and therefore there is more likely to be engagement with health-promotion activities that are enjoyable. Creativity may be required to maintain engagement with children. For example, it may be more appealing for a family to attend a 'fun' swim session than a lesson.

Challenges to family health promotion

This chapter highlights positive approaches to health promotion within a family unit. It is important for the healthcare professional to be aware of individual challenges that a family could be facing. These could include a single-parent or complex family, a family with minimal financial means, a family where one or more members have special needs, or a family that simply does not wish to engage with health promotion. Other potential stressors relate to children with disabilities, teenage years, family illness, divorce, and family chaos.

However, family health promotion provides the opportunity to adopt a more holistic and positive approach that embraces the needs of several family members.

Key points

- As a unit, the family is important in the public health strategy for goal-orientated health promotion.
- The children's nurse plays an important role in the facilitation of health promotion for the family unit.
- Understanding the family's views on health promotion is important when planning any type of education or health-promotion activity.

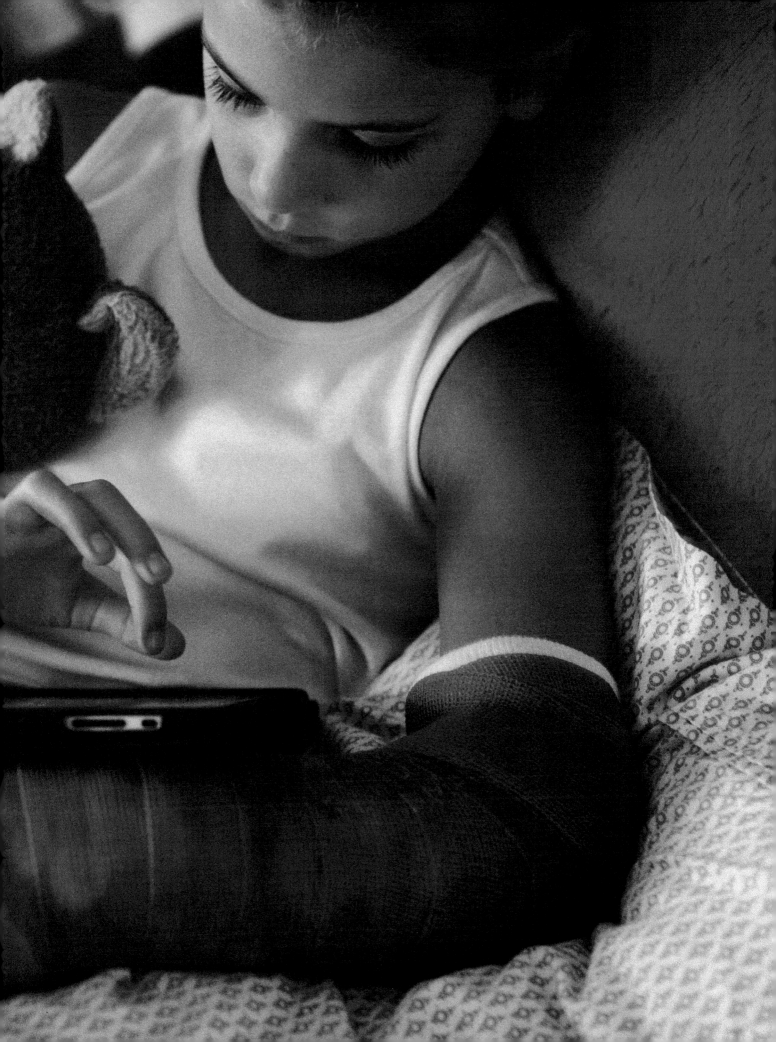

30 Communicating with children

Figure 30.1 Aspects to consider when communicating with children.

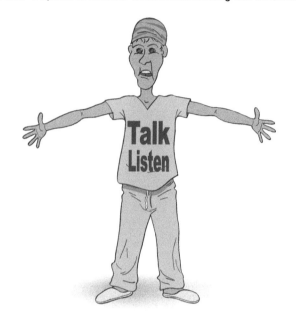

Talk
Listen

Purpose

- Sometimes it is just about talking to and interacting with children
- Establishing a therapeutic relationship
- Supporting children
- Eliciting and giving information
- Explaining procedures
- Listening to what they want to tell us
- Obtaining information about how they are feeling to help with diagnosis

When to talk and when to listen

- Circumstance will dictate when to talk or listen, but being aware of the child's needs is paramount
- Talking and questioning may be needed to elicit information
- Adopting an active listening approach is important when working with young people with mental health or social problems
- Employ active listening when hearing disclosures about abuse

Figure 30.2 The 7Cs of communication.

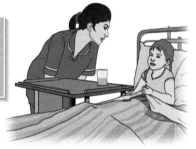

1. Confidence
2. Concise
3. Clear
4. Courteous
5. Correct
6. Coherent
7. Concrete

Figure 30.3 Six key active listening skills.

| Pay attention | Withhold judgement | Reflect | Clarify | Summarize | Share |

Barriers to effective communication:
Ambiguous messages
Complex message and jargon used
Body language of nurse contradicts what is being said.
Child and family not able to hear what is being said due to environmental noise

Child too unwell and parents too stressed to absorb what is being communicated
Patient's and family's beliefs about previous experiences or attitudes not checked and message is reframed
Nurse unable to communicate in appropriate manner for patent and family to understand what is being said

Communication with children and young people is both simple and complex, requiring the nurse to have a repertoire of skills to interact effectively (Figure 30.1). Good communication is essential for developing a positive relationship. The Nursing and Midwifery Council requires children's nurses to use a range of communication skills and technologies to support person-centred care and enhance quality and safety. They must ensure people receive all the information they need in a language and manner that allow them to make informed choices and share decision making. Many factors influence how, when, and why the healthcare practitioner will communicate with children and much of this is equally influenced by the presence of parents or other main carers.

Children's nurses will use a range of skills in providing care for children, but communication is the core skill of much that we do

Children and Young People's Nursing at a Glance, Second Edition. Edited by Elizabeth Gormley-Fleming and Sheila Roberts.
© 2023 John Wiley & Sons Ltd. Published 2023 by John Wiley & Sons Ltd.

and is the basis for demonstrating compassionate care. The wide range of arenas in which children's nurses work means that an equally wide range of skills and techniques are needed to meet specific situations. and some of these are considered here.

Factors influencing communication

One of the most obvious and crucial aspects of communication is the age of children, which determines their level of development. These two issues clearly determine how children communicate and understand those communicating with them.

Children

Until they are about 8 years old, children differ markedly in how they understand and communicate, ranging from the cry of babies to the more complex language of a school-aged child. Communication abilities emerge through psychomotor and cognitive development, such that the nurse should have a grasp of when and in what format children will usually communicate. Reference to speech and language charts can help to identify at what age a child can achieve certain skills, such as pronouncing their first words through to when they can formulate sentences. This knowledge would be helped by an awareness of the stages of development theorized by Piaget, Vygotsky, and Kohlberg. Thus, when communicating with children, the following principles are useful:

- Reflect on your professional style, attitude, and behaviour when communicating with children and their families.
- Infants rely on crying as their communication, but respond to touch, voice, and facial gestures, particularly from the mother. Responding to these forms in a similar way enables communication directly with the infant and this can be important when the parent is not present.
- Non-verbal communication and cues are important to children and they will identify and respond to these, so the nurse should be aware of how they project what it is they are trying to say and do.
- As children develop verbal language, there is increasing use of words, phrases, and sentences. However, they may not understand what these mean, so testing them out can help in communicating with children.
- Be aware of developmental concepts to understand what children are likely to understand at specific ages.
- Children need time and clear, appropriate explanations in order to understand communication, which can often be about doing things to them.
- Recognize the impact of the situation and the status of the child on their ability to understand what you are trying to communicate.
- Be aware of children's inability to communicate verbally because of disabilities, developmental delays, or traumatic scenarios, and adjust your approach to meet their needs.
- Children may change their style of interaction, being passive or active, which the nurse needs to be aware of when communicating.
- Adopting the SOLER approach (face people Squarely; Open body shape; Lean forward slightly; Eye contact; Relax) and then communicate using the 7C model (Figure 30.2).
- Active listening (Figure 30.3) is an important aspect of communication. Give the child your full attention and be prepared to come down to their level (e.g. sitting on the floor) when communicating directly with them.
- Repeat or reflect back what they have said or what they may be feeling to express that you understand.
- Use different approaches such as play, humour, or drawing to engage with children.

Young people

Communicating with young people over the age of 12 years requires not only a different approach, but the use of specific skills suited to their circumstance and the way in which they talk. This is particularly important for the 16+ age group, who may be adopting adult behaviours and language. Young people often communicate using their own codes of language, through different media, and in a style that adults do not understand. This is deepened through the influence of peers, the media, subcultures, and gang membership. Despite all this, young people have the same needs for communication as other age groups, with the additional crucial need for them to be listened to. We should listen to how they want to be communicated with and also the nurse sometimes needs just to listen – active listening is a crucial skill. It is preferable for the nurse not to attempt to adopt their language style, as this may obscure communication. In addition, the young person's sense of self means that the nurse should be aware of respecting personal space and adopting non-oppressive body language when interacting. The need for careful, clear, and informative explanation is important, as the young person may portray an attitude that suggests they understand when they do not. It is useful for the children's nurse to accept periods of silence during communication and to be comfortable with these.

Communicating in specific environments

While these approaches are useful when communicating with most children, there will be circumstances where they have to be altered to fit specific situations:

- Children undergoing procedures may be anxious, frightened, and defensive, so verbal and non-verbal communication is aimed at providing appropriate, supportive, and calming explanations.
- Undergoing surgery is a frightening prospect for children and their families. It may be necessary to prepare them through age- and development-appropriate language as well as alternative methods such as play, puppetry, drawing, and music.
- Children involved in trauma may be frightened as a result of the injury, what is happening, and being movement restricted where spinal injuries are concerned. Non-verbal behaviour is crucial in supporting the child and here therapeutic touch can be important. Explaining clearly and within eyesight of the child enables them to understand some of what is occurring.
- Young people with mental health issues may require communication that is therapeutic while inquisitive in terms of establishing problems and adverse situations.

Using reflection to show you are listening

Refection is a means of showing active listening. Repeating back what the child has said and summing up will confirm that their message has been received and understood. Try using similar words to the child, and either adding detail or shortening what they have said. This will promote confidence in the child and they may adopt a more open communication stance.

Key points

- Communication is necessary in all aspects of nursing practice if nursing care delivery is to be compassionate.
- Non-verbal communication is very important and the children's nurse needs to be attuned to this if they are to pick up vital cues about the child.
- Active listening will build trust and aid in the development of the therapeutic relationship.

31 Hospital play

Figure 31.1 Hospital play.

Having a health play specialist or another member of staff dedicated to leading and facilitating play in hospital offers many benefits to the child, family, and hospital staff

Play provides a link to home, aids normality, and enables the child to fulfil medical requirements in an enjoyable way, reduces stress and anxiety, and facilitates communication

The National Association of Health Play Specialists is a charity that promotes the physical and mental wellbeing of children and young people who are patients in hospital

An appropriate method of play should be selected, depending on the age and ability of the child

When children or young people are admitted to hospital, they are at their most vulnerable. They are not only ill, but are also separated from their friends and familiar surroundings. Play can really make a difference

Play is at the very centre of a healthy child's life. From the earliest age, playing helps children to learn, to relate to other people, and to have fun

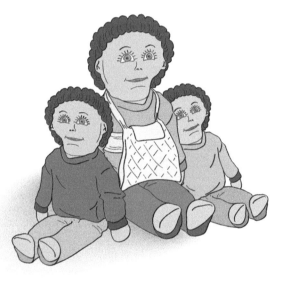

Timing of play preparation should be carefully considered. Younger children may not be able to retain the information if it is given too far in advance, whereas young people may benefit from preparation a few days before the procedure to allow them time to process it and develop any coping strategies

The role of the play specialist is to help children master and cope with anxieties and feelings using a variety of techniques, use play to prepare children for hospital procedures, support families and siblings, contribute to clinical judgements through their play-based observations, and act as the child's or young person's advocate

It is important to gain as much information from parents as possible at admission with regard to the child's special toy and any special vocabulary they may have. In addition, it is important to take into account any previous experiences the child may have had in hospital

All children's nurses should be able to assess a child's stage of development and level of understanding, which should be taken into consideration when giving a child information they need to be able to cope with a hospital procedure. This is because, for children, hospitals are filled with strange sights and sounds

Children and Young People's Nursing at a Glance, Second Edition. Edited by Elizabeth Gormley-Fleming and Sheila Roberts.
© 2023 John Wiley & Sons Ltd. Published 2023 by John Wiley & Sons Ltd.

What constitutes hospital play?

Therapeutic hospital play techniques can be hugely beneficial to all members of the multidisciplinary team. However, the techniques used are not often understood and therefore rarely used, unless a health play specialist is present to provide or facilitate such techniques. Therapeutic play is a framework of activities that are designed to take the psychological and cognitive development of the child into account. This will facilitate the child's emotional and physical wellbeing in hospital.

Play is essentially the language of children: through play they are able to learn about their environment and themselves.

Hospital play (Figure 31.1) provides the following opportunities:
- Provides a link to home – by being allowed 'normal' play, children are able to act out scenes from home (i.e. role play) and remember things from home that they may not have seen for some time (i.e. photos and sound games). This is particularly important for long-stay patients, where home familiarity should be introduced to ease the transition to home.
- Aids in fostering a feeling of normality.
- Boosts or helps regain confidence and self-esteem and allows children to take some control back into their life. This could include giving the child an active part in their treatment; for example, using role play to make a plan for a procedure involving children or young people so that they can make choices where appropriate.
- Minimizes regression.
- Improves concentration skills.
- Enables the child to fulfil medical requirements in an enjoyable way.
- Acts as an outlet for emotions – gives children the opportunity to express their feelings, frustrations, and tensions in an appropriate manner. For example, a child in traction might like to play with balloons, Velcro darts, or playdough to release tension.
- Reduces stress and anxiety.
- Facilitates communication.
- Enables information to be passed on in an appropriate and enjoyable manner – empowering the child and helping with informed consent.
- Allows games and activities to be adapted for all children, whatever their needs.
- Aids in all areas of development.
- Encourages parents and siblings to be involved.
- Provides much-needed boundaries. Without a 'normal' routine and in unusual circumstances, boundaries are slackened or lost completely, leaving children feeling unsure and out of control.
- Aids in compliance with medical procedures.
- Helps to divert thoughts that occupy and stimulate minds (distraction therapy) and provides fun – escapism!

Effects of a hospital admission

Every child responds to hospitalization in a different way: some will sail through, seemingly unaffected, while others will experience high levels of anxiety, distress, and other long-term effects. Healthcare play specialists can help avoid the negative aspects of hospitalization:
- Loss of concentration.
- Effect on relationships with peers and siblings.
- Temperament changes due to loss of boundaries and control.
- Loss of 'normal life' and what it entails (e.g. home, school, friends).
- Loss of confidence and self-esteem.
- Possible regression educationally and socially.
- Poor coping techniques when faced with strong feelings of fear and anxiety.
- Development of phobias.

Children are likely to be concerned about a hospital admission. Not only are they worried about the physical pain they may have to endure, they are also being confronted with a situation they are likely to know little about. Fear of the unknown will play a major part in the child's anxiety levels and illustrates the importance of preparation, sharing information, and addressing any misconceptions at the earliest opportunity.

Role of the healthcare play specialist

- Ensures a child-friendly environment.
- Organizes suitable activities and events.
- Promotes child development and minimizes regression.
- Develops and executes individual play programmes.
- Works as a part of the multidisciplinary team.
- Promotes and teaches others the value of hospital play.
- Contributes towards clinical judgements.
- Works with child psychologists as required.
- Facilitates informed consent and assent.
- Uses therapeutic play techniques to support children and their families – such as preparation, distraction, and post-procedural play.
- Helps children master and cope with anxieties.
- Is a child's advocate.

Healthcare play specialists are essential in creating a positive experience of hospital for the child and family and achieving this by the minimization of trauma.

Stages of hospital preparation

- *Pre-admission.* Preparation for hospital should begin in the home and there are many books and information in multimedia formats to help parents. Hospitals should ideally offer pre-admission visits and preparation programmes. Some of these can be in the format of online virtual tours that take the child through the stages of hospital admission.
- *On admission.* At this stage it is important to develop trust with the child and to ascertain what toys, games, or hobbies the child has and any special vocabulary they may have. In addition, it is important to take into account any previous experiences the child may have had in hospital. This period can be used by the play specialist to assess the child before any procedures are carried out, for example dolls can be adapted and used to prepare children for procedures. Dolls made from calico are easy to make.
- *During and after procedures.* Distraction techniques can be used to divert attention, help children to cope, and aid in compliance. Post-procedural play is important and this should always be offered to the child routinely. It can take practically any form and should include praise, certificates, and/or stickers. This form of play allows children to evaluate the procedure or experience by examining both the positive and the negative aspects.

Key points
- Play in hospital helps the child and family become familiar with the environment and the unknown.
- Children's nurses in collaboration with play specialists may use play as a strategy to prepare children for procedures.
- Play in hospital helps maintain continuity with the everyday life of the child.

32 Role of the community children's nurse

Figure 32.1 Role of the community children's nurse.

- The changing epidemiology of child health has resulted in a reduction in infectious disease and an increase in the numbers of children who live with a chronic illness
- Children with a chronic illness are more likely to be hospitalized, and repeated hospital admission can be detrimental to their psychological and physical health
- Provision of care at home by community children's nurses (CCNs) is less stressful to children and facilitates normality for the child and family
- The CCN is a knowledgeable practitioner who supports and empowers children to become competent to manage their chronic illness at home

- CCNs need good communication skills when working with children and families
- The CCN needs to develop a relationship with the child and family
- Children want CCNs who are kind, happy, and show an interest in their lives
- The CCN teaches children technical skills so that they can maintain their own health

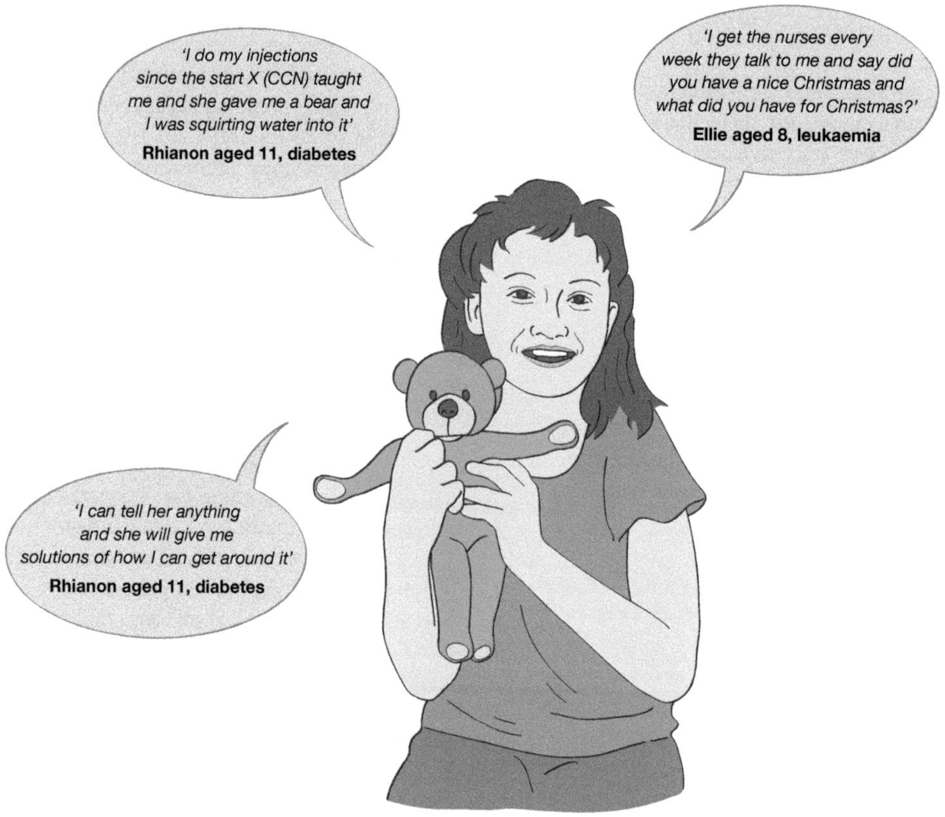

'I do my injections since the start X (CCN) taught me and she gave me a bear and I was squirting water into it'
Rhianon aged 11, diabetes

'I get the nurses every week they talk to me and say did you have a nice Christmas and what did you have for Christmas?'
Ellie aged 8, leukaemia

'I can tell her anything and she will give me solutions of how I can get around it'
Rhianon aged 11, diabetes

Prevalence of chronic illness in childhood

There is no definitive definition of chronic illness in childhood. However, certain aspects are included in most definitions: a condition that has lasted for longer than three months; that impacts the child's physical, cognitive, emotional, or social wellbeing; and that incurs periods of exacerbations that require hospitalization. There has been a significant increase in the number of children living with a long-term chronic health condition over the past 20 years. Major advances in medical technology, diagnosis, and treatment mean that conditions once thought of as fatal can be effectively managed. Children who would not previously have survived beyond childhood are now living and thriving well into adulthood, albeit with an increased need for supportive care.

Estimates suggest there are at least 1.7 million children living with a long-term chronic condition in the UK. The most common chronic illness in childhood is asthma; one in eleven children in the UK has asthma. It is a leading cause of urgent paediatric hospital admission and results in a small number of avoidable childhood deaths every year. Diabetes, another significant chronic condition in childhood, can lead to disability and premature death if not managed effectively. It is estimated that there are 36 000 children aged 0–19 years living with diabetes in the UK. Other long-term chronic conditions in childhood can include childhood cancers, cystic fibrosis, sickle cell disease, congenital heart disease, epilepsy, juvenile arthritis, Crohn's disease, mental health conditions, and emerging conditions such as long Covid.

Chronic long-term health conditions experienced during childhood are known to have a huge impact upon children and young people (CYP) and their families. All aspects of a CYP's life will be affected by a chronic long-term condition. Physical impacts on the CYP can include intense and/or invasive treatment regimes, side effects of medications, and pain, as well as limitations and restrictions in their physical ability. This can also have a negative impact upon their psychological and emotional wellbeing, which is further exacerbated by frequent and prolonged admissions to hospital. CYP suffering from a chronic long-term condition often feel isolated from society and their community. School absenteeism due to ill-health and exclusions from certain activities, for example children who are immunocompromised not being able to socialize with their peers, can compound these feelings. Caring for a sick child also has physical and social implications for parents, such as tiredness, stress, social isolation, and poorer health outcomes; in addition, the financial impact of a CYP's chronic long-term condition can be crippling. Some parents, and in particular those who are caring for a child with a complex health condition, may feel it necessary to give up their full-time employment in order to meet the significant care needs of their child, and will rely on social benefits and charity services for ongoing financial support as a result.

Benefits of home care for children with a chronic illness

For many years there has been a drive across the National Health Service (NHS) to move CYP healthcare provision to be more community based.

There are significant benefits to CYP and their families in receiving healthcare at home and/or closer to home within their community. It is recognized that CYP prefer to receive healthcare at home in comparison to hospital and that their quality of life is improved; in addition, families will suffer less of a financial burden and disruption for all family members will be minimized. Receiving care within the home environment can help to limit the impact of a health condition for CYP and their families, and is therefore a vital component of paediatric healthcare provision.

Role of the community children's nurse

Community children's nurses (CCNs; Figure 32.1) are registered children's nurses who hold a recordable specialist community nursing qualification. They have been described as the bedrock of care pathways for CYP who require nursing support at home and in their communities.

Four distinct groups of children who require CCN support have been identified:
- Children with acute and short-term conditions.
- Children with long-term conditions.
- Children with disabilities and complex conditions, including those requiring continuing care and neonates.
- Children with life-limiting and life-threatening illness, including those requiring palliative and end-of-life care.

Historically, CCN teams across the UK have developed according to the needs of their local populations. As a result, there are variations and inconsistencies in CCN service provision across the UK. In some areas, access to a CCN service is limited and CYP who meet the criteria set out by NHS England are unable to access support from a CCN team. Greater investment in CCN is required to ensure equity of provision across the country.

The skills required of a CCN are complex and multifaceted and incorporate clinical decision making, clinical diagnosis, and prescribing, as well as clinical skills such as administering medication, delivering treatment, and evaluating the holistic care needs of CYP and their families. The ability to think outside the box and be creative in solving problems is an essential requisite. CCNs must also possess more tacit skills, which enable them to listen to, support, and empower CYP and their families to manage chronic long-term and acute healthcare conditions at home.

Vital aspects of the role of the CCN include assessment, teaching, management, advocacy, and the facilitation of independence for CYP living with a chronic long-term health condition. Where possible CCNs will empower CYP to become self-caring individuals able to manage their own health needs with the help and support of their family. To gain independence, children need to be educated to understand their health condition, be able to recognize and take appropriate action to manage any deterioration in their condition, and master the skills required to maintain their optimum health. CCNs possess the knowledge and expertise to teach children the skills they require to become self-caring and independent. For example, children with type I diabetes must master injection techniques, take blood samples, and record their blood sugar levels. However, to be fully self-caring children must be able assimilate their knowledge and understand their condition, which will include knowledge in regard to what constitutes a normal blood sugar level, and what makes a healthy diet, as well as the ability to recognize the measures required to ensure their safely in the event of a hypoglycaemic or hyperglycaemic attack. Understanding these aspects will enable CYP to successfully manage their own health needs and make autonomous decisions about their ongoing health and treatment options.

The CCN will also provide ongoing support and education to parents, carers, and others involved in the care of the CYP to ensure the safe management of their health needs at home and within the community. This can include, but is not limited to, coordinating multiagency/multiprofessional meetings, writing reports, coordinating and/or contributing to continuing healthcare plans, contributing to education and healthcare plans, organizing and delivering competency-based training programmes, and referring the CYP and family to services such as those within the voluntary sector that can offer supplementary support. In addition, they will ensure that parents and CYP are supported to effectively navigate health, education, social care, and voluntary agencies in their local community. Effective partnership working between the CCN, parents, carers, and the wider multidisciplinary/multiprofessional team is therefore essential.

There are certain characteristics that CYP look for in a CCN: a happy disposition, respectfulness, and empathy. CYP want to be cared for by CCNs who provide more than just clinical care; they expect them to be interested in their everyday lives, and be willing to listen about issues that are important to them. They want to be valued for who they are, be seen as individuals in their own right, and be cared for by professionals who do not provide care that is solely based on their nursing needs. This makes the initial contact with a CCN of particular importance, as it provides the foundations for the development of a trusting. supportive relationship between the CYP, the family, and the CCN.

Key points
- Home care provides a better-quality life for the child or young person and their family.
- Children's community nurses are not only nurses but educators and advocators with excellent communication skills.
- Care at home enables children and young people to gain some control and independence in their life

33 Collaboration with schools

Figure 33.1 Hints and tips when engaging with schools and colleges.

- Engage other local health professionals: GPs, school nurses, ambulance service, emergency department staff, play specialists. It is helpful to offer a variety of professional experiences to share with children and young people

- Introduce professionals to children and young people and encourage the children and young people to introduce themselves too

- Find out what the children and young people already know about health and health services – listen and value their experiences and contributions. Many will have either personal experiences or family members and friends who use health services

- Use the available resources (e.g. NHS Institute Primary or Secondary School Lesson Plans), which include interactive activities such as the NHS song, films, and scenario cards (https://www.england.nhs.uk/publication/schools-resources-toolkit/)

- Signpost to other NHS services (e.g. NHS Choices, www.england.nhs.uk; and NHS Careers, https://monkeywellbeing.com/resources/)

- Gather and encourage feedback about local NHS services to assist in improving local services. Introduce websites such as www.patientopinion.org.uk

- Follow up with a letter of thanks to maintain links to secure assistance for future engagement and participation activities

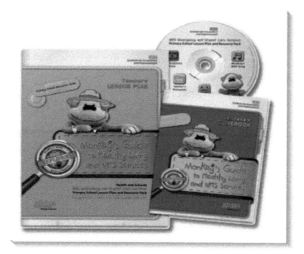

Examples of national resources available to support collaboration between health and education

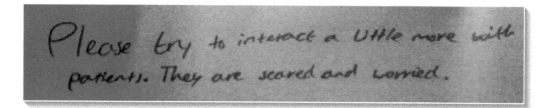

Personal, social, health, and economic (PSHE) education is an important part of all pupils' education. The Department for Education states that schools should seek to build on the statutory guidance in the national curriculum by offering input on drugs education, financial education, sex and relationships education, and the importance of physical activity and a healthy diet for a healthy lifestyle (Figure 33.1).

With the proportion of children experiencing a probable mental disorder increasing, from one in nine in 2017 to one in six in 2020, support relating to how to access physical and mental health services in schools is often lacking. Children and young people repeatedly give the feedback that no one educates them about prevention and how to access the National Health Service (NHS) until they are unwell, yet when they *are* given information and education they can make informed decisions about their health and healthcare.

The NHS is seeing an ever-increasing and, some would argue, unsustainable demand on its services. For example, there is increased attendance at Emergency Departments (EDs), although it is estimated that 40% of ED attendances could be avoided and early intervention when emotional wellbeing needs are identified could lead to better outcomes. Yet there remains limited public awareness about the range of healthcare services and alternatives available.

Engagement with children and young people

Engagement with children, young people, and families identified that schools are the ideal location to address these challenges. They offer an environment in which to educate and engage children and young people regarding health, while also building the knowledge of education staff about NHS services. The Children's Outcomes Forum reinforced this, highlighting that schools are very important places in which children's and young people's health and wellbeing can be supported and improved, and published a guide for school governors to assist them in holding schools to account regarding the physical and emotional health and wellbeing of their pupils.

Healthcare providers need to be innovative and go to where children and young people are, in environments where they are comfortable and secure. Partnerships with schools provide an ideal environment, and offer input from education professionals who are experts in communicating and engaging with a wide range of children and young people. School nursing, public health, primary, and hospital teams can all offer innovative approaches to building knowledge on the range of services available.

Collaboration between education and health professionals within the PSHE curriculum therefore offers a perfect opportunity to extend current health input to:
• Help children and young people understand personal actions they can take to promote their own health and wellbeing.
• Encourage children and young people to identify how to access the different health services available to them.
• Enhance the knowledge of education staff regarding health and wellbeing and health services.
• Help health professionals develop a culture of continuous involvement with existing and potential young service users.

Positive engagement and dialogue with children and young people about health services and the choices available to them can help encourage a change in their healthcare-seeking behaviour and relieve the strain on an overburdened NHS.

Resources to support teachers, educators, and health professionals

NHS England co-produced a resource for teachers, educators, and health professionals to help children and young people understand NHS services and the appropriate ways to access them.

The contents can be used flexibly, helping children and young people discover their local services, such as visiting a pharmacy, GP practice, or dentist, or informing them about how to access NHS 111, and what urgent treatment centres, EDs, and 999 offer. Structured resources such as these introduce children to the language of healthcare, local services, and mechanisms for providing feedback to the NHS about their experiences while within a familiar environment. Demonstrable benefits of close collaboration between schools and the NHS include the development of high-quality signposting information to children and families in school diaries highlighting the range of services available, such as the role of the local pharmacist, mental health services, and support lines such as ChildLine.

The Youth Health Champions programme, supported by the Royal Society of Public Health, is also embedded within schools and gives young people the skills, knowledge, and confidence to act as peer mentors, increasing their knowledge on health-related issues including accessing services, and resulting in them signposting their peers, family members, and locally community to relevant services. It has been shown that the programme ensures that young people are in more control of their health, boosts confidence, allows health messages to be conveyed in a youth-friendly way since public health campaigns are led by young people, and positively influences their local community. In a London Borough, 400 young people have completed this programme and are key health influencers in their local schools and communities.

Engaging vulnerable young people in conversations regarding accessing health services has been considered by the NHS Cadets programme, which is a partnership scheme between St John Ambulance and the NHS, aimed at 14–18-year-olds and offering opportunities to individuals from ethnic minority backgrounds, young carers, and those not in employment, education, or training, or at risk of becoming so. It provides an opportunity for young people to develop leadership and communication skills along with the provision of volunteering opportunities in the NHS. The NHS Cadets programme increases knowledge on employment opportunities in the NHS, the range of healthcare services, and how to access them.

The range of engagement activities between health and education continues to expand. As we see models of social prescribing now including children and the young, the availability of education programmes that integrate knowledge relating to accessing healthcare must increase. The NHS Constitution (https://www.gov.uk/government/publications/the-nhs-constitution-for-england) stressed that patient and public involvement should be part of the fabric of the NHS. Collaboration between health services and education can ensure that children and young people are actively engaged and participate in enhancing their own health and in using NHS services appropriately. The influence of children and young people within their own families and also as future parents and users of services should not be underestimated; we would do so at our peril.

Key points
• Children and young people recognize that there is a need for a preventative approach to their health needs and that information should be shared before it is too late.
• Schools are very important places in which children's and young people's health and wellbeing can be supported and improved.
• Positive engagement and dialogue with school-aged children and young people about health services and the choices available to them can enable change in their healthcare-seeking behaviour.

34 Family information leaflets

Figure 34.1 Developing family information leaflets.

Before you start writing the leaflet you need to:

- **consider the aims of your leaflet**
- **think about what you want your leaflet to achieve**
- realize the limitations of the leaflet

Who is the recipient of the leaflet?
- Decide who the leaflet is aimed at – this will influence the way you write
- If you anticipate that your target group will include a number of people whose first language is not English you should consider translation.
- Written leaflets do not suit everybody. You may need to consider other media

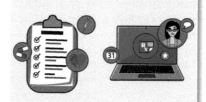

Evaluation and review:
All patient information must be evaluated to determine its usefulness. How this will be achieved should be determined as part of the ongoing quality monitoring process
All information leaflets should incorporate a review date. If clinical practice changes occur before the review date then this should see the review date brought forward

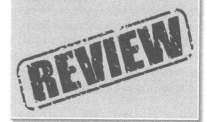

Stages in developing patient information

1. Gathering and sifting the information, which should be evidence based where possible
2. Writing the information – this will take time and should not be rushed.
3. Choose the font type and size and any images and prepare the information for publication
4. Approval process – end user testing and internal approval
5. Ordering the information
6. Designing the layout
7. Review date

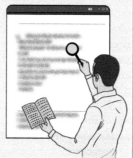

Designing patient information – Top tips

Make sure headings are placed consistently and stand out by using either a larger font or by emboldening the text
Careful use of colours, not too many, and contrasting colours are good to use
If information is going to be presented in a booklet format, use an index
Use a font size as large as possible
Make sure there is good use of white spaces. Dense text makes it more difficult for patients to find information
Avoid long lists of side effects: this can be frightening to patients. Use bullet points instead. Group side effects by order of occurrence or seriousness so patient knows to take action
Keep information located together and not split over different sections

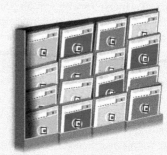

Success criteria for patient information: Readability scoring

90% of literate adults should be able to find the information and of these 90% should be able to understand the information
The Flesch Reading Ease Score test is a readability score for plain English that should be understood by the average 11-year-old

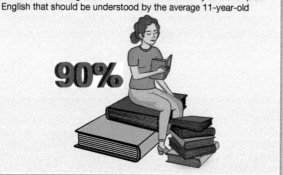

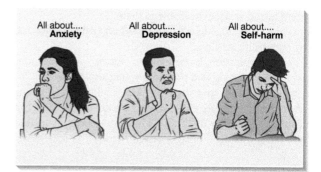

Children and Young People's Nursing at a Glance, Second Edition. Edited by Elizabeth Gormley-Fleming and Sheila Roberts.
© 2023 John Wiley & Sons Ltd. Published 2023 by John Wiley & Sons Ltd.

Families need information to help them make informed decisions about the care of their children. The development of information leaflets for families (Figure 34.1) is an important aspect of quality standards. Today a lot of information is available on hospital and other healthcare web pages, although it should be remembered that access to digital resources is not universal. The children and young person's nurse needs to appreciate this and should always check whether the family has internet access as part of the education and discharge process.

Efforts should be made to ensure that consistent advice and information is given to parents, carers, children, and young people across different care settings and agencies, and in forms that are accessible. Good-quality health information and education enhance patient cooperation and compliance with healthcare regimes. Additionally, good information may reduce patients' stress and anxiety, making it possible for the child and family to cope better with the procedure or experience.

Printed information may not answer all the questions the child may have about a condition or hospital stay, particularly if it is not well designed.

Giving information to some family groups can be especially challenging:
- Those with low literacy.
- Young children and adolescents.
- Those whose first language is not English.
- Individual children with learning disabilities and special needs, who may require materials that have been specially developed.

Writing patient information leaflets
- Who is it aimed at (child or carer or both)?
- Know the setting under which the target audience will read the leaflet.
- Know your purpose: ensure the information is relevant.
- Know your subject.
- Involve your audience.
- Get support in order to produce the leaflet.

Consider the content and style of the leaflet
- Make sure the title of the leaflet is clear.
- Use friendly, everyday language and plain English.
- Use clear and concise writing, keeping things brief and to the point.
- Use short sentences (an average of 15–20 words).
- Avoid jargon or abbreviations.
- Translate or explain essential terminology.
- Use friendly language and give the reader a sense of ownership by using words such as 'we', 'you', 'your'.
- Ensure information is accurate and up to date.
- Be evidence based where appropriate.
- To ensure a 'shelf-life' for the leaflet, avoid the use of names of staff where possible and use job titles instead.
- Be sensitive to religious, cultural, ethical, and gender issues.
- Explain where the reader can obtain more information such as useful websites, organizations, Patient Advice and Liaison Service (PALS), etc.
- Always give contact numbers.
- Think about the questions that the reader is likely to ask. Have you answered them?
- Clearly state the date the information was produced and when it will be reviewed.

Use the 10 principles of clear writing
1 Keep sentences short.
2 Use simple rather than complex explanations.
3 Use familiar words where possible.
4 Avoid unnecessary words.
5 Put action into verbs.
6 Write like you talk.
7 Use terms your reader can picture.
8 Link in with your readers' experience.
9 Use a wide variety of writing techniques.
10 Write to express, not impress.

If your leaflet includes treatment information, it should contain the following:
- An explanation of the procedure: remember parents may be very anxious.
- An explanation of the reason for consent.
- An explanation of the risks as well as the benefits.
- An explanation of any of the alternatives, including non-intervention; if there are no alternatives that would be as effective, this should be stated.
- Any areas of uncertainty surrounding the treatment.
- An explanation of the effects of treatment on the quality of life of the child.
- An invitation to ask questions about any areas of uncertainty.

Consider the order of the information in your leaflet
The order of your information is very important. It should reflect the child's healthcare journey and events and experiences the child or young person will encounter. For example, include what will happen before and after a procedure. Any information leaflets needs to be inclusive so should conform to local policy on the use of inclusive language.

Producing the leaflet
The leaflet should look professional and reflect a high standard of care provided. It should also be accessible to both parents and children. There are a number of ways in which this can be achieved:
- Pay attention to the layout of your leaflet.
- Use plenty of spaces so the page looks clean and uncluttered.
- Avoid large blocks of text: use short separated blocks.
- Use headings to break up text.
- A question-and-answer format can help to divide up text.
- Use bullets or numbering to make important information stand out.
- Use **bold** type for headings and for emphasis. Use UPPER CASE letters.
- Use *italics* and <u>underlining</u> sparingly, as they make the text more difficult to read.
- Align all text and subheadings to the left (justified text is harder to read).
- Font size: minimum 12 point. Use 14 point if you are writing information for visually impaired people.
- Use Arial or Frutiger font only. Times New Roman is particularly hard to read for visually impaired people and therefore should not be used.
- Do not write text over pictures or a design.

Key points
- If the leaflet is for NHS purposes, the NHS has specific guidance or standards for producing patient information in line with the standards set for the NHS brand.
- Approval should be sought before publishing any information for accuracy of content.
- All patient information leaflets should have a review date.

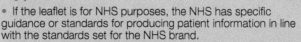

35 Safeguarding and child protection

Figure 35.1 Timeline of legislation and guidance on legislation.

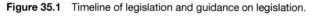

- Children and Young Persons Act 1933
- Sex Offenders Act 1997
- Children Act 1989
- The Children Act (1989) England and Wales
- The Children (Northern Ireland) Order 1995 and the Children (Scotland) Act 1995 share the same principles and have their own Guidance
- Department of Health (2000) Framework for the assessment of children in need and their families (non-statutory guidance)
- Department of Health, Social Services and Public Safety 2003 Cooperating to Safeguard Children
- Female Genital Mutilation Act 2003
- Domestic Violence Crime and Victims Act 2004
- Sexual Offences Act 2004 (2008 for Northern Ireland, 2009 for Scotland)
- Serious Organized Crime and Police Act 2005 set up Child Exploitation and Online Protection (CEOP)
- HM Government (2006) What to do if you're worried a child is being abused
- Scottish Government (2010) National guidance for child protection in Scotland
- Domestic Violence Crime and Victims (Amendment) Act 2012
- Female Genital Mutilation Act (2016)
- HM Government (2018) Working together to safeguard children: a guide to inter-agency working to safeguard and promote the welfare of children
- HM Government (2018) Information sharing advice for practitioners

Figure 35.2 Risk factors.

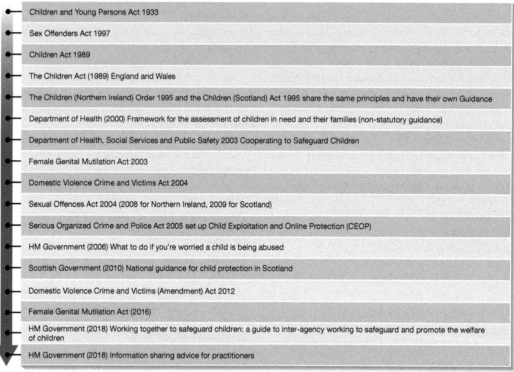

Child
<1 year of age
Disability or complex healthcare
need
Adolescence
Child who is a young carer
Looked-after child
Mental health needs
Developmental delay
Prematurity and low birth weight
Home-schooled children
Gang members as friends
Asylum seekers/refugees

Parents:
Domestic abuse
Substance misuse
Poor attachment with child and parents
Mental health needs
Very young parents
Poverty
Familial history of abuse/neglect or having
been in care system
Social isolation and lack of support
Significant life stress – divorce, injury,
bereavement.

Assessment framework

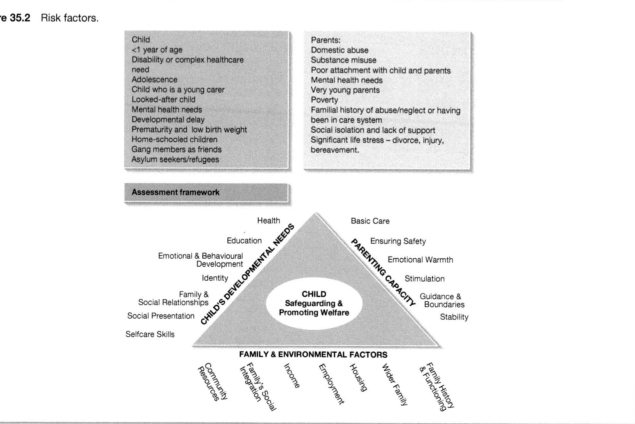

Health
Education
Emotional & Behavioural
Development
Identity
Family &
Social Relationships
Social Presentation
Selfcare Skills

CHILD'S DEVELOPMENTAL NEEDS

Basic Care
Ensuring Safety
Emotional Warmth
Stimulation
Guidance &
Boundaries
Stability

PARENTING CAPACITY

CHILD
Safeguarding &
Promoting Welfare

FAMILY & ENVIRONMENTAL FACTORS

Community Resources
Family's Social Integration
Income
Employment
Housing
Wider Family
Family History & Functioning

Children and Young People's Nursing at a Glance, Second Edition. Edited by Elizabeth Gormley-Fleming and Sheila Roberts.
© 2023 John Wiley & Sons Ltd. Published 2023 by John Wiley & Sons Ltd.

Introduction

Safeguarding children and young people means protecting them from harm and this is everyone's responsibility. All organizations and professionals must work in partnership to protect the children and young people in their care.

Actions are based on the belief that children have certain rights, they are vulnerable as they have not reached the age of maturity, and therefore they need to be protected in law.

Safeguarding refers to the 'continuum of care' for children and young people.

The aim of safeguarding is to:
• Protect children from maltreatment.
• Prevent impairment of the child's health or of their development.
• Ensure that children grow up in environments where care is safe and effective.
• Be proactive to enable all children to achieve the best outcome possible.

A child-centred approach is required if safeguarding services are to be effective, as all concerned need to understand the views and needs of the child.

Legal requirement and safeguarding children

There are a number of regulations that cover the protection of children in the UK (Figure 35.1). The four nations of the UK have their own legislation. All National Health Service (NHS) trusts and organizations that have any responsibility for children and young people will have their own safeguarding policies and procedures. Children's nurses should have an understanding of these. In addition, mandatory training on safeguarding is required for all healthcare staff.

Incidences

Many cases of child abuse go unreported and undetected, so accurate data are difficult to locate. Despite a number of serious case reviews, children continue to die at the hands of their parents/carers and others.

However, it is known that one to two children per week die at the hands of their carers in the UK. Approximately 50 000 children in England are subject to a child protection plan. This includes unborn infants. Boys are subject to more child protection plans than females, with more child protection plans for neglect than any other category. Emotional abuse is the second most reported category.

Risk factors

Risk factors are not indicators of abuse, but the more risk factors that are present, the more vulnerable the child is to maltreatment. The children's nurse must be able to assess the risk factors alongside the protective factors when planning care for the child. Children under 1 year of age are at more risk than other age groups and children with disabilities are also at increased risk of maltreatment. Figure 35.2 outlines other risk factors that the children's nurse must be aware of when assessing a child or young person.

Types of abuse

There are four main categories of abuse:
• Physical
• Emotional
• Sexual
• Emotional

Fabricated or induced illness has been added as a separate category of abuse. However, this landscape continues to change and the children's nurse must be aware of other areas of maltreatment. These include:
• Forced labour, modern slavery, and human trafficking
• Organ trafficking
• Female genital mutilation
• County lines
• Gangs
• Breast ironing
• Forced marriage
• Honour-based violence
• Radicalization

What should the children's nurse do?

Children's nurses have the autonomy and duty to report any suspected abuse. There are four stages to follow:
• *Identify* any safeguarding concern by assessing the child using the assessment framework.
• *Report* the concern. This should be to a senior staff member as identified in local policy.
• *Participate* in any enquiries. This includes debriefing and developing protection plans.
• *Reflect*: what new learning has occurred and will this change your practice?

The assessment framework

When assessing a child in need, a holistic approach is essential, and the assessment framework will be utilized as it will provide an understanding of the risk and protective factors that exist in the child's life.

The assessment framework consists of three domains:
• The child's developmental needs
• Parenting capacity
• Family and environmental factors

The aim of the framework is to promote equality of opportunity and has specific practice guidance on assessing children from black and minority ethnic backgrounds and children with a disability.

Intra-agency working

Many cases can involve a myriad of professionals. The key principle of the Children Act is to ensure that these agencies work in collaboration. This is important to ensure that the jigsaw is pieced together accurately. Based on this a plan can be identified. Failure to collaborate will not provide protection for the child.

Key points

• Be familiar with your organization's policies and procedures for safeguarding and promoting the welfare of children within the area of your practice.
• Remember that in many cases it is only when information from a number of sources is put together that a child can be seen to be in need or at risk of significant harm.

36 Gaining consent or assent

Box 36.1 Legal requirement for informed consent from children under 16 years of age

- Capacity of the child or young person to consent
- Voluntariness of the child or young person to consent
- Understanding of the risks and benefits involved

Box 36.2 Who has parental responsibility?

- The parents if married at the time of the child's conception or birth.
- For children born before 15 April 2002 (in Northern Ireland) or 1 December 2003 (in England and Wales) or 4 May 2006 (in Scotland), the mother, but not the father if they were unmarried at the time of birth, unless the couple subsequently marry or the father acquires parental responsibility via legal proceedings.
- Parents unmarried on or after 15 April 2002 (in Northern Ireland) or 1 December 2003 (in England and Wales) or 4 May 2006 (in Scotland), if they jointly register the birth with the father's name on the certificate.
- Same-sex partners will both have parental responsibility if they were civil partners at the time of treatment, e.g. *in vitro* fertilization.
- For non-civil partners or same-sex partners who are not civil partners, the second parent can get parental responsibility by applying for parental responsibility or becoming a civil partner of the other parent and making a parental responsibility agreement.
- A child's legally appointed guardian appointed by the courts or parents in the event of their own death.
- A person to whom the court has granted a Residence Order in favour of the child.

Children and Young People's Nursing at a Glance, Second Edition. Edited by Elizabeth Gormley-Fleming and Sheila Roberts.
© 2023 John Wiley & Sons Ltd. Published 2023 by John Wiley & Sons Ltd.

Consent is a legally defined decision that is made by a person who has been adequately informed and has adequate understanding without undue influence from another to enable them to make an informed decision (Box 36.1). The legal principles of consent are based on ethical considerations, thus the law on consent is based on the ethical consideration of autonomy.

English law states that consent must be freely given after explanation of the facts. However, the notion of informed consent has its roots in the American legal system and no doctrine of this nature exists in English law.

In the UK there is no set legal age at which children are determined to be competent to make decisions about their healthcare. The 'best interests' of the child apply in decision-making processes and should reflect a careful consideration of the rights of the child and reflect the wishes of that child. The ability to consent is currently based on the child's developmental stage and their expression of understanding of what it is they are consenting to.

Informed consent

Informed consent is a process and not a single event. It is considered good practice to invest time, effort, and care into ensuring that all decisions to be made are 'informed' choices and that the individual has an understanding of both the risks and benefits of any proposed treatment or intervention, and also of not receiving that treatment or intervention.

Refusal of consent

Refusal of consent occurs for varying reasons. It is particularly important to ensure that the 'informed consent' process has been respected and that sufficient time is given for the individual to consider the consequences of selecting various options – including refusal.

Parental consent

When a child refuses treatment in their 'best interests', then parental consent may take precedence over the child's refusal. Courts can also intervene when it is considered to be in the best interest of the child to have the treatment and also in cases where both the child and the parent refuse treatment.

Persons aged 18 years or over can always give consent for themselves unless they are deemed not competent to do so (England, Wales, and Northern Ireland).

Persons 16–18 years old are presumed in law to be competent and therefore can consent to treatment in the absence of parental consent. However, it is considered good practice to involve the family in decision making, unless there is reason to believe that it may not be in the best interest of that child to do so (England, Wales, and Northern Ireland).

Persons under 16 years of age cannot give consent unless deemed Gillick or Fraser competent – and this is a contentious area for some practitioners (England, Wales, and Northern Ireland). In Scotland, children of any age can consent to treatment unless they lack the capacity to do so.

The age of the child is not the sole indicator of whether they can make a decision. Information should be developmentally appropriate and delivered in a way that best suits the needs of the child (*Gillick* v. *West Norfolk and Wisbech AHA* (1985) 3 All ER 402 1985).

Parental responsibility

When a child is not competent to give consent for themselves, then the practitioner should seek consent from a person deemed to have 'parental responsibility' (Box 36.2). This may, or may not, be the child's parents. Legally, consent is required from one person with 'parental responsibility', but it is considered good practice at all times to seek the views of the child or those close to the child affected by the decision-making process.

Parental responsibility ends when the child is 18 years old (England, Wales, and Northern Ireland) and at 16 years in Scotland, though parents can still give 'guidance'.

Consent versus assent

The term assent is used to imply agreement with an opinion by a child or young person who is not legally empowered to give consent. It is just as important to give the child or young person all the required information that matches their capacity when seeking assent. To assent to something, you are agreeing with what has been said, for example if the nurse says 'May I take your pulse?' and the child offers their arm, then this is a signal that the child is in agreement to have their pulse measured. They are assenting to this procedure.

Consent means you are giving permission for treatment to happen.

Defining competence

Competence is a complex issue to define, assess, or even demonstrate. It is multifactorial, hence why it is challenging when applying it to decision-making ability with children and young people. The child's or young person's ability to and willingness to make choices and decisions about their healthcare will have been influenced by the lived experience of their health conditions and treatment. Competence relates to their ability to perform actions to make decisions. This can be decision specific and refers to the characteristics of a person.

Key points

- Children can consent to their healthcare treatment when it is considered that they have the ability to understand what they are consenting to, it is voluntary, and they can retain the information. This is referred to as capacity.
- The 'best interest' of the child is paramount when considering decisions about their healthcare needs.
- There are variations in the age of the child and their ability to legally consent to treatment in the four nations of the UK.

37 Parenting

Figure 37.1 Parenting styles.

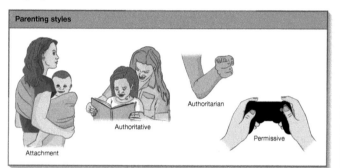

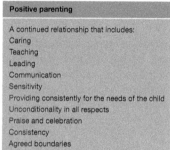

Parenting styles

Attachment
Authoritative
Authoritarian
Permissive

Positive parenting

A continued relationship that includes:
Caring
Teaching
Leading
Communication
Sensitivity
Providing consistently for the needs of the child
Unconditionality in all respects
Praise and celebration
Consistency
Agreed boundaries

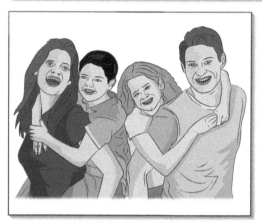

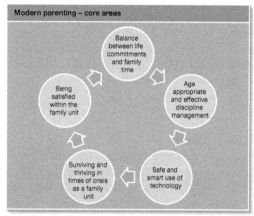

Modern parenting – core areas

Balance between life commitments and family time

Age appropriate and effective discipline management

Being satisfied within the family unit

Safe and smart use of technology

Surviving and thriving in times of crisis as a family unit

Actions for parents to take when children misbehave and they are stressed to avoid harm to their child

STOP

S – stop and pause, take stock, take deep breaths, and keep calm
T – think about what your actions will achieve. How will your child and others perceive your actions?
What will the outcome be now and in the longer term?
O – Options – you do have options. What are they? Where might you get support?
P – positive parenting – listen to your child. What is their story for their behaviour? Reinforce the boundaries.
Be consistent and follow through

What is parenting?

Parenting is the process of caring for and nurturing a child from birth to adulthood, with the aim of enabling the child to achieve their highest potential in life. The child's development is strongly influenced by the style of parenting, so the relationship between a child and their parents is of the utmost importance. The nature of the interaction between the child and their parents on matters such as discipline, behaviour, and dealing with emotions will have an explicit impact on shaping the child.

Through the ages, parenting has evolved.

Parents adjust their child-rearing behaviour to the risks that they perceive in the environment, the skills that they expect their children to acquire as adults, and the cultural and economic expectations they have of their children. Attitudes to parenting have changed in line with modernization (Figure 37.1):
- Less physical punishment.
- Less discipline and more tolerance.
- Acceptance of child's dependency.
- More affection and better relationships – particularly with fathers.
- More time spent together in recreation.

The home environment is crucial. Evidence has shown that the best outcomes (transition from childhood to being a responsible adult) for children are achieved when they are living in a home with both biological parents.

Young children who grow up in a home where there is stress, ineffective communication and discipline, and poor sibling relationships are more likely to have increased usage of drugs and alcohol in adolescence. It may be considered that society is now turning back to more parental control in the era of millennial parenting.

Changes to parenting in the 2000s

The role of women in society has changed significantly, with more mothers now in either full-time or part-time employment. Women are often the main earner in a family, and there has been a rise in the

Children and Young People's Nursing at a Glance, Second Edition. Edited by Elizabeth Gormley-Fleming and Sheila Roberts.
© 2023 John Wiley & Sons Ltd. Published 2023 by John Wiley & Sons Ltd.

Table 37.1 Parenting styles.

Parenting style	Description
Authoritarian	These parents are very directive and demanding, but not responsive. They expect their orders to be carried out without explanation and they provide structured environments with clear rules. Authoritarian parents use much more psychological control, expecting their children to accept their judgements and values without question. Authoritarian parents lead to children who perform well at school but have poorer social skills, lower self-esteem, and higher levels of depression.
Authoritative	These parents are both demanding and responsive. They are assertive, but not intrusive or restrictive. Their methods of discipline are supportive, not punitive. They outline clear expectations for a child's conduct and expect social responsibility and cooperation. Authoritative parents are more open to give and take. Authoritative parents lead to children who are able to balance external conformity with their own individuality and autonomy. These children are most likely to acquire self-confidence and self-esteem.
Permissive	These parents are more responsive than demanding. They are non-traditional and lenient, they do not require mature behaviour, and they set few demands for their children. They allow for self-regulation and avoid confrontation. Permissive parents lead to children who display problem behaviour, perform less well at school, but have higher self-esteem, better social skills, and lower levels of depression.
Neglectful	This parenting style is low in responsiveness and demandingness. In extreme cases this style might encompass rejecting and neglecting parents. Neglectful parents lead to children who are poorly adjusted, have a limited social conscience, and have low self-esteem, as well as the most problem behaviours.

number of men who remain at home as the full-time carer of their children. The social construct of a family has changed in recent times, with the traditional image of the heterosexual, married, two-child family in decline. Opposite-sex and same-sex married or civil partnerships represent two-thirds of all UK families. Same-sex married couples are the fastest-growing family type in the UK, with lone-parent families also increasing in number.

Parenting styles

The construct of parenting style is used to capture normal variations in the attempts of parents to control and socialize their children. Parenting style is a reflection of two elements:

- Parental responsiveness
- Parental demandingness

Parental responsiveness refers to the extent to which parents intentionally foster individuality, self-regulation, and self-assertion by being attuned, supportive, and acquiescent to the special needs and demands of their children.

Parental demandingness refers to the claims parents make on their children to become integrated into the family whole, by their demands of maturity, supervision, disciplinary efforts, and willingness to confront the child who disobeys.

The responsiveness and demandingness of parents help define distinct parenting styles.

There is no one correct type of parenting and many parents will exhibit more than one style when faced with their child's behaviours, actions, or requests. Each style reflects different patterns in values, practice, and parental behaviour.

The recognized parenting styles are (see Table 37.1):

- Authoritarian
- Authoritative
- Permissive
- Neglectful

Parenting factors that affect child development and behaviours

There are a number of factors that affect the child's development and behaviours in relation to how they have been parented:

- Family composition
- Family environment
- Mental health of parents

- Domestic violence
- Child abuse
- Parenting style

Parental responsibilities

Parental responsibilities were formalized by the Children Act 1989. Parenting is defined as 'all the rights, duties, powers, responsibility and authority which, by law, a parent of a child has in relation to the child and his/her property'. This empowers parents to make most decisions in a child's life – up to the child's 18th birthday. Parental responsibility is viewed as a continuum and is a diminishing concept as the child matures. The courts have the power to act in the child's best interests and order treatment despite parental wishes.

Support for parents

Parenting styles are generally learnt primarily from one's own experience of being parented and from observation of others: family members, friends, and social contacts. Many parents need support and guidance in how to parent.

Positive parenting

Positive parenting emphasizes the importance of mutual regard and the use of positive ways to discipline. It follows the principle that all children are born good. It considers the need to create a safe and stimulating environment. The learning environment should be positive and is premised on the fact that if the child approaches the parent for help, they are ready to learn. Disciple should be assertive and expectation should be realistic. Self-care for a parent is also an important and essential aspect of positive parenting.

Key points

- Parenting is an evolving construct that changes in response to societal changes.
- A child's development is strongly influenced by the style of parenting, so the relationship between a child and their parents is key if the child is to mature into a responsible citizen.
- Parenting style is influenced by one's own experience and through the observation of others and life events.
- Positive parenting emphasizes the importance of mutual regard and the use of positive ways to discipline a child.

38 Breaking bad or significant news

Figure 38.1 Factors influencing the process of breaking bad or significant news.

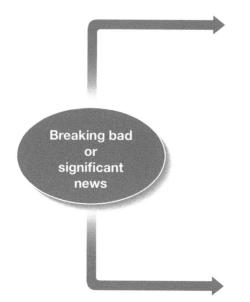

Barriers for the family

- Poor or inappropriate communication skills of professionals
- Lack of appropriate support
- Being given too much, conflicting, or confusing information
- Being given inadequate information
- Not understanding language or terms used
- Feeling uncomfortable in expressing emotions
- Not having time to ask questions

Barriers for professionals

- Lack of experience in breaking bad news
- Previous bad experiences in giving bad news
- Unsure of role in the process
- Poor or inexperienced communication skills
- Inadequate preparation for the event
- Having to use an inappropriate environment
- Not feeling able to respond appropriately to the family's emotion or subsequent behaviour
- Feeling inadequate in supporting the family after the news has been given

---

Box 38.1 Planning to break bad news

Ten steps
1. Prepare environment, staff, flow of information.
2. What is known already?
3. Consider what information is needed now.
4. Expect denial and plan for this.
5. Advise that this information is not good news – warning shot.
6. Explain: use findings to support message, e.g. the blood results have confirmed. . .
7. Listen to concerns.
8. Allow emotions and feelings to come to the fore.
9. Summarize, make a plan, what next?
10. Arrange support and be available in the immediate aftermath.

Box 38.2 The SPIKES mnemonic

S – setting
P – perception
I – invitation
K – knowledge
E – empathy
S – summary

Children and Young People's Nursing at a Glance, Second Edition. Edited by Elizabeth Gormley-Fleming and Sheila Roberts.
© 2023 John Wiley & Sons Ltd. Published 2023 by John Wiley & Sons Ltd.

For most health-care professionals one of the most challenging and stressful elements of their role is when they are required to give news to children, young people, their parents, and carers that they are likely to perceive as significant or bad. This is further exacerbated if the healthcare professional feels unprepared (Figure 38.1). This chapter offers a guide to the principles underpinning best practice for health professionals when breaking bad news to families.

Preparing to break bad news

Before giving bad or significant news to a child's family, careful preparation is needed. The children's and young person's nurse need to prepare. It is often beneficial to follow a stepped approach and rehearse to circumvent misinformation and to plan for possible reactions (Box 38.1). Prior to the meeting it is vital that the professionals involved discuss and plan their contribution together in delivering this news. In most cases, when the news is significant, such as the confirmation of a diagnosis or the news of a child's worsening illness or death, the news will be given by a doctor and the role of the children's nurse is to accompany the doctor and support the family.

It is imperative that the health professionals involved feel prepared with appropriate knowledge and skills and have any necessary information or evidence to share with the family that may be required at the time. If you are asked to accompany a doctor to do this, it is important to consider whether you feel you have the appropriate skills and experience to support the family. Ideally, if the family have already established a rapport or trusting relationship with another member of the nursing team, they would be the preferred professional to accompany the doctor.

Sometimes, the need to break bad news has some urgency (e.g. in the case of an emergency). However, whenever possible, the optimum time and appropriate place to give this news should be considered. The SPIKES mnemonic (Box 38.2) is a useful aide mémoire to help deliver bad or significant news. The environment should be selected in advance, ideally in a quiet room, never in the middle of a public place such as a corridor or busy practice area, with consideration given to the arrangement of furniture and ensuring water and tissues are discreetly placed in the room. It is important to ensure you will not be disturbed by distractions such as undue noise, a ringing telephone, or interruptions from other professionals.

When planning to deliver the bad news, it is important to ensure parents or carers will not be alone, that partners will be together to support each other, and that lone parents or carers have a family member or significant other with them. Every child has the right to be involved in decisions about their health, but in preparing parents to receive bad news it is important to establish whether they wish their child to be present at the disclosure. It should be remembered that children will respond to the emotions of their parents or carers, and for this reason parents often prefer their child not to be present at the initial interview. If this is the case, ensure the child is occupied and not left alone while the family is receiving the news.

Supporting the family when bad news is given

Good communication skills are pivotal to the process of breaking bad news. Parents often retain the memory of how bad news was broken rather than what was said. When talking to parents, use the child's name. It is important to explain the news clearly, using jargon-free language, giving the correct facts and not withholding information, but balancing this with not overloading the family with too much information.

It is important never to assume what the initial responses of parents or family members will be at the time of hearing bad news. The emotions they experience may be very complex and those they reveal may be very different from those they are feeling. Cultural and familial factors have a major influence on our public display of emotion and depend on factors such as personality, coping strategies, gender, role in the family, and the relationship with the professional breaking the news.

Emotions that may be demonstrated through their actions at the time include anger, disbelief, confusion, shock, denial, or, conversely, a lack of emotion or apparent acceptance. Depending on the circumstances prior to the disclosure (e.g. if the family have been worried about their child's unexplained illness, the diagnosis has been anticipated, the child or young person has a life-threatening or limiting illness or has been receiving palliative care for a long time), the news may come with a sense of relief, sometimes followed by a sense of guilt. The emotions experienced include outward displays of distress or grief, ranging from crying or shouting to silence, or disengagement. It is important to remember cultural differences in the display of emotions and not to show surprise at any of these emotions or the subsequent behaviour of those receiving the news. On hearing bad news, family members may use different coping strategies. Some parents may be immersed in their emotional responses whereas others will want to do something practical.

In supporting the family, your own body language should convey compassion and empathy, but also recognize the recipients' need for personal space and dignity. The use of appropriate non-verbal communication such as facial expressions and appropriate eye contact needs careful consideration. Touch can be therapeutic, but never assume it will be welcomed. In deciding whether to use this as a means of communication, it is important to take cues from family members and be guided by their body language. Do say you are sorry, but never say 'I know how you must feel'.

After the bad news has been broken

Give the family some time for the news to sink in. Silences are important and one should never feel the need to talk and fill the gap. Give the family an opportunity to ask further questions or reinforce the news if necessary. Ask if there is anyone you can call, anything they need, whether they would like some time alone, or if they would like you to stay for a while. They may need further information or referral to other professionals or services.

Breaking bad or significant news and supporting families through the process of receiving it are challenging elements of the children's nurse's role. It is vital for all professionals to collaborate with the goal of achieving best practice if children and their families are to feel well supported through the ordeal.

Key points
- Parents will often remember how bad news was broken rather than what was said.
- Consideration of culture is important, as this will impact on emotional behaviour.
- Planned support should be available and offered to family/carers.

39 Care of the dying child

Figure 39.1 Care of the dying child.

Context of caring for the dying child

- Fortunately, childhood death is rare
- Losing a child is a life-altering event for the family and defies the expected order of life
- Home, hospital, and hospice are potential locations for end-of-life care. Each family will have their own preference and their preference, where possible, should be facilitated
- The way a child dies has an impact on the family's response in bereavement
- Caring for a child at the end of life should centre on the individual needs of the child and family (including siblings and grandparents)
- Developmental factors influence the child's ability to understand illness and death, as well as their capacity to communicate anxieties and preferences regarding care

Assessing and planning care

- Professionals should be open and honest with families when the end of life is recognized
- Joint care planning with families should take place as soon as possible
- A written care plan should be agreed and made available to the multidisciplinary team
- A pathway like Together for Short Lives can provide the means of ensuring the end-of-life care needs and wishes of the dying child and their family are met effectively
- Ongoing assessment: care plans should be amended taking into account changes
- Provide clear and simple information and respect silences

Key components of care

- Compassionate child- and family-centred care
- Good communication
- Supporting the parents in decision making
- Pain and symptom management
- Culturally sensitive care
- Care responsive to changing needs
- Access to clinical expertise
- Emotional, psychological, and spiritual support for the child, the parents, and the siblings, including bereavement support
- Practical assistance with the care of the child including respite, equipment, and financial support
- Privacy, comfort, rest, nourishment
- Trust and hope
- Teamwork

Principles of symptom management

- Listen to the child and the parents
- Remember that symptom management not only promotes the child's comfort, but enhances quality of life for child and family
- Adopt a team approach
- Know your limitations and ask for help
- Continuous reassessment and review
- Consider pharmacological and non-pharmacological approaches
- A written plan detailing what to do and who to call if symptoms worsen
- Important to anticipate symptoms, provide information, and develop a plan
- Address parents' concerns and fears around morphine use

Symptoms experienced

Symptoms experienced depend on the child's underlying diagnosis. However, the following includes some commonly occurring symptoms:

- Nausea and vomiting
- Seizures
- Constipation
- Muscle spasm
- Fatigue
- Pain
- Agitation
- Dyspnoea
- Diarrhoea
- Anorexia

Needs of child and family

Last days of life

- Provide information: physical changes of the dying process, planning the funeral
- Perform regular mouth and eye care
- Attend to pressure area care
- Contact appropriate personnel: chaplain, social worker, family and friends
- Encourage sibling involvement
- Create memory opportunities: photographs, hand and foot prints (paint or plaster), memory book
- Cultural sensitivity is imperative when considering creative memories. Gain consent first

After the child dies

- Reassure the family there is no hurry – family can spend as much time with their child as they need
- Offer the family opportunity to bathe and dress their child in favourite clothes
- Offer opportunity to take child home if in hospital
- Ensure legal procedures are followed (e.g. certification)
- Address parents' issues about organ donation if raised

Flow diagram:

Recognition of end of life → Assessment of end-of-life needs and wishes → End-of-life plan ← The fifth standard

Family carers	Child/young person	Environment
Practical support	Pain/symptom control	Place of death
Sibling involvement	Quality of life	Ambience
Emotional support	Friends	Place after death
Spiritual issues	Emotional support	
Cultural/religious issues	Spiritual issues	
Funeral planning	Cultural/religious issues	
Organ donation	Funeral planning	
Grandparents	Organ donation	
	Resuscitation	
	Special wishes/visits	
	Memory box	

Death ← Organ donation

Family carers	Child/young person	Environment
Family support	Funeral	Place to be with the body
Practical help	Burial/cremation	Ambience
Sibling care		
Contacts		
Bereavement support		

Post death

Reproduced with kind permission of Together for Short Lives

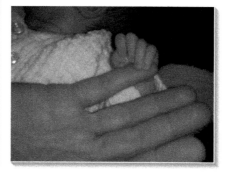

Ethical considerations

Ethical issues abound when caring for a dying child. Fostering a culture of honest and sensitive communication where ethical dilemmas can be openly discussed is crucial. Ethical issues include:

- Communication issues around truth telling
- Withdrawing treatment
- Long-term ventilation
- Provision of hydration and nutrition
- Medical ethics in different cultures

Quality care for the dying child and their family

Fortunately, childhood death is rare. However, when it does happen the death of a child represents a life-altering event for parents and the whole family. During end of life, the nurse plays a key role within the multidisciplinary team, in providing care and ensuring that the ideal of the good death is upheld. It is important to remember that the nurse and family may have different ideas of what is a good death. The composition of the team will differ depending on where the child's end-of-life care is being provided and the child's and family's individual needs. Care should be holistic and individualized, recognizing that the needs of each child and family at this time are different. Together for Short Lives encourages a care pathway approach for children with both life-limiting and life-threatening conditions. This is a framework for providing care for the child and their family from diagnosis through to bereavement care. In this chapter we examine each of the main aspects of quality care in turn, recognizing that these are interconnected (Figure 39.1).

Physical needs

The physical care of a dying child and their family greatly influences the quality of their lives and the ability of the parents/carers and siblings to cope with the child's death. Perceptions that a child is suffering impact greatly on both the child and the family unit. Good symptom management is a key component of care.

The first goal should be to address all distressing symptoms. Frequent assessment and review are imperative to ensure that the child does not become distressed. Commonly, one of the great fears for parents is that their child will suffer unrelieved pain at end of life. The assessment of pain in children, however, is influenced by the child's age and developmental stage. Underestimating pain is common, particularly among neonates and non-verbal children. Pain scales appropriate to the child's development stage, simple observation, and parental reporting are fundamental in good assessment. A detailed symptom management plan is essential. This plan should outline what to do and whom to call if symptoms worsen and anticipate and plan for other potential symptoms. Management should include access to specialized support 24 hours a day, regardless of the place of care.

Nursing care in the last days and hours of the child's life influences the family's experience of death and impacts their bereavement. Involving parents, carers, siblings, extended family, and friends in care can create a sense of order and understanding. This can help families exert some control on their situation. Information regarding the physical changes that can occur to the child as death approaches should be shared freely and normalized. Restlessness, agitation, noisy or rattly breathing, incontinence, eye changes, and circulatory changes are common symptoms experienced. Restlessness and agitation should be managed in accordance with the symptom management plan to avoid further distress. The family should be reassured that although noisy breathing is distressing for them, the distress to the child is thought to be minimal or non-existent.

While many families will choose to care for their child at home on grounds of familiarity and family togetherness, it is important that families understand that they can change their mind at any time. Plans should include options for seamless transition between home, hospital, and hospice where appropriate.

Psychosocial needs

The psychosocial needs of the child and their parents are inextricably linked and hence so is the resultant support. Knowing that their child is dying can result in major emotional, practical, and financial stressors for parents and the entire family. Parents report that they are often caught up in juggling the competing demands of family life while attempting to remain focused on being there for their dying child. They find themselves overwhelmed by uncertainty, decision making, caregiving, guilt, and grief. Sharing time with the child's siblings can become difficult. Each individual child, parent, and family unit have their own ways of coping, therefore the psychosocial support required from professionals is unique to each individual and family. The focus of psychosocial support should be quality of life for child and family, despite the nearness of death. Provision of reassurance, comfort, creating some sense of normality, and making memories are fundamental aspects of providing care for a dying child.

Whether or not the child is aware of the fact that they are dying can further complicate the psychological care that can be offered. While it is thought that many children, especially those who have lived through a long-term illness, have an awareness that they are dying, many parents assume that their child will not understand the issues surrounding death and are therefore reluctant to broach the subject in an attempt to protect them. This can cause tensions between professionals and parents: professionals may feel that giving children the opportunity to communicate may allay their fears regarding dying.

Regardless of where the child's care is being provided, it is often the nurse who is most frequently with the child and family providing personal and sensitive, individualized care. The children's nurse should listen to the child's and family's feelings carefully and respectfully, as well as their individual needs and wishes. The nurse will also need to ensure that good levels of communication are maintained and that information is given in an easily understood format and reinforced over time as required. This information will enable parents and, if appropriate, children to make decisions regarding care. Given the complexity of such decisions, communication between parents and healthcare professionals should be characterized not as a one-off activity, but rather as an ongoing process within which discussion takes place. Such support is essential in allaying fears, permitting a sense of control, and facilitating anticipatory grieving. The use of play as a strategy to help the child express their feelings should not be understated. The nurse should identify their limitations and refer the child and family on for specialized support with a play therapist/specialist as appropriate.

Spiritual needs

Spirituality will have a different meaning for every family and, as with physical and psychosocial needs, requires ongoing assessment. More than simply ensuring that a family's religious practices are upheld, spirituality is about expressing oneself, meaning and purpose, individual values, self-worth, and faith in self, others, or a higher power. Therefore, spiritual care is care that is responsive to the human spirit and the nurse should endeavour to provide opportunities for what is important to the individual child and family. For some it may be arranging a visit from the chaplain or administering a sacrament. For others it could be creating some meaning through rituals or creative memories. Rituals can provide the opportunity for the child, parents, siblings, and other family members to express their love and sadness and create precious memories.

Key points

- All children, young people, and families are unique and have their own individual needs right to the end.
- Good communication is key to understanding these individual needs.
- Distressing symptoms such as pain and agitation need to be managed at all times.

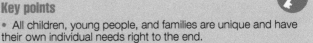

40 Dealing with aggression

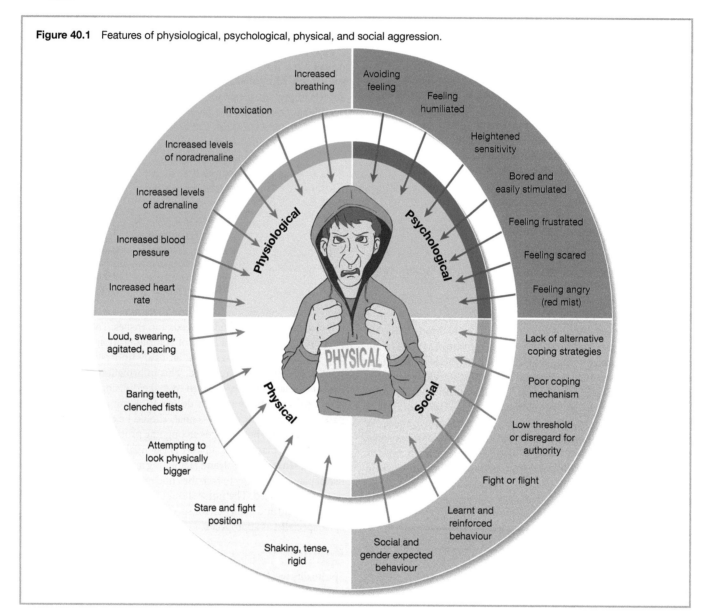

Figure 40.1 Features of physiological, psychological, physical, and social aggression.

What is aggression?

There are a number of competing theories about what aggression is and the purpose it serves. Social psychologists define aggression as behaviour that is intended to harm another individual who does not wish to be harmed. Dealing with aggression can be scary for professionals and other service users working in young people's healthcare settings. Aggression in the theoretical sense has a number of subsets, which range from all-out 'violence' to 'verbal threats' and 'irritating annoyance'. Thus, not all acts of aggression are intended to cause physical damage, but rather serve as a warning and a response to frustration.

Quite often aggression is the result of 'hot-headed', non-thinking reactions to either threatening or frustrating situations young people find themselves in. Examples ranging from road rage to temper tantrums serve to remind us that aggression is a complex phenomenon that impacts a number of domains and bodily systems (physiological, physical, psychological, and social; Figure 40.1). If you think about the times you have been aggressive, it would probably be when you were tired, angry, upset, frustrated, scared, or feeling ill. You would remember feeling agitated, short-tempered, tense, loud, and maybe tearful and later regretful. In the heat of the moment you would probably have little regard for other people and not be responsive to reason. Physiologically, your heart would be pumping fast; you would be breathing hard and in a state of fight or flight. These are the symptom of aggression and a result of aversive

Children and Young People's Nursing at a Glance, Second Edition. Edited by Elizabeth Gormley-Fleming and Sheila Roberts.
© 2023 John Wiley & Sons Ltd. Published 2023 by John Wiley & Sons Ltd.

events, our thoughts (cognitions), and the release of and response to chemicals, including alcohol, but in particularly the male sex hormone testosterone.

What causes aggression?

Physiologically, aggression is caused by hormones and evolutionary factors. Physically, it is wired into the deepest and oldest parts of our brain and has the aim of protecting ourselves as much as giving us means of surviving. In the past 20 years or so, there has been a recognition of dietary factors and that some children are aggressive as a result of specific childhood psychological conditions such as attention deficit hyperactivity disorder (ADHD). Socially, aggression has been valued in some cultures and is often unwittingly reinforced in gender stereotyping and cultural variables. As children mature and develop, it is through social learning that they begin to refrain from tantrums, gain a sense of self, and cognitively begin to moderate their behaviour.

Dealing with aggression is a personal thing. Most children and young people display aggressive outbursts when they feel threatened by others or are frustrated and cannot get their own way. Thus, most aggressive outbursts are dependent on situation, circumstance, the cognitive awareness of the child, and associated trigger factors. This means that much aggression can be planned for and strategically reduced. Personality variables that relate to perceived threat also predict aggression.

Emotional or impulsive aggression

Impulsive aggression occurs with no or only a small amount of forethought or intent. It is usually defined by a short, loud outburst that has an obvious cause and can be easily contained. A typical example is the child who embarrassingly cries, or screams in a fit of tantrum in a supermarket, or the infant who never wants to go to bed. At this younger age aggression serves a purpose for the child of expressing unhappiness and desire or wants. Over a period of time with consistent reinforcement, routine, and supportive parenting, most children can overcome these types of emotionally triggered aggressive outbursts.

For teenagers and the healthcare professionals who work with them, aggression has different connotations related more to cognitive triggers that are characterized by more intentional planning, forethought, and frustration. Aggression in this respect shows itself in at least two ways: physical or non-physical.

• *Physical aggression* is aggression that involves harming others physically – for instance spitting, hitting, or kicking in more than self-defence. Physical aggression is immediate, violent, and requires urgent de-escalation interventions to reduce arousal.

• *Non-physical aggression* is often referred to as passive or verbal aggression. It does not involve physical outbursts, but rather verbal aggression such as threats, shouting, screaming, name calling, and in some cases 'social aggression'. This is active participation in the intentional harming of others' social relationships by spreading rumours and other behaviours such as blanking, silent treatment, name calling, racist and sexually stereotypical jokes, and spreading gossip. Social aggression is becoming an increasing concern in cyberspace with cyberbullying.

Triggers of aggression

The best approach to understanding the triggers of aggression is prevention. This means planning ahead and also having a predetermined plan for dealing with aggression as a team when it occurs.

This means being aware of policy, attending relevant training, and knowing your clients. The primary triggers for most young people are when they are frustrated or disappointed or feel undermined or unfairly treated. Whether this is the case or not, if that is their perception and they have a 'nothing to lose' feeling and if the young person has a history of having a short fuse, then planning ahead and having strategies for dealing with potential outbursts need to be a consideration. These include having a stringent routine, a full programme of activities to prevent boredom, a transparent sense of equity between all young people being cared for, and rewards for good behaviour. Other strategies include role modelling expected behaviours around disappointment, having a reward to work towards at the end of the shift, easily achievable small tasks, and, in nearly all cases, the development of an authentic, caring relationship to help the young person ventilate feelings appropriately.

De-escalating physical aggression

Aggression can be explained in terms of learning, reinforcement, modelling, punishment, arousal, and cognition, but this is rarely relevant when a young person becomes physically aggressive in a healthcare setting. Dealing with physical aggression in a team approach requires the implementation of predesigned policy and training of all involved. The metaphor of the escalator serves well to emphasize that the quicker a team can prevent and then stop the escalator rising with the young person on it, the better the outcome of any incident. The following is an outline of the key points when dealing with a physically aggressive incident:

1 *Safety*: of self, the aggressor, and others. Seek assistance and clear the immediate area. If the child is endangering themselves or others, attempt to remove harmful objects safely.

2 *Wait*: if you try to engage in conversation with the aggressive person, it will probably escalate the incident. Wait. They will run out of steam eventually. Then try to talk calmly about the issue.

3 *Gently engage*: deal with the immediate situation by remaining calm and employing non-verbal cues (pay particular attention to proximity, volume of voice, open posture, and non-threating stance). Keep verbal clues simple to reduce stimulation and, for now, avoid judgement, moralizing, or giving an opinion. Give reassurance and clear instructions as to your intentions and expectations. Offer compromise and limited alternatives. Only as a last resort should you grapple with and attempt to physically restrain the child.

4 *Post-incident issues*: apply consequences (remember to teach compromise). Consider the personal triggers for the child and work towards addressing creative ways of confronting these in the future.

Put into place an incident debrief and paperwork. Consult policy and guidelines. Ensure that team training is in place.

Key points
- Aggression is either physical or non-physical. Physical aggression involves harming others and non-physical aggression may be verbal or passive.
- Your own safety is paramount, so the children's and young person's nurse needs to seek assistance immediately
- Triggers that may precipitate aggression in the child or young person need to be understood by the healthcare team.

41 Minimizing the effects of hospitalization

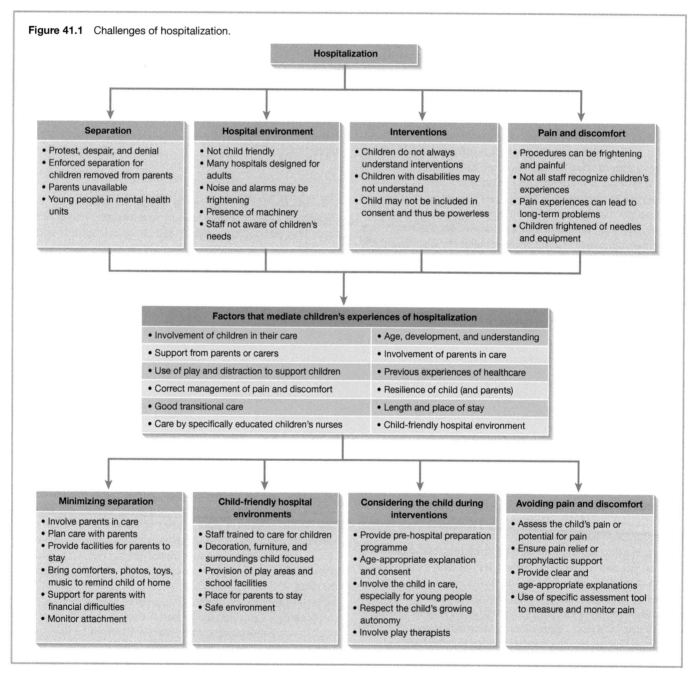

Figure 41.1 Challenges of hospitalization.

Hospitalization

Separation
- Protest, despair, and denial
- Enforced separation for children removed from parents
- Parents unavailable
- Young people in mental health units

Hospital environment
- Not child friendly
- Many hospitals designed for adults
- Noise and alarms may be frightening
- Presence of machinery
- Staff not aware of children's needs

Interventions
- Children do not always understand interventions
- Children with disabilities may not understand
- Child may not be included in consent and thus be powerless

Pain and discomfort
- Procedures can be frightening and painful
- Not all staff recognize children's experiences
- Pain experiences can lead to long-term problems
- Children frightened of needles and equipment

Factors that mediate children's experiences of hospitalization
- Involvement of children in their care
- Support from parents or carers
- Use of play and distraction to support children
- Correct management of pain and discomfort
- Good transitional care
- Care by specifically educated children's nurses
- Age, development, and understanding
- Involvement of parents in care
- Previous experiences of healthcare
- Resilience of child (and parents)
- Length and place of stay
- Child-friendly hospital environment

Minimizing separation
- Involve parents in care
- Plan care with parents
- Provide facilities for parents to stay
- Bring comforters, photos, toys, music to remind child of home
- Support for parents with financial difficulties
- Monitor attachment

Child-friendly hospital environments
- Staff trained to care for children
- Decoration, furniture, and surroundings child focused
- Provision of play areas and school facilities
- Place for parents to stay
- Safe environment

Considering the child during interventions
- Provide pre-hospital preparation programme
- Age-appropriate explanation and consent
- Involve the child in care, especially for young people
- Respect the child's growing autonomy
- Involve play therapists

Avoiding pain and discomfort
- Assess the child's pain or potential for pain
- Ensure pain relief or prophylactic support
- Provide clear and age-appropriate explanations
- Use of specific assessment tool to measure and monitor pain

Hospitals can be threatening, frightening, and painful environments where children are faced with strangers who want to 'do' things to them. Illness, trauma, and hospital care are often the most traumatic things children experience, even with the presence of their parents. In addition, hospitals present a conflict for children who are taught about ownership of their body and to be wary of strangers. Nonetheless, changes in the way healthcare is provided, giving rights to patients, improvement in staff knowledge, and increasing knowledge of children and parents about medical issues, mediated through the internet, have impacted how hospitalization is experienced. Similarly, the concept of hospitalization has changed with shorter bed stays, development of primary care, avoidance of hospital care, and overall improved health of children.

Children and Young People's Nursing at a Glance, Second Edition. Edited by Elizabeth Gormley-Fleming and Sheila Roberts.
© 2023 John Wiley & Sons Ltd. Published 2023 by John Wiley & Sons Ltd.

The experience of hospitalization

Hospitals used to be places of long stays, routine, rigidity, restricted visiting, limited emotional care, and often painful experiences for children. Much of this has changed; however, it does not necessarily alleviate how children experience what is happening to them (Figure 41.1). What is trivial to an adult can be a major stressor to a child.

Experience of the child

While much of the hospital environment is anxiety producing, one experience has the potential to cause trauma for children and this is separation from their parents. Parents can usually stay with their children, but other responsibilities may prevent this and so the child becomes separated. The impact of separation is dependent on circumstances, age and development, but may be displayed in specific stages:

1 *Protest*: The child actively searches for their parents and protests through clinging to them, crying, screaming, rejecting staff, and possibly being aggressive.

2 *Despair*: The child is exhausting their ability to protest and so enters a stage of despair about the situation. This may result in withdrawal, sadness, non-communication, and possible regression to earlier behavioural stages of development.

3 *Denial or detachment*: The child's attachment is focused on those around them rather than on the parents. They seek out, interact with, and respond to staff and may even reject their parents. This stage is rarely seen now, except in children who have been abused or neglected.

Experience of parents

Much research has identified the adverse experience of hospitalization on children. However, there can be impacts on parents that in turn affect the child:

- Anxiety when separated from their child.
- Feelings of guilt.
- Conflict between parents if they are not able to stay with their child.
- Emotional impact of the ill child on their ability to cope.
- Physical demands of maintaining life and being at the hospital.
- Development of postnatal depression.

Interventions and adverse experiences of hospital

Experiencing hospital care can lead to a range of situations and interventions that are potentially traumatic for the child, although this is not always the case, as children are resilient and can cope with many stressors. Stressors for the child include the following factors.

Environment

- Strange, clinical, and often frightening environments that may not necessarily be child friendly.
- Adult-orientated environments.
- Machinery and equipment that are large and frightening in comparison to the size of the child.
- Noise, lights, and alarms.
- Loss of control as they are not in their usual environment.

Staff

- Having to interact with strangers.
- Staff who are more orientated towards adults.
- Not considering the specific needs of children and families.
- Staff who do not understand the child's developmental needs for support, preparation, and care.

Circumstances

- Emergency situations in which the survival needs override those of the child.
- When the child has experienced trauma.
- Safety of the child when there is a concern about abuse.
- The child requires interventions that they do not want.

Interventions

- Loss of control resulting from the specific intervention.
- Pain resulting from the intervention, lack of preparation, staff not following analgesia pathways.
- Procedures over which the child has no control or input.
- The child is restrained in order to undertake a procedure.

Interventions to alleviate the impact of hospitalization

Hospitals and children's units

Hospitals admitting children should have policies about their rights, issues of consent, safeguarding, and nursing and medical procedures, so that the deleterious impacts of hospital are minimized.

Staff

Children should be cared for by professional staff who have in-depth knowledge of children, development, and conditions that affect them. Staff must provide care that is child centred while being sensitive to their rights and wishes. Nurses particularly must advocate on behalf of children in order that no harm is done and the child does not suffer, particularly when painful procedures are performed.

Interventions

Throughout all interventions children's needs must be the central concern and the aims to appropriately prepare them, obtain their consent, ensure analgesia or anaesthetic is provided, communicate effectively about what is happening, and support them, bearing in mind the child's age, development, and status.

Key points

- The effects of hospitalization on the child and family are many and can be far-reaching.
- The children's and young person's nurse must advocate for the child to ensure they come to no harm during their hospitalization.
- Loss of control from the child's and family's perspective due to ill-health results in stress, so information is essential at all stages of their hospitalization.

42 Transition from hospital to home

Figure 42.1 Care issues for consideration when the family with a child with complex care needs are transitioning from the acute hospital setting to home.

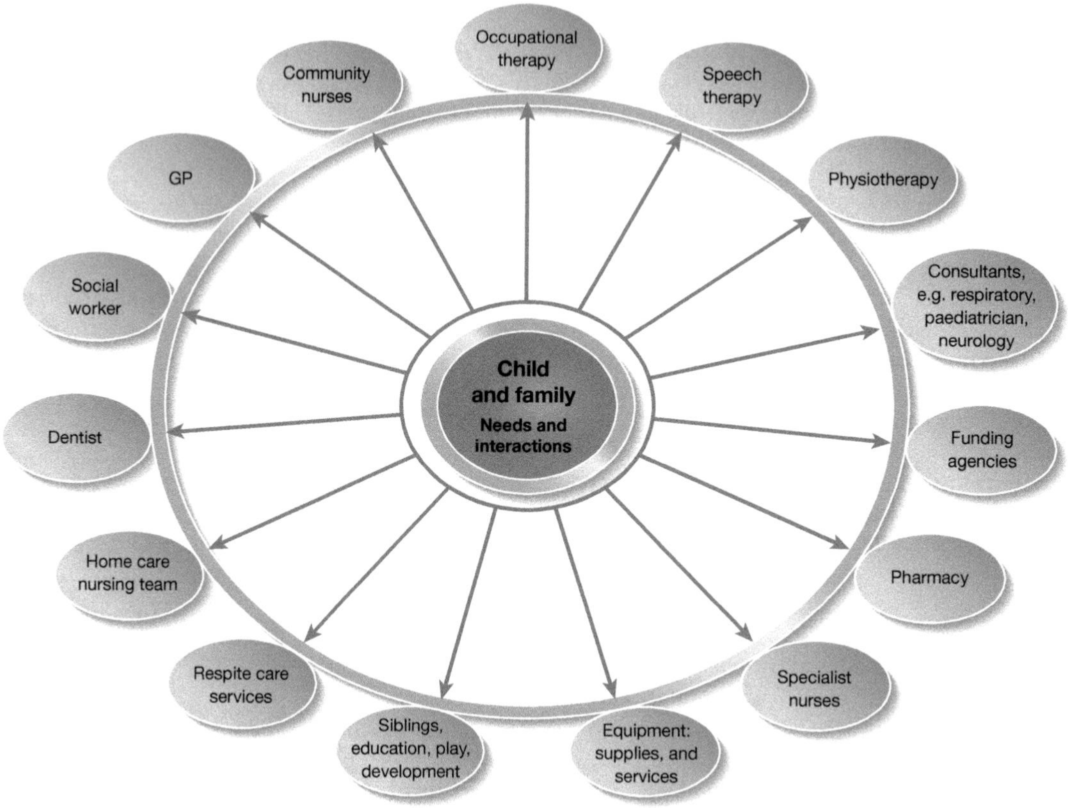

- Occupational therapy
- Community nurses
- Speech therapy
- GP
- Physiotherapy
- Social worker
- Consultants, e.g. respiratory, paediatrician, neurology
- Dentist
- Funding agencies
- Home care nursing team
- Pharmacy
- Respite care services
- Specialist nurses
- Siblings, education, play, development
- Equipment: supplies, and services

Child and family
Needs and interactions

Figure 42.2 Hospital to home.

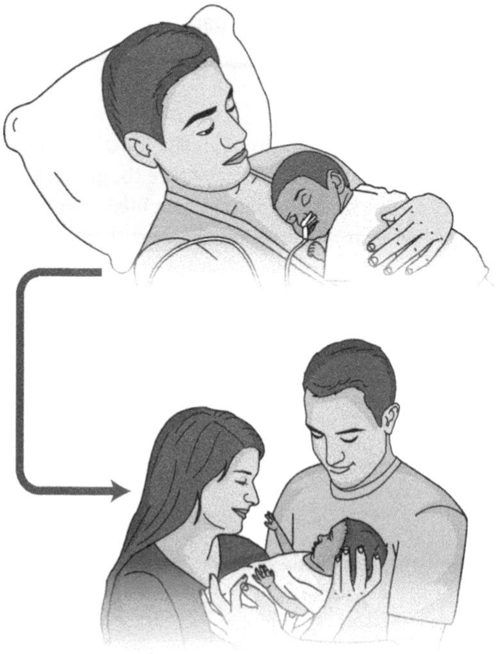

Figure 42.3 Strategy for continuing care at home.

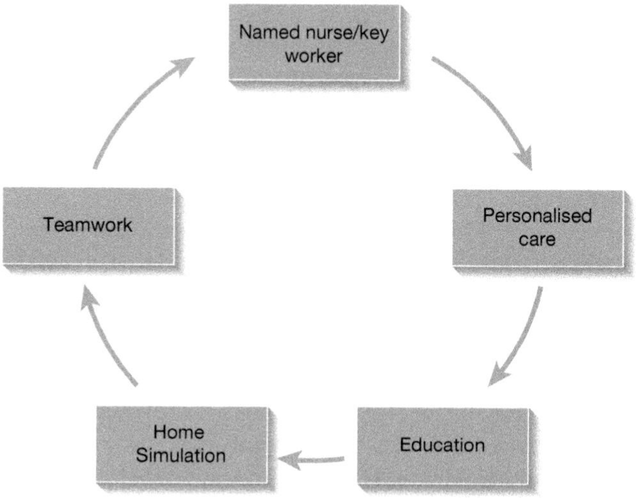

- Named nurse/key worker
- Teamwork
- Personalised care
- Home Simulation
- Education

Children and Young People's Nursing at a Glance, Second Edition. Edited by Elizabeth Gormley-Fleming and Sheila Roberts.
© 2023 John Wiley & Sons Ltd. Published 2023 by John Wiley & Sons Ltd.

This chapter presents care issues that emerge for consideration when the family with a child with complex care needs are transitioning from the acute hospital setting to home. This includes children with chronic conditions and those who are technology dependent, where ongoing care necessitates the involvement of multiple providers. Figure 42.1 identifies many of the needs and interactions of the family with a child with complex care needs.

Children should be cared for, where possible, with their family, in their own home. However, if the family are to cope with being the primary carers, then a number of structures need to be in place to ensure a dynamic partnership between service providers and the child's family. Knowledge of the needs of each individual family is required to identify the strengths of each family and to identify and address their specific physical, emotional, financial, and social needs, to ensure they can adapt their lives in a positive way to their changing circumstances.

Challenges to transitioning to home

Many children and their families (Figure 42.2) may wait protracted periods of time in acute hospitals while negotiation ensues between the acute and community services over a wide range of transitional care needs:

- Absence of a coordinated vision for discharge in the tertiary care setting and no clear time frame for discharge.
- Lack of leadership and clear negotiation and communication between the parents and primary, secondary, and tertiary care services.
- No clear funding arrangements.
- Absence of organized home-care service delivery.
- Delayed modifications to the child's home.
- Procurement of adequate technology for home care.
- Parents' financial challenges in changing work patterns.
- Preparation of parents for the physical care of the child at home.

Assessing needs for discharge to home

There is a requirement for a thorough and accurate assessment of the needs of the child and family. Ideally, planning the discharge home of a child with complex care needs begins once it is established that the child, with some accommodation, could be cared for in their own home (Figure 42.3). This initially requires the tertiary care centre, together with the family, to widely consult with the multidisciplinary team to identify the extent of support services required for the child's care at home. This consultation phase is key to beginning the process of planning for home care and establishing a trusting relationship between the parents and the primary, secondary, and tertiary care services, as the parents begin to transition to being the primary carers.

Specific needs

Education needs

Parents need to know how to care for the child, how to identify changes in the child's condition, how to respond to any changing conditions, and how to access relevant support services in relation to equipment.

For example:

- Airway management and dealing with airway emergencies.
- Care of a tracheotomy.
- Care of the ventilated child and care of associated technology.
- Care of the immobilized child, including cleansing and dressing and pressure sore prevention or management.
- Drug therapies, dosage, and adverse effects.
- Communication – specific aids required.
- Pain assessment and management.

Care support

The family may also require home-care nursing, respite services, and access to ongoing health support services such as GP, community nurses, physiotherapy, speech therapy, and psychological support to help parents cope.

Social needs

Housing modifications may be required. Parents will require financial advice and support in relation to the cost of caring for a child with complex needs at home, as well as support to access education and developmental care where necessary.

Integrated care pathway

An agreed discharge plan and a specific care package should emerge from the assessment phase. The implementation of this plan requires a key worker or named coordinator, who has responsibility for acting as a dynamic service coordinator for the family. This means that they will have oversight of the family's interaction with hospital and community services, financial advice, procurement and servicing of equipment, and the ongoing review and refinement of the family's needs. This should include maintenance of a record of all appointments, funding plans, and budget allowances, with responsibility for identifying and accessing services to support any changing needs of the family.

Key points

- A wide range of supports need to be in place to ensure a dynamic partnership between service providers and the child's family.
- Planning for transitioning to home should start very early.
- Parents of a child with complex care needs have education, social, emotional, and financial requirements.
- An integrated care pathway guided by a named coordinator can support the child and parents through their transition to home.

43 Safety in children and young people's nursing

Figure 43.1 Improving patient safety.

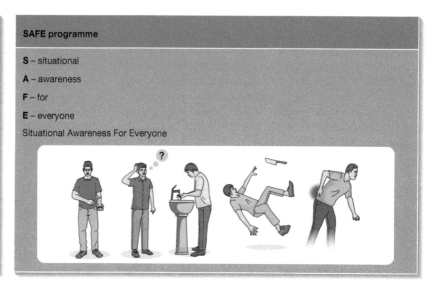

NHS strategic aim to improve patient safety: 3Is

- **Insight:** improved understanding of safety by drawing on multiple sources of patient safety information
- **Involvement:** equipping patients, staff, and partners with the right skills and opportunities to improve safety throughout the system
- **Improvement:** designing and supporting programmes that deliver effective and sustainable change in the most important areas

SAFE programme

S – situational

A – awareness

F – for

E – everyone

Situational Awareness For Everyone

Fundamental safety principles:

- Prevention
- Detection
- Mitigation
- Escalation

SAFETY FIRST

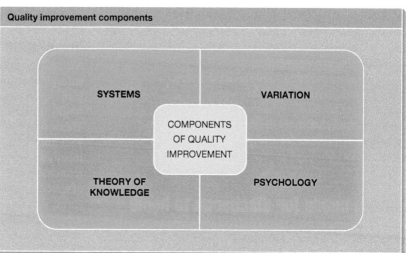

Quality improvement components

SYSTEMS

VARIATION

COMPONENTS OF QUALITY IMPROVEMENT

THEORY OF KNOWLEDGE

PSYCHOLOGY

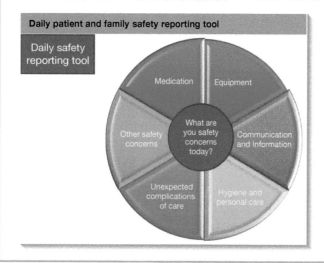

Daily patient and family safety reporting tool

Daily safety reporting tool

Medication
Equipment
What are you safety concerns today?
Other safety concerns
Communication and Information
Unexpected complications of care
Hygiene and personal care

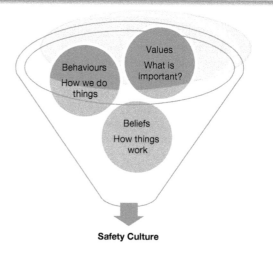

Behaviours — How we do things

Values — What is important?

Beliefs — How things work

Safety Culture

Children and Young People's Nursing at a Glance, Second Edition. Edited by Elizabeth Gormley-Fleming and Sheila Roberts.
© 2023 John Wiley & Sons Ltd. Published 2023 by John Wiley & Sons Ltd.

Introduction

The safety of children and young people (CYP) in hospital is everyone's business and the last decade has seen this topic gain prominence in all areas: national strategy, research, and the development of systems and tools for use in practice.

It is currently estimated that there are 2000 preventable deaths in UK hospitals annually. Some 10–15% of all patients are harmed every year. The CYP nurse must be able to make positive contributions to improve safety and the quality of care and treatment they deliver to achieve effective and enhanced health outcomes. To do this they are required to assess the risks to the safety of the patient experience and take appropriate action to manage those risks, always putting the patient's best interests, needs, and preferences first.

What is patient safety?

Safety is the ability of a system to sustain its normal function under expected and unexpected conditions. Patient safety relies on harm being designed out and barriers being put in place to prevent harm (Figure 43.1). However, when these barriers are breached, harm is likely to occur as the successive layers of defence are weakened or disappear.

Why does harm happen?

There are a number of factors that need to be understood about why harm happens. It is usually an amalgamation of factors that will lead to harm occurring. These factors are:
• Organization and culture (management decisions and organizational processes) – latent failures.
• Contributory factors (environmental factors, team/staff factors, task factors, patient factors) – human failure.
• Care delivery problems (unsafe practice, omissions, errors, and violations) – active failure.

When any of the above types of failure occur, defences and barriers are transgressed, and harm occurs to the patient. Some of the recent public inquiries have been able to evidence organizational and culture elements that led to contributory factors and then active failure at the point of patient care, resulting in significant harm to patients, including death.

Systems thinking and improving safety

The vast majority of patient safety cases are as a result of the systems, conditions, environments, constraints, and procedures that exist in the National Health Service (NHS). They are not as a result of an individual's action. In order to improve patient safety, an understanding of the complexity of the constituent aspects of a system is required: clinical care, hospital, and the NHS as a whole. This approach is referred to as systems thinking. This is a holistic approach to analysing those interrelated parts to identify how systems work over time. Data and observation are methods used to better understand how systems think. The four main components of systems thinking are:
• Understanding of the system in which one works.
• Examining the way people think and behave – what are their beliefs and attitudes?
• Knowing the variations in the system.
• Being aware of what theory or method of change is best used for change.

Situational awareness

Situational awareness is having an awareness (perception) of the activities or elements of an environment within a period of time and space, and understanding how those elements may impact on others (patients) in the immediate future. It is knowing what is going on in real time. This requires decisions to be made that are then translated into action.

The three main components of situational awareness are:
• Perception – gathering information.
• Comprehension – recognizing and understanding what is happening in the environment.
• Projection – anticipating what will happen,

Situation awareness for everyone

The Situation Awareness for Everyone (SAFE) programme was developed following a collaboration with 28 hospitals and a series of quality improvement projects were implemented and evaluated. From this, a pack of six discrete resources were produced.

The primary aim of the SAFE programme is to reduce avoidable error and harm to sick children in hospital by building a safety-based culture. In addition to this, it also sought to do the following:
• Reduce *variation* in treatment so that all children and families receive care of a comparable standard.
• Improve *communication* between all healthcare professionals and support staff involved in the care of the child and their family.
• Involve parents and *empower* children and young people to be more involved in their own care.

Situational awareness considers the perspective of everyone involved in the care of the child, including the child and their family, as well as doctors, nurses, allied health professionals, and support staff, with a view to enabling the correct clinical decisions to be made.

Huddles

A huddle is an open exchange of information between all staff members in a ward/department/theatre, where information is shared to equip staff with the knowledge and skill required to identify patients who may be at risk of deterioration or where there are concerns of harm. The safety of the ward in terms of safety theory and frameworks is a talking point, as is the prediction of safety for the next period of time between huddles. The reliability of care is also a discussion point. Huddles are of short duration, usually 10–15 minutes, and occur at regular intervals during the shift, usually every 6–8 hours. All members of the ward team – registered nurse, doctors, nursing associate, medial students, physiotherapist, cleaning and catering staff, healthcare support workers, play specialist – should be in attendance.

The aim of a huddle is to improve situational awareness and to empower staff to raise concerns by:
• Identification
• Mitigation
• Escalation

The challenges and barriers to the implementation and sustaining of huddles often relate to lack of time and capacity, lack of senior leadership, and the capacity of staff to embrace change and understand where it fits within existing practices. The benefits of huddles, in addition to improved patient care and safety, are improved teamwork and efficiency in care delivery.

Leadership and patient safety

All CYP nurses have a leadership role when caring for sick children and young people. Leadership is an essential aspect of nursing, as it serves as a way of encouraging others to deliver effective care through role modelling good practice. When caring for a sick child who may be a deteriorating patient, the CYP nurse must advocate for the child and their family and lead on communicating all concerns effectively using recognized safety tools, such as the SBAR (Situation, Background, Assessment, Recommendation) process. This will allow priority clinical reviews that are based on accurate assessment using recognized tools, for instance PEWS (Paediatric Early Warning Score). This will result in precise and timely interventions. The leadership role of CYP nurses in delivering healthcare should be visible in all aspect of their work. This means they are aware of what works effectively and what needs improvement. When caring for the deteriorating child, leadership should focus on effective assessment, situational awareness, effective team communication, and effective clinical interventions based on the patient's unique needs at that time.

As an advocate for the patient, the role of the CYP nurse is to ensure that a safe and effective clinical environment is maintained. This will include leading on areas for development by implementing quality improvement initiatives and encouraging and developing colleagues to follow.

How can we keep children and young people safe in practice?

The path to patient safety requires the CYP nurse to challenge their own beliefs and those of others if behaviour is to change. Continuously checking and reflecting on practice are essential.

Knowing what works well is as important as knowing what went wrong if risk is to be mitigated. Reporting incidents is key to the future of patient safety. It is only by analysing data that trends can be identified and therefore this evidence can be used as a vehicle for change and quality improvement.

The use of recognized risk assessment tools should be standard practice and part of the quality improvement plan. These include SBAR, PEWS, and huddles. You should also ask the child and family if they are feeling safe. This can be achieved through daily safety reporting tools.

Safety netting advice is another aspect of improving patient safety. Safety netting is providing parents with information that is designed to help them seek further medical help if their child's condition fails to improve, or suddenly changes, or if they have ongoing concerns about their child's health. The aim of safety netting is to ensure timely review and reassessment of the child to mitigate against harm.

Patient safety alerts are provided from a central source. These offer vital safety information about medical devices and medication that must be adhered to.

Key points
- Patient safety is everyone's responsibility, and the CYP nurse must engage in quality improvement initiatives to improve standards of care.
- Checking and questioning the reliability of the systems and processes in use should become daily questions.
- Integration of learning into practice is required to respond to challenges and to improve patient safety.

Part 3

Chapters

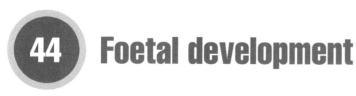

44 Foetal development

Figure 44.1 Foetal development.

Fertilized egg   2-cell stage   4-cell stage   8-cell stage   16-cell stage   Blastocyst

Foetus – 4 weeks   Foetus – 10 weeks   Foetus – 16 weeks   Foetus – 20 weeks

Figure 44.2 Adaptation of the foetal circulation system.

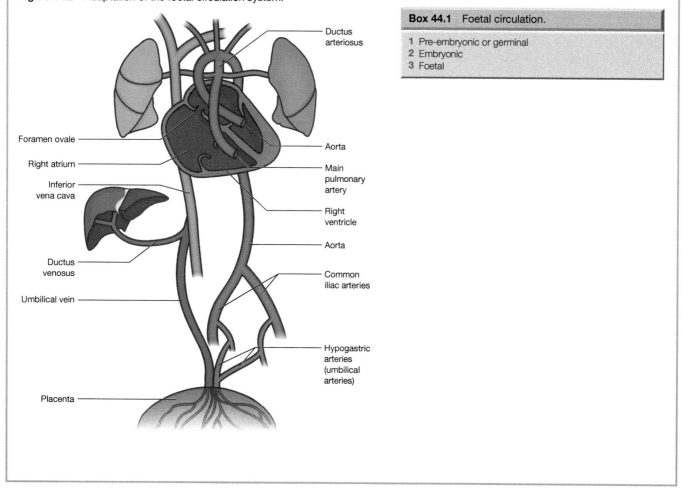

Ductus arteriosus
Foramen ovale
Right atrium
Inferior vena cava
Ductus venosus
Umbilical vein
Placenta
Aorta
Main pulmonary artery
Right ventricle
Aorta
Common iliac arteries
Hypogastric arteries (umbilical arteries)

Box 44.1 Foetal circulation.

1 Pre-embryonic or germinal
2 Embryonic
3 Foetal

Children and Young People's Nursing at a Glance, Second Edition. Edited by Elizabeth Gormley-Fleming and Sheila Roberts.
© 2023 John Wiley & Sons Ltd. Published 2023 by John Wiley & Sons Ltd.

Pre-embryonic development

All human life commences from one single cell produced from the union of a male and a female. This union marks the beginning of the prenatal period. The first two weeks post conception are known as the pre-embryonic or germinal stage. The fertilized ovum undergoes mitotic division, resulting in a zygote then a morula. Within four days it becomes a blastocyst, which implants into the uterine endometrium.

Embryonic development

The process of embryonic development occurs in three main stages (Box 44.1). The first two weeks post conception are known as the germinal stage. This is followed by the embryonic stage of eight weeks' gestation, and the third stage is called the foetal period.

Three germ layers – ectoderm, mesoderm, and endoderm – form the main tissues and organs in the developing embryo. By four weeks the embryo has a head, a trunk, and tiny limb buds. Blood is also circulating around the embryonic body at this stage. By four to eight weeks, the embryo measures 2.5 cm and has recognizable facial features and major sensory organs are developing, such as eyes, ears, nose, lips, and tongue. The cardiovascular system, kidneys, and liver are functional and the lungs are developing. Skeletal growth is cartilaginous and the limbs begin to lengthen.

Foetal development

See Figure 44.1.
- *8 weeks. The embryo becomes the foetus.*
- *9–12 weeks.* The eyelids close, the oral palate fuses, urine is produced, and genitals are established. Red blood cells are produced in the liver. The foetus measures approximately 6.5 cm and weighs around 18 g.
- *13–20 weeks.* Ossification of the skeleton begins and limbs reach their final proportions. Head hair is visible and lanugo is present over the body, as is vernix. The liver and pancreas secrete enzymes and the foetus is capable of sucking. The foetus measures around 15 cm at this stage.
- *21–28 weeks.* Lungs mature with alveoli visible. Fat deposits increase and lanugo begins to disappear. There is rapid brain growth at this stage.
- *28–32 weeks.* Skin is pink but lacking in subcutaneous fat, although brown fat deposits increase. The main organs are functional and cerebral development increases as the brain grows. Length is approximately 38 cm and weight around 1800 g.
- *34–37 weeks.* Fat deposits increase and the foetus becomes 'chubby'. The foetus 'practises' breathing movements – the lungs are now capable of breathing spontaneously. Genitalia are visible on ultrasound scan and the foetus is seen sucking and swallowing fluid. Fine tuning of the brain and neural system continues till birth. Length is approximately 45–50 cm.
- *37–40 weeks.* The foetus is now capable of surviving at birth without intensive care. Movements felt by the mother are less intense as the growing foetus has less room to move around and the foetal head descends into the mother's pelvis. Lanugo has disappeared and the lungs are fully functional. The foetus will be able to breathe, suck milk, digest, absorb and excrete products. The central nervous system is fully functional, exhibiting numerous reflexes and behaviours. Length is approximately 50 cm and weight 3–4 kg.

Foetal circulation

The main differences between foetal and adult circulation are as follows:
- Low pulmonary blood flow → pulmonary vascular resistance (PVR) high.
- Low placental resistance → systemic vascular resistance (SVR) low.
- Shunting of blood from right to left side of circulation through foetal shunts.

Foetal blood flow

Blood containing nutrients and oxygen flows from the placenta into the umbilical cord via the umbilical vein, which goes to the liver, where it branches off to the left lobe and receives the venous blood from the portal vein (Figure 44.2). This mixed blood bypasses the liver via the ductus venosus to enter the inferior vena cava, where it travels to the right atrium of the heart. Approximately 75% of this mixed blood is diverted through an opening in the septum called the foramen ovale and into the left atrium. The remaining 25% of the blood is pumped into the right ventricle and pulmonary artery – some will go to the lungs, but most will go into the ductus arteriosus, which bypasses the lungs to deliver blood to the aortic arch. All of this is influenced by the high resistance in the right ventricle and pulmonary artery. The blood from the left atrium passes into the left ventricle, then enters the aorta, passing along its branches to supply head, neck, and arms, before travelling through the vessels in the chest and abdomen. The aorta divides into the common iliac arteries, small streams passing down into the legs, but the main streams pass into the hypogastric arteries. These arteries arise in the pelvis and pass through the umbilicus and enter the cord as the two umbilical arteries, which return deoxygenated blood back to the placenta for oxygenation. In the foetal circulation, the right side of the circulation is dominant due to high PVR, so any shunting will be from right to left. The left side is less dominant due to low SVR, because the placenta is a low-resistance organ.

Adaptation at birth

Once the umbilical cord is clamped the umbilical vein ceases to pump blood and collapses – the umbilical arteries and veins constrict, and low resistance from the placenta is removed. There is a rise in SVR leading to increased pressure (SVR) in the left atrium, as well as a fall in pressure in the right atrium, resulting in blood trying to move from left to right across the septum and closure of the foramen ovale. The baby breathes, the airways open, and pulmonary circulation improves, increased oxygen levels close the ductus arteriosus (a reduction in prostaglandin levels also assists), and there is greater blood flow to the lungs. Blood flow in the hypogastric arteries ceases and these become ligaments.

Key points
- Knowledge and understanding of prenatal development are important for the children's nurse when caring for the preterm infant or the child with a congenital birth defect, as they can give an informed explanation to parents to help them understand when and why the defect occurred.
- At any stage in embryonic development, planned and expected events may not occur and this can lead to a range of congenital conditions that will impact on the life of the child and family.
- The intrauterine environment can impact on foetal development and any risk to the developing foetus must be avoided where possible.
- Failure of adaptions at birth can lead to significant health problems, particularly those of a cardiac nature.

45 Examination of the newborn

Figure 45.1 Examination of the newborn – what is included.

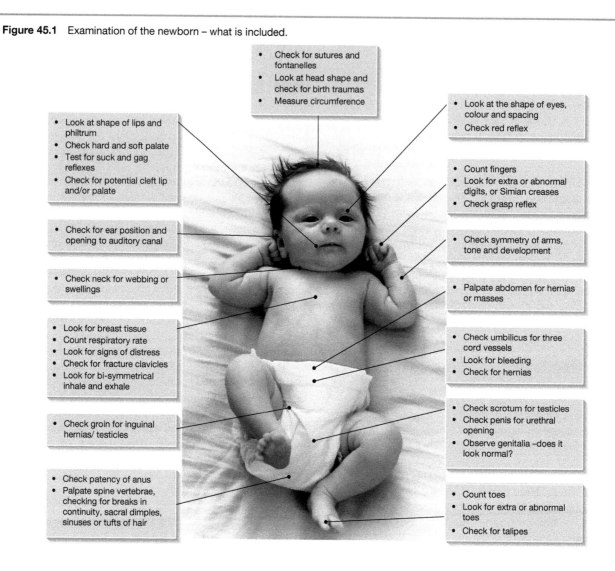

- Check for sutures and fontanelles
- Look at head shape and check for birth traumas
- Measure circumference

- Look at the shape of eyes, colour and spacing
- Check red reflex

- Look at shape of lips and philtrum
- Check hard and soft palate
- Test for suck and gag reflexes
- Check for potential cleft lip and/or palate

- Count fingers
- Look for extra or abnormal digits, or Simian creases
- Check grasp reflex

- Check for ear position and opening to auditory canal

- Check symmetry of arms, tone and development

- Check neck for webbing or swellings

- Palpate abdomen for hernias or masses

- Look for breast tissue
- Count respiratory rate
- Look for signs of distress
- Check for fracture clavicles
- Look for bi-symmetrical inhale and exhale

- Check umbilicus for three cord vessels
- Look for bleeding
- Check for hernias

- Check scrotum for testicles
- Check penis for urethral opening
- Observe genitalia –does it look normal?

- Check groin for inguinal hernias/ testicles

- Check patency of anus
- Palpate spine vertebrae, checking for breaks in continuity, sacral dimples, sinuses or tufts of hair

- Count toes
- Look for extra or abnormal toes
- Check for talipes

Box 45.1   Nursing A–E assessment.

Airway (A):
- Check for airway patency
- Check for crying with no abnormal sounds

Breathing (B):
- Check respiratory rate (RR): between 40 and 60/min
- Check the chest is rising symmetrically

Circulation (C):
- Check heart rate (HR): between 110 and 160/min
- Check the colour of the skin and mucous membranes: consider skin tone and ethnicity. Potential blue in the hands and feet (acrocyanosis)

Disability (D):
- Check that eyes are PEARL (pupils equal and reactive to light)
- Check for grasp reflex

Environment (E):
- Apyrexial. Between 36.4 and 37 °C

Children and Young People's Nursing at a Glance, Second Edition. Edited by Elizabeth Gormley-Fleming and Sheila Roberts.
© 2023 John Wiley & Sons Ltd. Published 2023 by John Wiley & Sons Ltd.

Overview of newborn examination

Newborn physical examination aims to identify and refer babies born with congenital abnormalities (for example of the eyes, heart, hips, and [in males] testes), where these are detectable, within 72 hours of birth and any further abnormalities that may become detectable by 6–8 weeks of age, so reducing morbidity and mortality. Links between neonatal assessment and neurosensory and motor impairments in high-risk infants have been relatively well established. The initial examination carried out after birth is to identify any deviations from normal, but it should be pointed out to parents that some conditions only become apparent days and weeks after birth, and so this examination cannot rule out problems later on.

A general physical examination of the baby is carried out by the midwife or paediatrician soon after birth. At this time, the weight, head circumference, and length are measured and recorded in the baby's Personal Child Health Record Book ('red book'). These measurements are plotted on a centile chart. Average head circumference for a term baby is in the range 35–38 cm; length is usually 46–55 cm in term babies.

Term babies normally lie in a flexed position, moving their arms and legs occasionally. The practitioner should look for symmetry when considering movement, posture, and the overall appearance of the baby. Each part of the baby is examined systematically.

Using a systematic approach

Examining a baby can be done using a systems approach (Figure 45.1) and/or an ABCDE approach (Airway/Breathing/Circulation/Disability/Exposure) (Box 45.1). Both illustrate a systematic approach to examination, which is important for a thorough assessment to avoid any omissions. However, the systems approach is akin to the guidelines for the UK Newborn and Infant Physical Examination (NIPE) screening programme, which is completed on all babies between 6 and 72 hours of age. This includes the following:

- *Skin*: Look at colour. Term babies have thicker skin, which looks creamy pink; preterm babies have thinner skin, which looks more reddish in colour and may be covered in vernix (a white waxy substance) or lanugo (fine hairs). Check for rashes or birth traumas.
- *Head*: Feel around the skull for the suture lines as well as the anterior and posterior fontanelles, checking for the normality of these. Often there is moulding (overlapping). Check for large swellings, which can either be cephalhaematoma (bleeding between two layers of bone) or caput succedaneum (oedema), both of which can be painful and require analgesia. Measure the head circumference.
- *Eyes*: Make sure eyes are present; look at spacing, shape, and iris for deviations from normal. Check the colour of the sclera for jaundice, blueness (osteogenesis imperfecta), or infection. Red reflex should be checked for presence – also that pupils are reactive to light (PEARL).
- *Nose*: Check for shape and bridge configuration – also patency of nostrils.
- *Mouth*: Feel the hard and soft palate for clefts and look for premature teeth or tongue ties. Check that suck and gag reflexes are present.
- *Ears*: Tops of ears should be level with eyes. Look for rotation: low-set, rotated ears can be indicative of chromosomal abnormalities. Check for an opening to the auditory canal. Lack of cartilage suggests prematurity. Hearing should be tested prior to discharge.
- *Neck*: Look for webbing (chromosomal defect) and cystic hygromas (swellings), which can block the airway.
- *Spine*: Feel the spine from the base of the skull right down to the anal sphincter. Check for breaks in the continuity of spinal column. Look for tufts of hair or sinuses, both of which may be indicative of occult spina bifida.
- *Chest wall*: Look for symmetry, breast tissues, and nipples (absence indicates prematurity). Observe breathing rate (40–60/min) and look for respiratory distress (indrawing, tachypnoea). Check clavicles for fractures – common in large babies or difficult deliveries.
- *Arms and hands*: Check for symmetry in length and shape as well as the range of movement of arms. Count the fingers and look for webbing, or extra or overlapping digits, which may indicate genetic defects. Look for simian crease (single deep crease on palm), which is linked to trisomy 21 (Down's syndrome). Check the colour of fingernails – blueness may indicate cardiac disease.
- *Abdominal wall*: Gently palpate for any lumps (hernias), particularly around the umbilicus or groin area. Check the umbilicus for three cord vessels before shortening the cord and applying the clamp.
- *Genitalia*: Girls – look for labia majora and minora, clitoris, and urethra. Labia majora covers these structures in term babies, but gapes open exposing them in preterm babies. Boys – check penis for urethral opening (abnormal opening on the underside – hypospadias) and the scrotal sac for two testicles – may be undescended. Both these conditions require referral and follow-up.
- *Anal sphincter*: Check that it is patent. The baby should pass meconium within 24–48 h after birth. Failure to do so may indicate meconium ileus, bowel obstruction, or imperforate anus. The baby should also pass urine – 3 mL/kg/h.
- *Legs and feet*: Check for symmetry in length and shape as well as the range of movement. Count the toes and look for webbing, or extra or overlapping digits, which may indicate genetic defects. Look for inverted feet (talipes) – can be positional or true talipes, both of which will require physiotherapy or orthopaedic treatment.

Other observations

The baby should have colour, heart rate, respiratory rate, and temperature checked before leaving the delivery suite to ensure that these fall within the normal parameters. Colour should be cream-pink, but the baby may still look a little blue in the hands and feet (acrocyanosis) for up to 24 h. Heart rate should be 110–160/min; respiratory rate should be 40–60/min. Temperature should be 36.4–37 °C. The umbilical cord should be checked at intervals for bleeding. Normally, the heart sounds, femoral pulses, neurological reflexes, red reflex, and hips are checked when the baby is having the final examination prior to discharge home. Hearing tests are carried out within the first few weeks of life.

Key points

- The link between neonatal assessment and neurosensory and motor impairments in high-risk infants is relatively well established.
- Some conditions are not identifiable at birth and parents need to know this.

46 Neonatal screening tests

Figure 46.1 Neonatal screening tests.

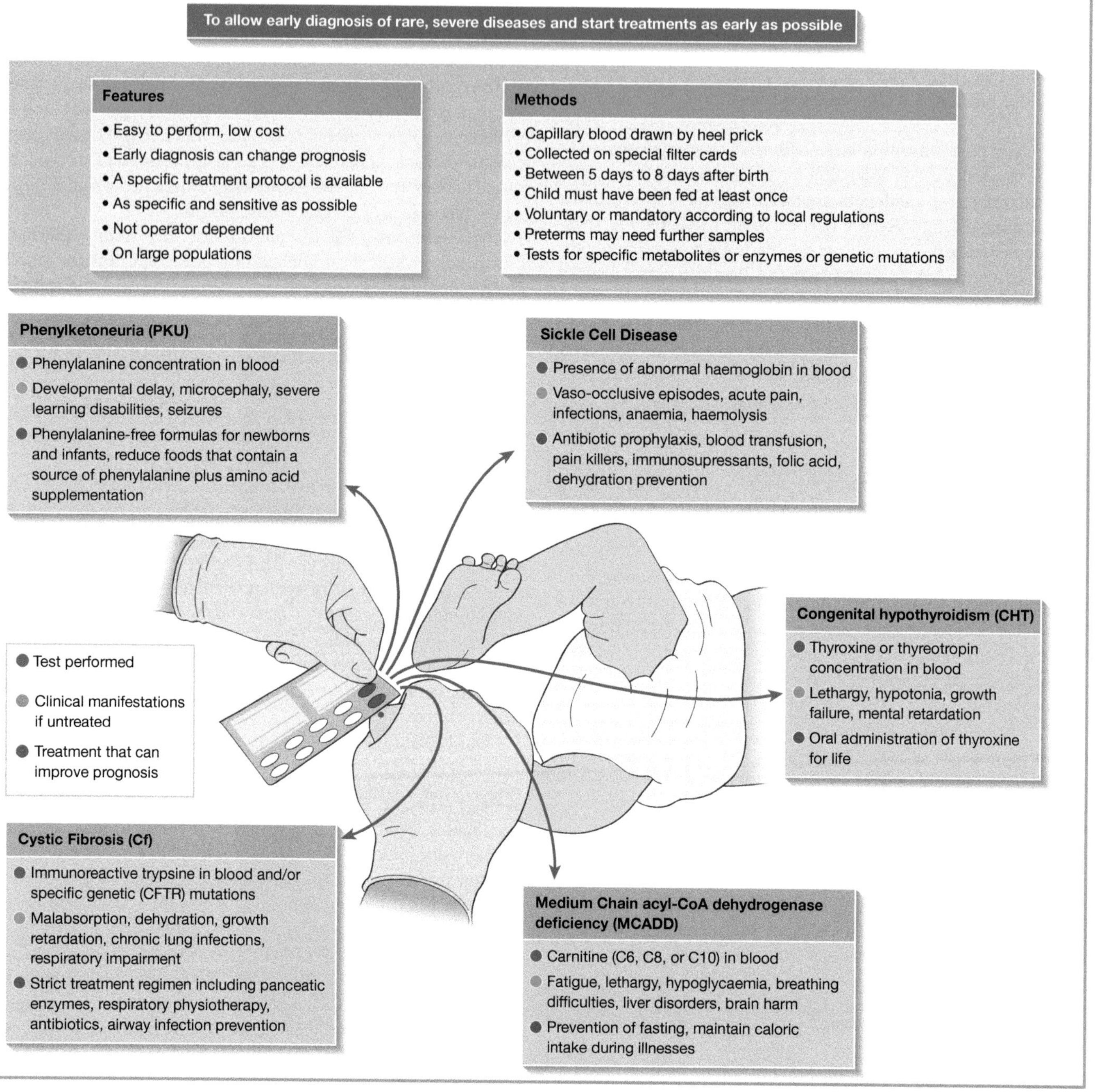

> To allow early diagnosis of rare, severe diseases and start treatments as early as possible

Features
- Easy to perform, low cost
- Early diagnosis can change prognosis
- A specific treatment protocol is available
- As specific and sensitive as possible
- Not operator dependent
- On large populations

Methods
- Capillary blood drawn by heel prick
- Collected on special filter cards
- Between 5 days to 8 days after birth
- Child must have been fed at least once
- Voluntary or mandatory according to local regulations
- Preterms may need further samples
- Tests for specific metabolites or enzymes or genetic mutations

Phenylketoneuria (PKU)
- Phenylalanine concentration in blood
- Developmental delay, microcephaly, severe learning disabilities, seizures
- Phenylalanine-free formulas for newborns and infants, reduce foods that contain a source of phenylalanine plus amino acid supplementation

Sickle Cell Disease
- Presence of abnormal haemoglobin in blood
- Vaso-occlusive episodes, acute pain, infections, anaemia, haemolysis
- Antibiotic prophylaxis, blood transfusion, pain killers, immunosupressants, folic acid, dehydration prevention

- Test performed
- Clinical manifestations if untreated
- Treatment that can improve prognosis

Congenital hypothyroidism (CHT)
- Thyroxine or thyreotropin concentration in blood
- Lethargy, hypotonia, growth failure, mental retardation
- Oral administration of thyroxine for life

Cystic Fibrosis (Cf)
- Immunoreactive trypsine in blood and/or specific genetic (CFTR) mutations
- Malabsorption, dehydration, growth retardation, chronic lung infections, respiratory impairment
- Strict treatment regimen including panceatic enzymes, respiratory physiotherapy, antibiotics, airway infection prevention

Medium Chain acyl-CoA dehydrogenase deficiency (MCADD)
- Carnitine (C6, C8, or C10) in blood
- Fatigue, lethargy, hypoglycaemia, breathing difficulties, liver disorders, brain harm
- Prevention of fasting, maintain caloric intake during illnesses

Neonatal screening programmes

The neonatal screening programme (NSP) allows the early detection of uncommon and severe congenital diseases that are not clinically evident at birth, but in which the prognosis can be significantly influenced by starting specific treatments very early in life. Within the neonatal screening programme newborn blood spot (NBS) screening enables early identification, referral, and treatment of babies with nine rare but serious conditions, including sickle cell disease (SCD), cystic fibrosis (CF), congenital hypothyroidism (CHT), and phenylketonuria (PKU). Maple syrup urine disease (MSUD), isovaleric acidaemia (IVA), glutaric aciduria type 1 (GA1), and homocystinuria (HCU).

Children and Young People's Nursing at a Glance, Second Edition. Edited by Elizabeth Gormley-Fleming and Sheila Roberts.
© 2023 John Wiley & Sons Ltd. Published 2023 by John Wiley & Sons Ltd.

The NSP helps to improve the baby's health and prevent severe disability or even death. For each condition, the benefits of screening outweigh the risks. The newborn babies who have positive results to the screening test (usually about 1%) undergo further diagnostic tests to exclude or confirm the diagnosis (Figure 46.1).

It is important that babies are offered timely screening; parents are supported to make an informed choice about screening for their baby; all screen-positive babies are referred to diagnostic and clinical care promptly; equal access is provided for high-quality screening across England; all screening results are recorded on a child health information system and parents given a copy; and harmful effects of screening, including anxiety, inaccurate information, and unnecessary investigation, are minimized.

Sample collection and analysis

Neonatal screening tests are usually performed on the newborn infant's capillary blood drawn by heel prick. Several blood spots are collected on special filter cards and allowed to dry. The cards also contain information regarding the newborn baby. Collection of blood spots should be performed when the baby is 5 days old but can be up to 8 days old. Babies born at less than 32 completed weeks' gestation (less than or equal to 31 weeks + 6 days) need a second blood spot sample taken, in addition to the day 5 sample, to screen for CHT. Blood is analysed for the presence of specific metabolites, enzymes, or genetic mutations.

Conditions commonly screened

Phenylketonuria

PKU is an autosomal recessive genetic disease that prevents metabolization of phenylalanine (Phe), an amino acid introduced in the body with several proteic foods (incidence 1 in 10 000). At birth children are 'normal', but if untreated they develop severe learning difficulties, microcephaly, electroencephalogram (EEG) alterations, and seizures. Children with PKU tend to hypopigmentation of hair and skin and a characteristic musty odour of sweat and urine. Treatment consists of reducing foods that contain a source of Phe (e.g. eggs, fish, dairy products, meat, nuts, legumes, some artificial sweeteners) and in administering amino acid supplementation. Special Phe-free formula feeds are given to infants. The screening test measures Phe concentration in blood.

Congenital hypothyroidism

CHT is an endocrinopathy that affects 1 in every 3000–4000 newborn babies and is mainly caused by a defect of development of the thyroid gland. If untreated, within a few weeks from birth the child develops growth failure and irreversible severe learning difficulties. Typically, an infant with CHT appears sleepy, hypotonic, colder than normal, and uninterested in feeding. The treatment is oral administration of thyroxine for life, which is sufficient to prevent the onset of symptoms. Regularity in thyroxine administration and adherence to a follow-up programme are paramount. Body weight and heart rate should be periodically checked. The onset of fatigue may indicate the need to adjust the drug dosage.

Cystic fibrosis

CF is an autosomal recessive disease (incidence varies in ethnic groups, 1 in 2500–100 000) that determines a malfunction of mucous cell membrane ion exchange, resulting in an excessive thickness of all exocrine secretions. Babies with CF present with malabsorption due to exocrine pancreatic insufficiency, chronic lung infections with progressive respiratory impairment, and many other clinical manifestations that reduce life expectancy. However, CF may remain asymptomatic long after birth. No cure is currently available, but an early treatment regimen has shown to be effective in reducing disease progression, delaying lung infections, and increasing lifespan. CF screening is based on measuring immunoreactive trypsine (IRT), which is higher in children with CF, and/or on the research of a panel of genetic mutations coding for CF. Children found positive by screening undergo the sweat test (titration of chloride in sweat) to confirm diagnosis.

Sickle cell disease

SCD is an autosomic recessive disease of blood, with higher incidence in tropical and Mediterranean populations. It is caused by defective haemoglobin; red blood cells assume a sickle shape and lose elasticity, causing acute vaso-occlusive episodes with acute pain, infections, anaemia, haemolysis, and several other manifestations and long-term complications. Treatment is complex and includes blood transfusions, antibiotic prophylaxis, immunosuppressants, pain killers, folic acid, preventing cold and dehydration, and many other measures. Early detection of SCD reduces the risk of some complications (in particular pneumococcal infections) and may improve patients' quality of life. A screening test investigates for the presence of abnormal haemoglobin in the newborn infant's capillary blood. If the test is positive, a second blood test is performed to confirm the diagnosis within the second month of life. SCD screening may also detect subjects with beta-thalassaemia disorders.

Medium-Chain Acyl-CoA dehydrogenase deficiency

Medium-chain acyl-CoA dehydrogenase deficiency (MCADD) is an autosomal recessive disease (incidence 1 in 4000–4 017 000) that impedes the conversion of some body fats into energy, in particular during fasting. This may cause fatigue, lethargy, and hypoglycaemia. Symptoms appear early in life and if left untreated, MCADD can lead to severe complications such as seizures, breathing difficulties, liver disorders, brain damage, coma, and death. Early diagnosis improves prognosis as it allows prevention of risky situations, such as fasting – in particular during illnesses – and other circumstances where body energy production requires fatty acid oxidation.

Maple syrup urine disease

This is a genetic condition that occurs if the baby inherits two faulty copies of the branched-chain alpha-keto acid dehydrogenase (BCKAD) gene, one from each parent. (incidence 1 in 150 000). The BCKAD gene provides instructions to make the BCKAD enzyme, which is required to break down some of the amino acids found in food and milk (including breast milk and normal infant formula). Without the BCKAD enzyme the baby is unable to completely break down the keto acids, resulting in a build-up of amino acids and keto acids that are harmful to the brain. Symptoms include vomiting or difficulty feeding, abnormal movement of the arms and legs, lethargy, progressive neurological deterioration, sweet-smelling urine and sweat, poor feeding or loss of appetite, and weight loss. Symptoms usually appear within the first few days or weeks after birth. Treatment consists of a special low-protein diet and dietary supplements that reduce the build-up of leucine, valine, isoleucine, and alloisoleucine. Without early treatment, babies can develop brain damage, due to high levels of harmful substances in the body that can be life threatening.

Isovaleric acidaemia

IVA is a genetic condition where the baby inherits two faulty copies of the isovaleryl-CoA dehydrogenase (IVD) gene, one from each parent (incidence 1 in 150 000 babies born in the UK). The IVD gene provides instructions to make the IVD enzyme, which is used to fully break down an amino acid called leucine found in food and milk (including breast milk and normal infant formula). Normally, leucine is broken down into a substance called isovaleric acid. Babies with IVA are unable to break down isovaleric acid, which leads to a harmful build-up of the acid in the blood and urine. Symptoms sometimes appear within the first few days or weeks after birth and may include developing a distinctive odour of 'sweaty feet', poor feeding or loss of appetite, and weight loss; Without early treatment, babies can develop brain damage, including learning difficulties due to high levels of harmful substances in the body, which can be life threatening.

Glutaric aciduria type 1

Babies with GA1 inherit two faulty copies of the glutaryl-CoA dehydrogenase (GCDH) gene, one from each parent (incidence 1 in 300 000 babies born in the UK). The GCDH gene provides instructions to make the GCDH enzyme, which is required to break down glutaric acid derived from amino acids (lysine, hydroxyl-lysine, and tryptophan) found in food and milk, including breast milk and normal infant formulas. Without this enzyme harmful levels of some substances accumulate in the blood and can make the child unwell. Symptoms of GA1 usually do not appear until a few months after birth. Increased concentration of harmful substances including glutarate and 3-hydroxyglutarate raises the risk of a metabolic crisis. If GA1 is not treated it can cause long-term brain damage. Treatment consists of a special low-protein diet and dietary supplement, which can reduce the build-up of harmful substances and helps to reduce the risk of a metabolic crisis and brain damage.

Homocystinuria (pyridoxine unresponsive)

Babies are born with HCU if they inherit two faulty copies of the cystathionine β-synthase (CBS) gene, one from each parent. The CBS gene provides instructions to make the CBS enzyme, which converts homocysteine into cystathionine. Homocysteine is made from the amino acid methionine, which is found in food and milk, including breast milk and normal infant formula. Babies with HCU lack the CBS enzyme, resulting in the build-up of both homocysteine and methionine. Symptoms usually do not appear until a few months or years after birth. Some babies can develop problems with their eyes, including severe short-sightedness and dislocation of the lens, which may cause blurred vision. Without early treatment, babies can develop brain damage, including learning difficulties, and other complications can develop such as bone and joint problems, and blood clots or strokes. In a small portion of babies, the level of homocysteine can be controlled by giving pyridoxine (vitamin B6). A special low-protein diet with the aim to reduce the intake of methionine and the build-up of homocysteine, which lead to brain damage.

Key points

- Newborn screening tests enable early detection of a range of conditional conditions.
- Early detection ensures early medical input to not only treat the condition, but prevent complications.
- Parents need to be provided with all the facts to make an informed choice to have their baby screened.

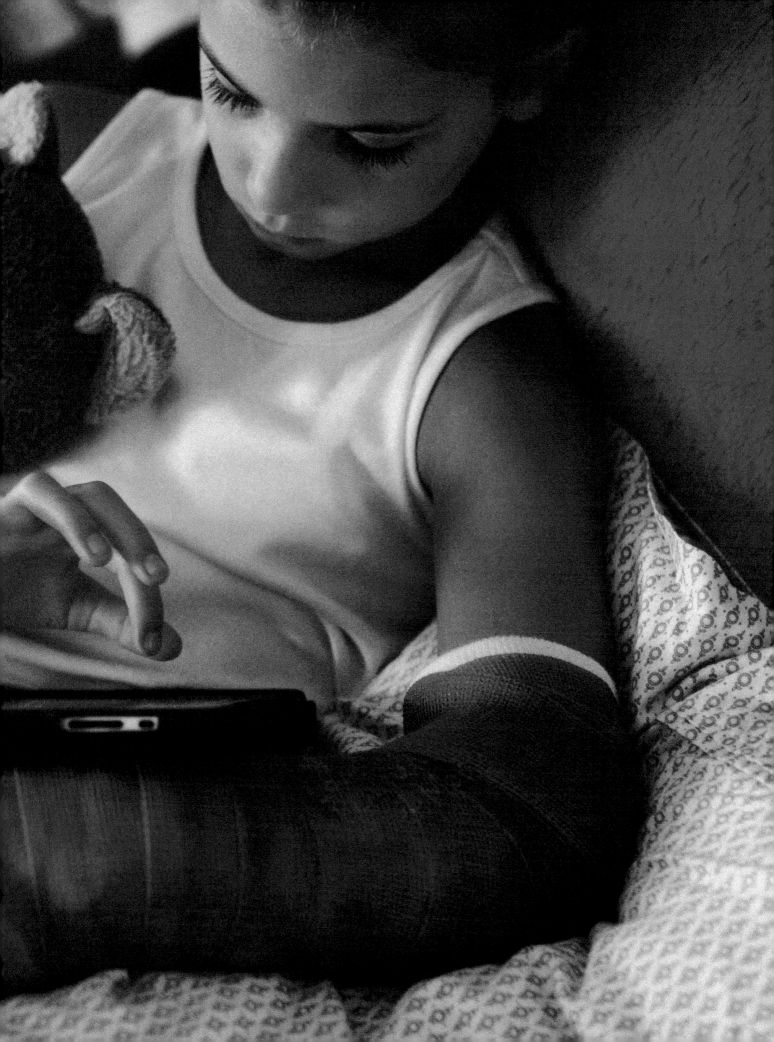

47 The premature baby

Figure 47.1 Late premature baby.

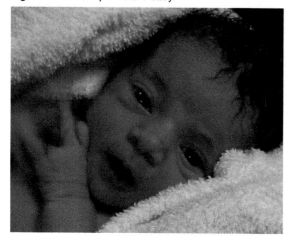

Figure 47.3 Very premature baby.

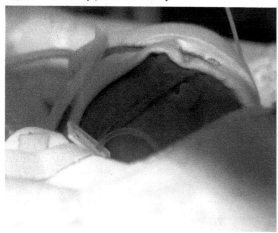

Figure 47.5 Premature baby with feeding tube.

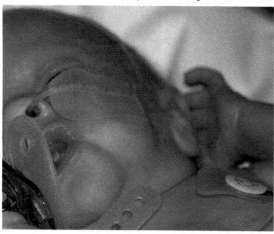

Figure 47.2 Moderately premature baby.

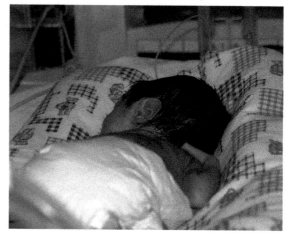

Figure 47.4 Premature baby in incubator.

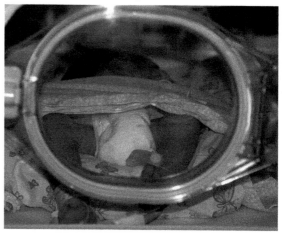

Figure 47.6 Premature twins receiving skin-to-skin contact. *Source:* DFID – UK Department for International Development/ Wikimedia Commons / CC BY 2.0.

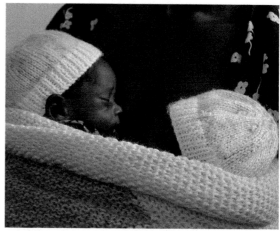

Children and Young People's Nursing at a Glance, Second Edition. Edited by Elizabeth Gormley-Fleming and Sheila Roberts.
© 2023 John Wiley & Sons Ltd. Published 2023 by John Wiley & Sons Ltd.

Premature birth

Premature birth is defined as delivery at less than 37 completed weeks' gestation. There are different degrees of prematurity, namely late premature (32–37 weeks), moderately premature (28–32 weeks), and very premature (less than 28 weeks). Babies born in the first of these groups (Figure 47.1) generally do not present significant problems and may be cared for within the special care or transitional care unit for relatively short time periods before discharge. Babies in the latter two groups (Figures 47.2 and 47.3), however, are more likely to have greater care needs and will require admission to a neonatal unit depending on the presenting condition(s) and severity. These babies will remain on the unit for a longer period, for respiratory support, thermal care (Figure 47.4), and nasogastric/orogastric feeding (Figure 47.5), until they are sufficiently mature and stable to be discharged home.

Causes of prematurity

The causes of early onset of labour and premature delivery are uncertain and often unexplained, probably due to a combination of maternal and foetal risk factors rather than one single cause. Risk factors include the following, some of which can be identified antenatally:

• Maternal conditions or illness such as pre-eclampsia, placental abruption, antepartum haemorrhage, infection, diabetes, hypertension.
• Premature prolonged rupture of membranes (P-PROM).
• Maternal alcohol or substance abuse.
• Multiple pregnancies (Figure 47.6) and polyhydramnios.
• Poor obstetric history, including cervical incompetence.

Assessing gestational age

Antenatally, gestation and estimated date of delivery (EDD) are usually predicted from the date of the last menstrual period, if the dates are known, early ultrasound scan measurements, and uterine growth. If information is unknown about a baby on admission, tools exist to assess gestational age – for example, the Dubowitz tool and Ballard's tool both assesses babies on a range of criteria to determine gestational age through neuromuscular and physical assessment. Overall, these scoring systems require that there is a careful examination of the baby, looking at characteristics of appearance, reflexes, and behaviour, which provide an indication of whether the baby is just small or premature.

Characteristics of the premature baby

Specific key features on assessment indicate that babies are immature and form an essential part of the subjective assessment at birth and/or on admission to transitional or special care:

• The head is large in proportion to the body.
• The face is small with a pointed chin and, if very immature, the eyelids may be fused.
• Cranial sutures and fontanelles are widely spaced, and the skull bones are soft.
• Due to lack of subcutaneous fat, the skin is pinkish/red, and surface veins are prominent.
• The body is covered with soft downy (lanugo) hair in the mid-trimester.
• Limbs are thin, extended, and muscle tone is underdeveloped.
• The chest is small, narrow, and the abdomen large.
• Genitalia are not fully developed, the labia majora do not cover the labia minora (female), and the testes may not have descended (male).
• Suck and swallow reflexes are uncoordinated.

Problems of the preterm baby

In the first weeks, short-term complications of premature birth may arise relating to the immature body systems:

• *Respiratory*: a premature baby will have an immature respiratory system that lacks surfactant, a substance that allows the lungs to expand. Consequently, the baby may develop respiratory distress syndrome and, later, a chronic lung disorder known as bronchopulmonary dysplasia.
• *Cardiac*: Common cardiac problems in prematurity are patent ductus arteriosus (PDA) and low blood pressure (hypotension). PDA is a persistent opening between the aorta and pulmonary artery and often closes on its own; however, if left untreated, it can lead to a heart murmur, heart failure, and respiratory distress.
• *Neurological*: The earlier a baby is born, the greater the risk of bleeding in the brain, known as an intraventricular haemorrhage. Most haemorrhages are mild and resolve with little short-term impact, but some babies may have significant bleeding that causes permanent brain injury.
• *Thermoregulation*: Premature babies can lose body heat rapidly, have limited stored body fat, and cannot generate enough heat. A low core body temperature (hypothermia) can result, leading to breathing problems and low blood sugar levels.
• *Gastrointestinal*: Premature babies are more likely to have immature gastrointestinal systems, resulting in complications such as necrotizing enterocolitis (NEC), a serious condition in which the bowel wall becomes inflamed, particularly after they start feeding. Those who receive only breast milk have a much lower risk of NEC.
• *Blood*: Premature babies are at risk of anaemia and newborn jaundice. The drop in red blood cell count during the first months of life is greater in premature babies compared to term. Similarly, jaundice is more common in preterm babies due to liver immaturity, reduced red blood cell lifespan, and slow establishment of feeding.
• *Metabolism*: Low blood sugar (hypoglycaemia) can occur due to reduced stored glucose (glycogen) and greater difficulty converting glycogen into active forms of glucose.
• *Immunity*: An underdeveloped immune system can lead to a higher risk of infection and, in the worst instance, sepsis.

In the longer term, premature babies have an increased risk of sudden infant death syndrome (SIDS), motor deficits and poorer cognitive skills, neurological abnormalities, long-term oxygen requirement, visual and/or hearing loss, cerebral palsy, and chronic lung disease. However, with recent advances in neonatal care, babies born prematurely now have a much greater chance of intact survival than previously. For those babies born at extremes of prematurity who are discharged from hospital, the risk of some degree of long-term morbidity needs to be assessed and considered in any follow-up, relating to outcomes for the baby and family. Finally, the admission of a premature baby to the neonatal unit poses a significant stressor to parents. Many preterm babies are in the hospital for several weeks or months until they are ready to be discharged home. Ultimately, the aim would be to prevent preterm birth to avert this situation in the first place. Interventions to prevent preterm onset of labour are the subject of ongoing research.

Key points

• The causes of early onset of labour and premature delivery are uncertain and often unexplained.
• Premature birth is defined as delivery at less than 37 completed weeks' gestation.
• Being born prematurely may lead to a range of potential problems relating to physical immaturity and significant stress to parents.

48 Neonatal transport

Figure 48.1 Transfer of baby out of incubator. *Source:* Maria mono / Flickr.

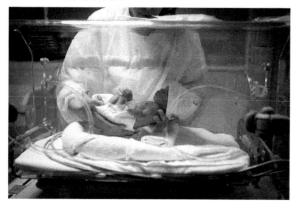

Figure 48.3 Transport incubator (2). *Source:* Connect NW Neonatal Transport Team.

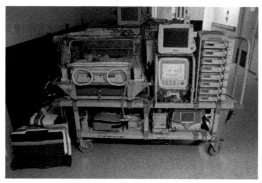

Figure 48.5 Transfer of baby and transport incubator into the ambulance. *Source:* With permission from Patrick Turton, Lead Nurse for Neonatal Transport Service at University Hospitals Bristol and Weston NHS Foundation Trust.

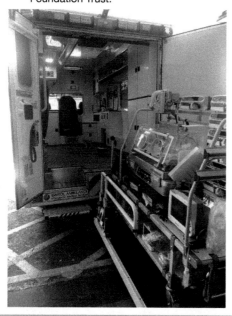

Figure 48.2 Transport incubator (1). *Source:* Philipp Lensing / Wikimedia Commons / CC SA 1.0.

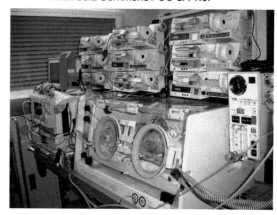

Figure 48.4 Transport incubator (3). *Source:* What's the rush / Flickr.

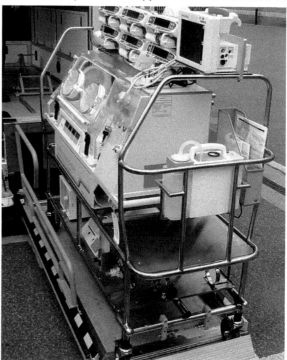

Figure 48.6 Ambulance in transit. *Source:* Manhattan Research Inc. / Wikimedia Commons / CC BY 2.0.

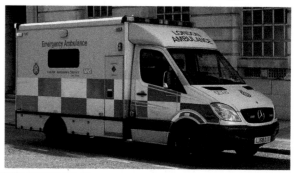

Critically ill babies are a highly vulnerable and unique population who for optimal outcomes require specialized teams for stabilization and transport. There are many reasons why a neonate may need to be transferred from one unit, department, or hospital to another. They may be extremely preterm, require surgical assessment, or may need further management and/or specialized intervention that cannot be offered in the home unit. Whatever the reason, transfers require careful preparation and planning in order to minimize any potential risks to the baby and team involved.

Transporting a sick neonate can be a complex procedure, involving preparing the neonate for movement from their static incubator (Figure 48.1) into a portable transport incubator (Figures 48.2–48.4), and loading of the equipment into a vehicle for transfer such as an ambulance (Figures 48.5 and 48.6), helicopter or fixed-wing plane.

The neonatal transport processes

The logistic and clinical complexities of all transfers will vary. Moreover, organization and management involve many phases, which include:

- *Referral* or request for transfer by the referring unit.
- *Activation* of the transferring team.
- *Handover* of baby details and *communication*.
- *Stabilization* and *preparation* for transfer.
- *Journey* and subsequent *arrival* at receiving unit.
- *Handover* of baby details.
- *Return* of transferring team to base.

First, assessment of the baby and the relevant clinical history ascertains the need to be transferred for further management. Considerations are whether transfer is appropriate for the baby, if they are too unstable for transfer, and, if so, whether a specialist can review the baby in the referral unit. Following a decision to transfer, the referral is made to the neonatal transfer service and activation of the transfer process commences.

Handover and communication are essential. The clinician or advanced neonatal nurse practitioner following the decision to transfer the neonate will liaise with the transport service and the receiving unit. A succinct summary of the problem should be relayed to the transport team, and again later to the receiving unit. This will enable a decision to be made on the most appropriate mode of transport and receiving unit. The information that should be relayed to the transport team is as follows:

- Description of the problem: history, clinical condition, vital signs, laboratory results, interventions, including what has been done or is needed and what the effect has been. This information will aid in diagnosis and future management.
- What further management is needed? This will facilitate appropriate management during transport and on arrival at the receiving unit.

A transport lead is delegated to provide advice prior to and during transport and to delegate tasks. At all stages of the transport, communication is crucial, relating to:

- *Parents*: update on their baby's condition, reasons for transfer, and information about the receiving unit such as location and visiting.
- *Colleagues*: concise information throughout the transfer relayed among the referral unit, transport team, and receiving unit.
- *Documentation*: pre-transport, during transport, and on arrival at the receiving unit, including vital signs, all interventions, effects, and changes in management.
- *Identification* and documentation of problems at each stage of the transfer.

Stabilization and preparation before transfer require rapid assessment and management of life-threatening problems (ABC):

- *Airway*: must be patent and stable throughout the transfer.
- *Breathing*: it may be necessary to intubate prior to transfer.
- *Circulation*: vascular access secured and dependent on severity of baby's condition.

Equipment checks prior to departure may include a pre-departure checklist, a final review of ABC, selection of mode of transport as the most appropriate for the baby and circumstances, and the safety of the baby and staff. During the actual journey, environmental influences such as fluctuations in temperature, noise, movement, vibration, G forces, and barometric pressure can potentially be areas of stress, pain, and discomfort to the neonate. Continued communication and documentation should occur during the journey and on arrival at the receiving unit, including another detailed handover to appropriate staff, before the transfer team returns to base.

Teamwork

Advances in management within neonatal care have necessitated the development of specialized teams of clinicians and nurses to manage neonatal transfers safely and in a timely manner. The nature of working in a small team means that there can be an overlap of the roles of the team members. Common tasks of transferring monitoring, infusions, documentation, checking and troubleshooting equipment, and restocking equipment can be undertaken by all team members. However, there needs to be a clear understanding about the allocation and distribution of roles that considers the varying levels of skill and experience of the team members.

Equipment

Delivering a neonatal transport service means having the ability to provide a mobile intensive care unit. The transport incubator is housed on a trolley with attachments for the associated equipment. While there are commonalities (Figures 48.2–48.4) across various services, the configuration of each system is slightly different, and familiarity with one's own system is essential. In addition, designing and purchasing a transport incubator must be undertaken with consideration to agreed standards. Whichever system is used, appropriate fixation of equipment to the trolley, and of the trolley to the ambulance, is critical in maintaining baby and team safety inside the ambulance. It is also preferable to have an ambulance specifically designed to transfer babies (Figure 48.5), so that the team will be aware of the layout of their vehicle and the specific safety and manual handling constraints. The team should also be familiar with the storage of their equipment and supplies so that they can respond quickly and efficiently should they need to. It is also important to be aware of the loading mechanisms of the vehicles, as well as the electrical and gas supplies, to help in troubleshooting and problem-solving if required. A range of equipment and disposables, to deal with any potential interventions, also need to be available. Safety is a priority throughout all stages of the transport process and is crucial for an effective and risk-free transfer. Clear and ongoing communication with the baby's parents is paramount too.

Key points

- Transporting a sick neonate can be a complex procedure.
- Continued assessment, communication and safety considerations should occur through all stages of the transport process.
- Parents should receive updates on their baby's condition at all stages of the transport, where possible.

49 Jaundice and hyperbilirubinaemia

Figure 49.1 Haemoglobin and bilirubin metabolism. *Source:* Johndheathcote / Wikimedia Commons / CC BY-SA 3.0.

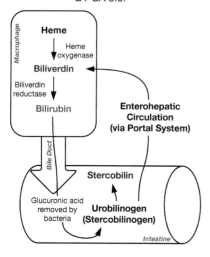

Figure 49.2 An incubator where phototherapy is in progress.

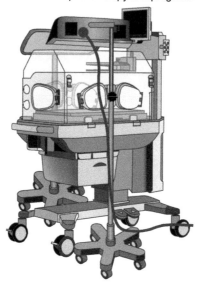

Figure 49.3 A baby on a phototherapy mattress. *Source:* Davidlevilindsay / Flickr / CC BY-SA 2.0.

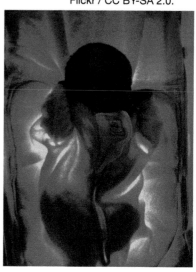

Figure 49.4 Phototherapy lights (1). *Source:* SilentObserver / Flickr / CC BY 2.0.

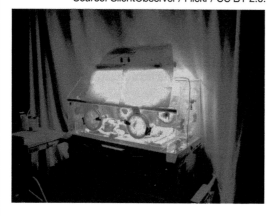

Figure 49.5 Phototherapy lights (2).

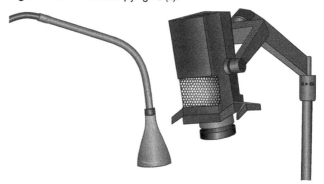

Figure 49.6 A baby receiving phototherapy with eye shields.

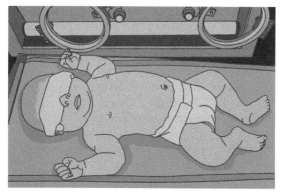

Figure 49.7 Treatment threshold graph.

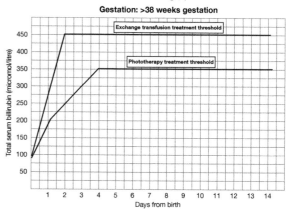

Children and Young People's Nursing at a Glance, Second Edition. Edited by Elizabeth Gormley-Fleming and Sheila Roberts.
© 2023 John Wiley & Sons Ltd. Published 2023 by John Wiley & Sons Ltd.

Physiology of bilirubin

All babies have high haemoglobin levels at birth and in the early days their foetal red blood cells are haemolysed. This results in increased levels of bilirubin in the plasma, formed from the iron-containing heme molecule (Figure 49.1). This is unconjugated bilirubin, which is fat soluble and cannot be excreted by the body, so it attaches itself to albumin-binding sites and travels to the liver. If the bilirubin becomes detached, it circulates as free unconjugated bilirubin and can cross the blood–brain barrier, resulting in encephalopathy or brain damage, known as 'kernicterus'. Once it reaches the liver the unconjugated bilirubin is acted on by the liver enzymes glucuroneryl transferase and glucuronic acid. Oxygen and glucose are required for this to happen. Once conjugated, the bilirubin leaves the liver as water-soluble bilirubin, which can now be excreted by the body. Approximately 80% of this bilirubin travels down the common bile duct to the small intestine, where it is excreted in the stools as stercobilinogen. Approximately 15% enters the bloodstream and travels to the gut and kidneys, where it is excreted as urobilinogen; the remainder continues to circulate in the enterohepatic circulation.

Hyperbilirubinaemia

Hyperbilirubinaemia, also known as jaundice, is an excess of bilirubin in the blood, that results in serum bilirubin (SBR) levels higher than 300 pmmol/L in term babies and 200 pmmol/L in preterm babies. Babies become jaundiced when plasma bilirubin exceeds the albumin-binding sites or the ability of the liver to conjugate and excrete bilirubin from the body by normal means. Babies appear yellow, particularly the skin, sclera of eyes, and mucous membranes of the mouth, as bilirubin is deposited in the tissues.

Causes

- *Physiological*: Normal breakdown of red blood cells resulting in high levels of unconjugated bilirubin in the first 3–4 days of life; usually resolves within 7–10 days.
- *Pathological*: may appear within the first 24–48 hours of life and indicates ongoing haemolysis. Causes include rhesus or ABO incompatibility, or congenital or acquired sepsis.
- *Prolonged*: Jaundice that persists for longer than two weeks. This is caused by metabolic conditions such as galactosaemia or hypothyroidism, infections such as urinary tract infections, or breast-milk jaundice.
- *Obstructive*: This is caused by an obstruction of the common bile duct. Conjugated bilirubin cannot travel to the gut for excretion and so builds up in the liver and there will be a high direct bilirubin level (>20% of total SBR level), the baby's stools will be pale in colour, they will appear very jaundiced, may be sleepy, and do not feed well. Any baby who remains jaundiced for >2 weeks after birth should have a repeat SBR level checked as well as liver function tests to exclude biliary atresia, which is a life-threatening condition.

Assessment of jaundice

The mother's history should be checked for details of previous pregnancies, blood group and rhesus factor status, medications, labour/delivery, and method of feeding. The baby's condition since birth is also observed, including skin colour and the sclera of the eyes and mucous membranes; all may appear yellow. The baby's alertness is important, as very jaundiced babies tend to be sleepy and difficult to feed. The colour of stools and urine is also checked; pale or grey stools may be a result of biliary atresia. Urine may be a little darker than normal. A transcutaneous bilirubin meter can be used in the first instance in babies born at more than 35 weeks' gestation after the first 24 hours of life. If the result is >250 μmmol/L,

in younger gestations and in the first 24 hours, a blood sample is required for SBR measurement. For SBR levels, an indirect (unconjugated) + direct (conjugated) level can be requested. Anaemia and/or sepsis should be ruled out. Babies with prolonged jaundice should also have fractioned SBR levels checked as well as liver function tests to rule out biliary atresia.

Management of jaundice

Depending on the cause, treatment usually takes place on a neonatal unit (Figure 49.2) or in transitional care. Management may include additional feeding for physiological jaundice, phototherapy (Figures 49.3–49.6), albumin transfusions, or exchange transfusions for the more serious cases. In all cases of jaundice, the SBR levels must be monitored very closely, with results being plotted on a graph (Figure 49.7) to indicate the rate of increase; the graph also provides indicators to how the condition should be managed.

Phototherapy

Phototherapy is the use of light in the blue-green spectrum, to break down and begin the process of treating unconjugated bilirubin in the plasma, reducing the workload of the immature liver. The lights are directed onto the naked baby's skin in an effort to conjugate the bilirubin in the subcutaneous tissues. Phototherapy can be administered via biliblankets, mattresses (Figure 49.3), overhead lamps (Figures 49.2, 49.4 and 49.5), or spotlights, with conventional or fibreoptic light. Overhead lamps are the more common form used and consist of a specific spectrum of light; blue light, for example, is known to be effective at reducing SBR levels. The lamp should be the recommended distance from the baby and can be used over incubators or cots.

Care of a baby having phototherapy

The baby should be nursed naked, and enteral feeds and/or fluids should be calculated to ensure adequate fluid and protein intake. There is no indication for increasing intravenous fluids for phototherapy treatment. Eyes should be covered while under phototherapy to prevent retinal damage (Figure 49.6). Temperature should be recorded regularly to prevent hypothermia as the baby is nursed naked. Skin rashes can occur due to photosensitivity – no treatment is necessary and nothing should be applied to the skin during phototherapy. The nappy area should be checked for excoriation, as stools containing bile salts can burn the skin, resulting in red, sore areas that require specialized treatment. It is important to ensure that the baby has 'time out' of phototherapy for feeding as and when appropriate, when the eye pads are removed and physical contact with the parents is established. Babies may be more unsettled in an incubator with eye pads on – the use of soft rolls around the baby may be useful when positioning supine. It may be difficult to observe cyanosis when babies are nursed under blue lights, so oxygen saturation monitors may be necessary for clinically unstable babies. Breastfeeding may be challenging because of the need to remove the baby from underneath the lights, but biliblankets, if available, can be used during feeds; breast-feeding should always be encouraged if possible and the baby's condition allows.

Key points

- Hyperbilirubinaemia may be due to physiological, pathological, prolonged, or obstructive causes.
- All babies with jaundice will need close clinical assessment and regular serum bilirubin level checks to guide management.
- Breastfeeding should be encouraged when treating a baby receiving phototherapy.

50 Congenital heart disease

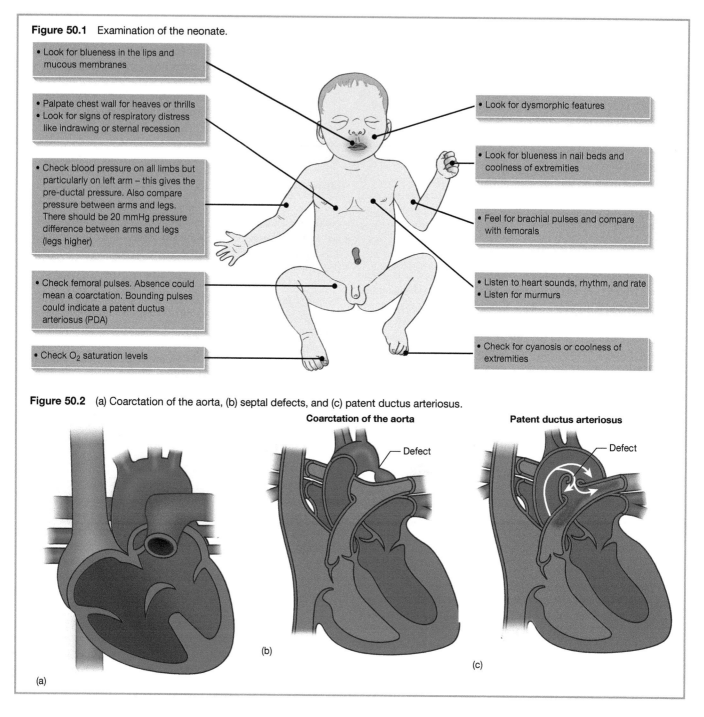

Figure 50.1 Examination of the neonate.

- Look for blueness in the lips and mucous membranes

- Palpate chest wall for heaves or thrills
- Look for signs of respiratory distress like indrawing or sternal recession

- Check blood pressure on all limbs but particularly on left arm – this gives the pre-ductal pressure. Also compare pressure between arms and legs. There should be 20 mmHg pressure difference between arms and legs (legs higher)

- Check femoral pulses. Absence could mean a coarctation. Bounding pulses could indicate a patent ductus arteriosus (PDA)

- Check O₂ saturation levels

- Look for dysmorphic features

- Look for blueness in nail beds and coolness of extremities

- Feel for brachial pulses and compare with femorals

- Listen to heart sounds, rhythm, and rate
- Listen for murmurs

- Check for cyanosis or coolness of extremities

Figure 50.2 (a) Coarctation of the aorta, (b) septal defects, and (c) patent ductus arteriosus.

Coarctation of the aorta

Patent ductus arteriosus

Defect

Defect

(a)

(b)

(c)

Pathophysiology

The embryonic cardiovascular system is functional by 21 days. Cardiac anomalies can be congenital or acquired, but this system is highly susceptible to abnormalities when exposed to teratogens in early pregnancy. Congenital heart disease (CHD) affects about 1 in 145 babies, but half of these will not require treatment; others will be treated with medication and/or surgery. Congenital heart defects are usually described as cyanotic or acyanotic:

- *Acyanotic*: Left-to-right shunting will not cause cyanosis, because blood flows from the systemic to the pulmonary system.
- *Cyanotic*: Right-to-left shunting results in blood flowing from the right side of the circulation to the systemic circulation

Children and Young People's Nursing at a Glance, Second Edition. Edited by Elizabeth Gormley-Fleming and Sheila Roberts.
© 2023 John Wiley & Sons Ltd. Published 2023 by John Wiley & Sons Ltd.

(i.e. deoxygenated blood mixes with oxygenated blood causing cyanosis, even when nursed in 100% oxygen).

Diagnosis

Taking a detailed history is vital: family history (other siblings); prenatal history, any maternal illnesses, medications, complications in pregnancy, labour, or delivery; and the baby's condition since birth in relation to feeding, observations, weight gain, and general health.

Cardiac problems can present in four ways (Figure 50.1): colour change (cyanosis), respiratory distress, collapse, or the baby may be asymptomatic.

• *Genetic syndromes*: Babies with trisomy 21 (Down's syndrome) have a higher risk of multiple cardiac defects. Look for unusual features.

• *Colour*: Central cyanosis – blue lips, mucous membranes, and nail beds. If colour improves with oxygen, the condition is more likely to be respiratory. Heart failure usually results in increasing pallor as the blood pressure falls and peripheries become cold.

• *Respiration*: Respiratory rate increases, as does effort. Flared nostrils, subcostal and intracostal retractions, grunting, and/or wheezing sounds.

• *Capillary refill time* (CRT): CRT of >3 s can be indicative of poor peripheral circulation. Babies may look mottled and pale.

• *Auscultation*: Listen for 'lub-dub' heart sounds, rhythm, and regularity. Listen for murmurs, which indicate turbulence of the blood at some juncture in the heart. They can be classified according to their location, intensity, quality, and timing (systolic or diastolic).

• *Palpation*: Pulses should be checked for presence and strength (brachial and femoral). Absence of femoral pulses may be indicative of coarctation of aorta or left ventricular outflow conditions. The chest wall should be palpated for precordial activity (heaves and thrills), which indicates reduced pulmonary or aortic outflow.

• *Blood pressure readings*: Four-limb blood pressure readings can highlight differing pressures between upper and lower limbs. A systolic difference of 15–20 mmHg between upper and lower limbs is indicative of coarctation of the aorta (pressure in legs should be higher).

• *Oxygen saturation levels*: O_2 saturation readings should be >95%, so readings <90% indicate either cardiac or respiratory illness.

• *Chest X-ray*: Identifies respiratory disease or enlarged heart size.

• *Electrocardiogram* (ECG): Will assess atrial and ventricular function and should be interpreted by an appropriately skilled professional.

• *Echocardiogram*: Provides information on cardiac structures, pressures and gradients within the heart, and overall function.

• *Cardiac catheterization*: An invasive procedure that provides diagnostic or therapeutic treatment such as balloon septostomy.

Common conditions

There are over 30 types of CHD. Listed here are some of the more common cardiac conditions:

Patent ductus arteriosus

Before birth, this foetal shunt (ductus arteriosus) enables blood to bypass the lungs as the foetus obtains its oxygen through the placenta. The ductus normally closes soon after birth, allowing blood to travel to the lungs and pick up oxygen. In patent ductus arteriosus (Figure 50.2c) it remains open, resulting in potential respiratory and cardiac problems for the baby (most frequently in premature babies). Treatment with ibuprofen or indometacin during the early days of life often closes the ductus; failing that, surgery may be required.

Septal defects

A hole in the separating central wall (septum) between the two atria or the two ventricles causes blood to circulate improperly, so the heart has to work harder. Atrial or ventricular septal defects (Figure 50.2a) can be repaired by sewing or patching the hole.

Coarctation of the aorta

A narrowing of the aorta (Figure 50.2b), usually occurring in the descending section, results in a reduced flow of blood to the lower parts of the body. Femoral pulses may be absent. A surgeon resects the narrowed section, replacing it with manmade material or part of a grafted blood vessel. The narrowed section can sometimes be widened by inflating a balloon on the tip of a catheter inserted through an artery.

Management of cardiac disease

The infant should be nursed in a quiet, comfortable environment with reduced stimuli or stress. Crying increases O_2 requirements. Be aware of the following:

• *Continuous monitoring* is required of colour, heart rate, respiratory rate, blood pressure, oxygen saturations, TCO_2 and CO_2 levels, as well as fluid intake and output.

• *Blood gas analysis*, with frequency depending on the baby's ongoing condition. Oxygen requirements alter according to results.

• *Daily blood tests* including full blood picture (FBP), urea and electrolytes (U&E), and any other necessary investigations such as drug levels.

• *Temperature regulation* – nurse in a neutral thermal environment. Maintain normal temperature, minimizing use of oxygen and calories.

• *Calculation of intravenous fluids, feeds, and nutrients* to ensure growth, normal U&E levels, avoiding metabolic disturbances. Monitor blood glucose.

• *Feeding* – deliver feeds (preferably breast milk) in a way that minimizes effort and calorie consumption. Tube feeds may be necessary.

• *Administration of medications* must be timely, with observation for effects and adverse effects recorded, particularly digitalis and inotropes.

• *Minimizing the risk of infection* is vital because of the risk of sepsis in this vulnerable group. Prevention of infection protocols must be adhered to.

• *Family support* is vital as cardiac conditions will result in anxiety for all concerned. Information and good communication are essential.

Follow-up and prognosis

Due to advances in heart surgery, 85% of children with CHD will survive into adulthood. All babies and young children will be reviewed by the surgeon who carried out their surgery or the cardiologist who will manage their condition into childhood or adulthood.

Key points

• Diagnosis of CHD may be *in utero*, at birth, or within early infancy.
• The associated symptoms of CHD are colour change, respiratory distress, sudden collapse, or the baby may be asymptomatic
• Survival rates post cardiac surgery are very high.

51 Neonatal resuscitation

Figure 51.1 Newborn life support (NLS) algorithm. *Source:* Adapted from UK Resuscitation Council (2021) NLS guidance.

Preparation:

- Have you introduced yourself to the parents?
- Checked obstetric notes?
- Washed hands?
- Is equipment working?
- A warm flat surface; good lighting; clock?

Preterm <32 weeks:

- **Place undried in plastic wrap + radiant heat**
- Inspired oxygen (28 – 31 weeks = 21 – 30% and <28 weeks = 30%)
- If giving inflations, start with 25 cm H_2O

Acceptable pre-ductal SpO$_2$:

2 min – 65%
5 min – 85%
10 min – 90%

Key Points:

- At all times ask, '**Is help needed?**'
- Maintain temperature throughout the event
- Titrate oxygen to achieve target saturations throughout the event

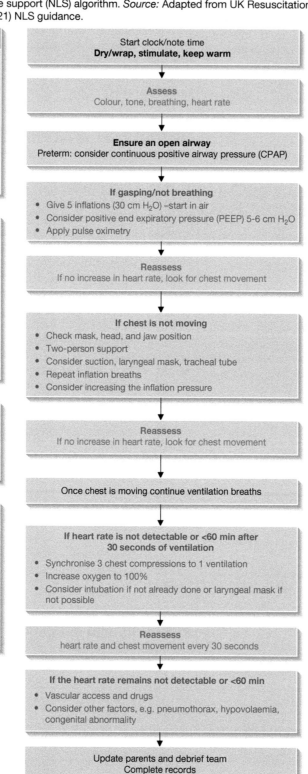

Start clock/note time
Dry/wrap, stimulate, keep warm

Assess
Colour, tone, breathing, heart rate

Ensure an open airway
Preterm: consider continuous positive airway pressure (CPAP)

If gasping/not breathing
- Give 5 inflations (30 cm H_2O) –start in air
- Consider positive end expiratory pressure (PEEP) 5-6 cm H_2O
- Apply pulse oximetry

Reassess
If no increase in heart rate, look for chest movement

If chest is not moving
- Check mask, head, and jaw position
- Two-person support
- Consider suction, laryngeal mask, tracheal tube
- Repeat inflation breaths
- Consider increasing the inflation pressure

Reassess
If no increase in heart rate, look for chest movement

Once chest is moving continue ventilation breaths

If heart rate is not detectable or <60 min after 30 seconds of ventilation
- Synchronise 3 chest compressions to 1 ventilation
- Increase oxygen to 100%
- Consider intubation if not already done or laryngeal mask if not possible

Reassess
heart rate and chest movement every 30 seconds

If the heart rate remains not detectable or <60 min
- Vascular access and drugs
- Consider other factors, e.g. pneumothorax, hypovolaemia, congenital abnormality

Update parents and debrief team
Complete records

Figure 51.2 Neutral position.

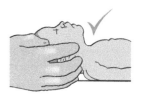

Head is placed in a neutral position

Figure 51.3 Face mask position.

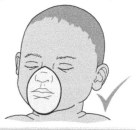

Covers mouth, nose, and chin but not eyes

Figure 51.4 Landmarks for chest compression.

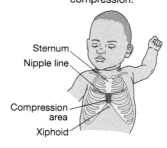

Sternum
Nipple line

Compression area
Xiphoid

Resuscitation in newborn babies, and within the neonatal unit if required after delivery, is undertaken using the UK Resuscitation Council 2021 guidelines. Any resuscitation should follow a structured approach using an algorithm (Figure 51.1). The well-known ABCDE (Airway – Breathing – Circulation – Drugs/Disability – Environment/Equipment) approach can be adapted and applied to neonatal resuscitation as follows:

Airway

- Check the airway is patent (clear).
- Obstruction is usually caused by a flexed head or tongue position rather than blood, mucous plugs, or secretions. Suction only if needed and under direct vision.
- Place the baby's head in a neutral position (Figure 51.2). Avoid overextension or flexing the baby's head.
- If the baby is floppy, a haw thrust may be needed to bring the tongue forward.
- To perform a jaw thrust, place one or two fingers under each side of the jaw and push the jaw forwards.
- Inserting a laryngeal mask under direct vision (laryngoscope) in the anatomically correct position will assist in keeping the airway patent. To select the correct size of laryngeal mask, use the formula for LMA size (patient weight [kg]/5) × 0.5. For example, LMA size 1 = <5 kg.

Breathing

- Check for regular, bilaterally even chest movements.
- If breathing or chest movement is absent, inflation breaths will be needed to aerate the lungs.
- Using a correctly fitted mask (Figure 51.3) and T-piece or mask and bag, give five inflation breaths of two to three seconds each (use appropriate cm H_2O pressure) and reassess the baby's response (check for spontaneous breathing).
- If there is no response, recheck the head and airway position and for any obstructions.

Circulation

- Check for a strong pulse, warm peripheries, and a 'pink' skin colour.
- If the heart rate remains slow and fails to increase with effective aeration of the lungs, commence chest compressions.
- The aim is to move oxygenated blood from the pulmonary veins to the coronary arteries.
- Chest compressions will only be useful if the lungs have been aerated first.
- Chest compression technique: place two thumbs or fingers on the baby's chest using correct landmarks for positioning (Figure 51.4). Then apply pressure to the lower third of the sternum. Avoid the xiphoid. Depress to reduce the anteroposterior diameter of the chest by one-third with no bounce. The thumb technique is more effective than the two-finger technique, but is useful if you are alone or have small hands. Give three compressions to one breath. Allow the chest to recoil between compressions to allow blood to fill the heart. With good-quality compressions, the heart will respond quickly. Stop and recheck the heart rate after every 30 seconds. When heart rate rises (>60 bpm) stop chest compressions. Monitor the baby's progress and if the heart remains slow or undetectable, then escalate to a senior member and do not stop resuscitation.

Drugs/disability

- On rare occasions, the baby may not demonstrate the expected response to the ABC parts of the algorithm; therefore, it is necessary to consider 'D'.

- If effective ventilation and good-quality cardiac compressions have been delivered yet cardiac output remains poor or absent, then drugs may be needed to reverse intracardiac acidosis. In such circumstances the prognosis is generally poor.
- Insertion of an umbilical venous catheter provides a quick and effective means to administer drugs close to the heart.
- Sodium bicarbonate 4.2%: dose 2–4 mL/kg.
- Adrenaline 1 : 10 000: dose 0.2 mL/kg.
- Dextrose 10%: dose 2.5 mL/kg.
- In some situations, a neurological assessment is required in the neonatal period. Check for AVPU (Alert – Voice – Pain – Unresponsive) response. If head trauma is suspected in older neonates, the paediatric version of the Glasgow Coma Score (GCS) may be undertaken.

Environment/equipment

- A baby needing support in transition to extrauterine life may be transferred to a neonatal unit. This may include premature babies or term babies that have encountered a problem during the perinatal period and labour (e.g. hypoxia, infection).
- Use local policy for admissions criteria.
- A Resuscitaire® (Drager, Hemel Hempstead, UK) with gas supply, pressure relief valve, and T-piece circuit. If a Resuscitaire is not available, you will need a warm, flat surface with good lighting and a clock or watch to record the timing of events.
- Suction apparatus – Yanker sucker, catheter sizes 12–14 French.
- Laryngeal mask.
- Stethoscope – neonatal/paediatric.
- Saturation probe and oximeter.
- Warm towels and wraps.
- Round, soft silicone face masks. The correct mask size should cover the mouth, nose, and chin. Sizes are 00, 0/1, 2.
- Mask ventilation via T-piece. Connect to air using a pressure-limited circuit. Oxygen is rarely required but, if given, use a blender and monitor the baby's response using pulse oximetry. Avoid oxygen saturation >95% in very premature babies due to the risk of retinal damage at low gestations.
- Self-inflating bags are useful if piped gas is not available. It is only on rare occasions that babies need endotracheal intubation.

Other important points

- Direct information should be given primarily to the parents of the baby. Once the baby responds and spontaneously maintains respiratory and cardiac output, the baby should be handed to the parents.
- To communicate structured, clear, and factual information in a resuscitation event, use the SBAR (Situation – Background – Assessment – Recommendation) approach.
- All resuscitation events must be recorded in the notes. Avoid subjective statements and include what time you were called and when you arrived; the baby's tone, breathing, heart rate; action taken and the baby's response; arterial/venous cord blood pH, base excess; who participated in the resuscitation and what was said to the parents.

Key points

- Any resuscitation should follow a structured approach using an algorithm and following current guidelines.
- Equipment must be available, and staff must be competent in its use.
- Communication with parents is vital and details of what was said should be documented.

52 Incubator/Overhead heater care

Figure 52.1 Overhead heater.

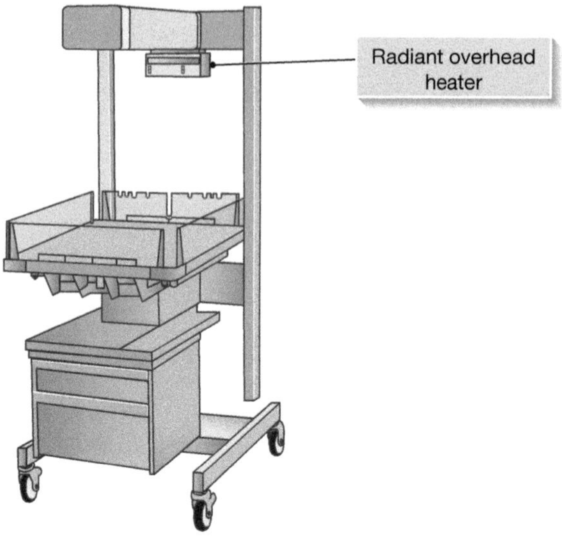

Radiant overhead heater

Figure 52.2 Resuscitaire®.

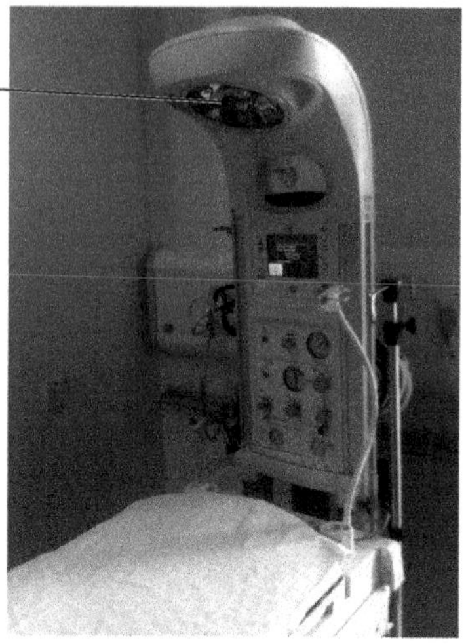

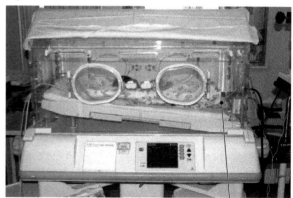

Figure 52.3 Incubator 1.

Perspex sides

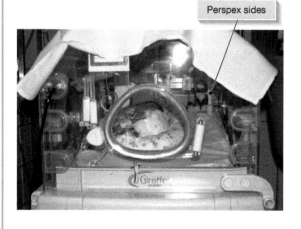

Figure 52.4 Incubator 2.

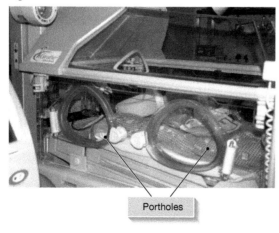

Double-panelled walls

Figure 52.5 Incubator 3.

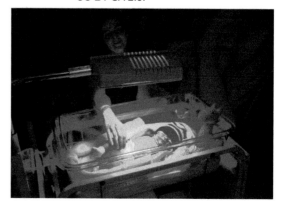

Portholes

Figure 52.6 Open bassinette. Treehouse1977 / Flickr / CC BY-SA 2.0.

Children and Young People's Nursing at a Glance, Second Edition. Edited by Elizabeth Gormley-Fleming and Sheila Roberts.

Heat balance

The goal in controlling a baby's thermal environment is to minimize the energy and oxygen expenditure in order to maintain a normal central body temperature and prevent hypothermia, ensuring that cardiac output is maintained and thermal stress is eliminated. Due to key physiological differences between neonates and older children and adults, babies rely on non-shivering chemical thermogenesis to produce heat. Oxygen and glucose are consumed during this process; therefore, the baby may become hypoxaemic or hypoglycaemic when faced with added thermal stress. Measures to keep the environment normo-thermic are paramount in order to maintain homeostasis and prevent heat loss. Various interventions are known to be effective: ensuring the environmental temperature is optimum and, if possible, facilitating skin-to-skin contact between baby and parents. However, if a baby is admitted to a neonatal unit, plastic wraps or bags may be used at birth, particularly for extremely preterm infants, as well as various devices, including overhead heat sources (Figure 52.1) such as a Babytherm® (Dräger, Hemel Hempstead, UK) and/or a Resuscitaire® (Dräger; Figure 52.2), and incubators with essential features, namely Perspex sides (Figure 52.3), double-panelled walls (Figure 52.4), and portholes (Figure 52.5). These are used to nurse babies until they are stable enough to be transferred to an open cot, bassinette (Figure 52.6), and/or thermal mattress.

Heat loss

It is vital that care providers understand the principles of heat balance in order to be able to provide a normothermic environment for the baby. The two key principles are to block avenues of heat loss (via the four mechanisms of heat transfer) and to provide heat and environmental support to maintain a normal temperature.

Four mechanisms of heat transfer

• *Radiation*: Heat loss in the form of a warm skin surface near to a cooler object that is not in contact with the baby – inside the incubator or window. Radiation is a significant source of heat loss because of the infant's large surface area to volume ratio.
• *Conduction*: The loss of heat due to a cooler object being in direct contact with the newborn baby (e.g. cold scales, stethoscope).
• *Convection*: The loss of heat to moving air at the skin surface, which is dependent on the air's velocity and temperature (e.g. cold drafts).
• *Evaporation*: Water from the skin or mucous membranes lost to the air. Term babies should be dried at delivery and management of insensible losses is vital at any gestation. In very premature babies, the use of plastic wrapping at birth and subsequent humidification is essential.

Incubator and overhead heater management and care

Incubators provide a controlled, enclosed environment that is convectively heated with warm air. The temperature is set to a certain reading / level according to the baby's gestation, age, and central body temperature. This could somewhere within a range, for example between 29 and 34 °Celcius and adjusted accordingly. Incubator control units gradually increase or decrease the heat output to maintain the temperature constantly, without significant fluctuations. An incubator is preferred and most likely to be used for neonates of <1.5 kg and/or a gestational age of <30 weeks.

Babytherms® and overhead heaters are more open and are radiantly heated by an overhead heater and gel mattress. Overhead heat devices are beneficial for those infants who require multiple interventions and treatment, and who are slightly larger. When considering which is the more suitable environment for the infant, careful attention should be paid to the following factors.

Incubator

• Once switched on, it takes approximately 30 minutes for the optimum temperature to be reached.
• If 'baby' monitoring is used, care must be taken not to place thermal skin sensors, if used, over areas of brown fat (found mostly in the nape of the neck, axilla, and between the scapulae). Brown fat is a specialized type of fat that contains thermogenin, a key enzyme in the regulation of non-shivering thermogenesis.
• Incorrect readings will take place if thermal skin sensors are covered or become disconnected.
• The portholes should not be open for too long.
• Accurate baby and air temperature monitoring and recording should be performed regularly, according to local policy and condition of the baby.
• The incubator should be kept away from air-conditioning ducts, direct sunlight, windows, and drafts.
• If humidification is required for very preterm babies the percentage humidity should be set according to local policy and the baby's gestation/age. Sterile water should be used and the water level should be checked hourly.
• Daily cleaning should be undertaken as per local policy and every seven days the incubator should be changed for a clean one.

Babytherm® or overhead heater

• Once switched on, the mattress takes approximately one hour, and the overhead heater takes approximately 30 minutes, for the set temperature to be reached.
• Each level of the overhead heater is 10% higher or lower than the next, so careful attention should be paid when adjusting the temperature of the overhead heater.
• As with incubators, regular monitoring and documentation of the baby's temperature should be performed.

Transferring from an incubator or overhead heater

Transferring a baby from an incubator or overhead heater to an open cot (bassinette) is essential in preparing the baby and the family for discharge. The baby's temperature should be monitored regularly to ensure the baby is regulating their temperature satisfactorily. Care must be taken to ensure thermal stability during care and interventions. Teaching and support should be given to the parents about the signs and symptoms of heat loss and heat retention and what to do if they are concerned. Furthermore, the importance of the parents maintaining a home environment that prevents heat and cold stress should be discussed before the baby is discharged home.

Other considerations

Incubators and overhead heaters were developed to maintain thermal stability in low birth weight and sick newborns, thus improving their chances of survival. While positive progress has been made in the production of these technological devices, there are still important aspects of care to consider. A potential challenge is exposure to high noise levels in the Neonatal Intensive Care Unit (NICU). Strategies aimed at modifying the NICU environment, along with structural improvements in incubator design, are required to reduce noise exposure. A very bright environment may also adversely affect the rest–activity patterns of the baby. Accordingly, the use of both incubator covers and circadian lighting in the NICU might attenuate these effects.

Key points
• Babies rely on non-shivering chemical thermogenesis to produce heat due to their physiological differences to older children.
• Competence in setting up and nursing neonates in incubators and/or overhead heaters is required.
• Care must be taken to ensure thermal stability during episodes of care.

53 Sudden infant death syndrome

Figure 53.1 Sudden infant death syndrome.

Sudden infant death syndrome, or sudden unexpected death in infancy, is a term commonly used to describe an unexpected death in infancy:

- Uncommon under the age of 1 month
- Peaks at 2 months
- 90% occur by 6 months
- Very few occur over 1 year

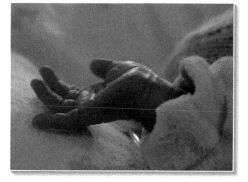

Cause of sudden infant death syndrome include:

- Accidents
- Infection
- Congenital abnormality
- Metabolic disorder
- Combination of factors
- Undiscovered causes

Risk factors

- Premature infants
- Low birth weight infants
- Male infants
- Infants born to mothers who are still young

Smoking

Infants whose parents smoke or who are cared for in a smoky environment are at a much higher risk of a sudden infant death. Health promotion is paramount to help reduce this risk

Sudden infant death syndrome can occur:

- In a cot
- In a pram
- In a car seat
- In parent's arms
- In parent's bed

It usually occurs during a period of sleep

Reducing the risk of cot deaths

- Cut smoking in pregnancy
- Do not allow anyone to smoke in the same room as the infant
- Put the infant to sleep on their back and not on their front
- Place the infant with their feet at the bottom of the cot to prevent wriggling down under the covers
- Never sleep with an infant on a sofa or armchair

Never sleep with an infant in bed

Children and Young People's Nursing at a Glance, Second Edition. Edited by Elizabeth Gormley-Fleming and Sheila Roberts.
© 2023 John Wiley & Sons Ltd. Published 2023 by John Wiley & Sons Ltd.

Definition

Cot death is the sudden, unexpected, and unexplained death of an apparently healthy baby. Some sudden and unexpected deaths can be explained by the post-mortem examination, revealing, for example, an unforeseen infection or metabolic disorder. Those that remain unexplained after post-mortem examination may be registered as sudden infant death syndrome (SIDS), sudden infant death, sudden unexpected death in infancy, unascertained death, or cot death.

Incidence

The latest figures for SIDS were documented in 2019: 170 unexplained infant deaths occurred in England and Wales in 2019, a rate of 0.27 deaths per 1000 live births, and a decrease from 0.32 deaths per 1000 live births in 2018.

Although the SIDS rate has declined since the 1990s, significant racial and ethnic differences continue. There is also a higher incidence in boys (0.29 deaths per 1000 live births), accounting for 55.3% of all unexplained infant deaths in 2019, a decrease from 57.6% in 2018.

It is very uncommon for an infant less than 1 month old or over the age of 1 year to die of SIDS: 90% of those who die are 6 months old or younger, with a peak incidence of 2 months of age, accounting for 72% of all unexplained deaths to have occurred in infants less than 4 months of age. However, in the UK in 2018, 6.5% of sudden unexplained deaths of children under 2 years were among children aged 12–24 months (Figure 53.1).

Infants with a low birth weight (<2.5 kg) are over four times more likely to die from SIDS than an infant born with a birth weight >2.5 kg.

In 2019, the unexplained infant mortality rate was highest for mothers aged under 20 years of age, at 0.96 deaths per 1000 live births. There has been a decrease in numbers for mothers of all age groups since 2004.

Causes of SIDS

The exact cause of SIDS remains unknown; however, there are a variety of theories. It is thought to be down to a combination of factors, mainly environmental factors such as tobacco smoke, getting tangled in bedding, a minor illness, or breathing obstruction. There is also an association with parents co-sleeping with their baby. Babies who become overheated when sleeping are at increased risk of SIDS, as are babies who sleep on soft surfaces. Another theory is associated with babies sleeping on their fronts and being unable to rouse themselves when their oxygen levels decrease and their carbon dioxide levels increase. The rising carbon dioxide level is the trigger that rouses the baby to ensure they turn their head and breathe more rapidly to increase oxygen intake.

Measures in place to reduce the risk

The Back to Sleep Campaign was launched in the early 1990s and this has had a positive impact. In 2012, the Safe to Sleep campaign replaced it to help emphasize a 'continued focus on safe sleep environments and back sleeping as ways to reduce the risk of SIDS and other sleep-related causes of infant death'. The number of SIDS deaths has fallen by over 85% since the introduction of the Back to Sleep and Safe to Sleep campaigns. Both of these campaigns widely advertised the risk that parents and carers were taking by placing their infants to sleep on their stomachs.

Historically, this is how infants had always been put to sleep, and may have been the advice of grandparents and healthcare professionals.

Advice to parents to help reduce the risks

There are a number of risk factors that can contribute to SIDS. The education of parents is paramount in helping to reduce the numbers of infant deaths that still occur:

- Always put the infant to sleep on their back.
- Keep the cot in the adults' room for the first six months of life.
- Recommend the baby is placed with their feet near to the bottom of the cot to prevent them getting underneath bedding.
- Duvets, pillows, and quilts should not be used.
- The mattress should be firm.
- Do not share a bed with an infant.
- Do not sleep with an infant in an armchair or on a sofa.
- Do not allow the infant to become too hot – keep bedding and clothing to a minimum and keep the room they are sleeping in cool rather than overheated. Room temperature should be 16–20°C.
- Breastfeed if possible.
- Do not smoke during pregnancy or after the birth of the infant.
- Do not allow anyone to smoke in the same room as the infant.
- Be more vigilant if taking drugs or alcohol.
- If the infant was born prematurely, was born with a low birth weight, or born to a mother under the age of 20 years, the infant will have an increased risk. These infants should be observed more frequently.

Smoking

There is evidence to support that smoking can significantly increase the risk of SIDS. This applies to mothers who smoke during pregnancy or after pregnancy, and any other adults who smoke around an infant. The environment an infant is in should be completely smoke free, as an infant in a smoky environment is eight times more likely to die from SIDS.

Support for parents

When a baby dies suddenly and unexpectedly, the death will have to be investigated to try to establish the cause of death. A post-mortem examination will be performed. The multi-agency guidelines for care and investigation into sudden unexpected death must be followed. This will be very distressing for the family and support needs to be identified very early in the bereavement process. Sharing information with parents at every step of the process is important. Siblings at home at the time of death will need support on an ongoing basis. Multiple agencies will be involved in the investigation and aftercare of the family. The situation must be handled sensitively, as it is traumatic for all involved, family and professionals.

Key points

- SIDS remains the biggest killer for infants less than 1 year old.
- Placing infants on their backs in a smoke-free environment can significantly reduce the risk of death.
- A healthcare professional has a huge responsibility in educating parents and carers.

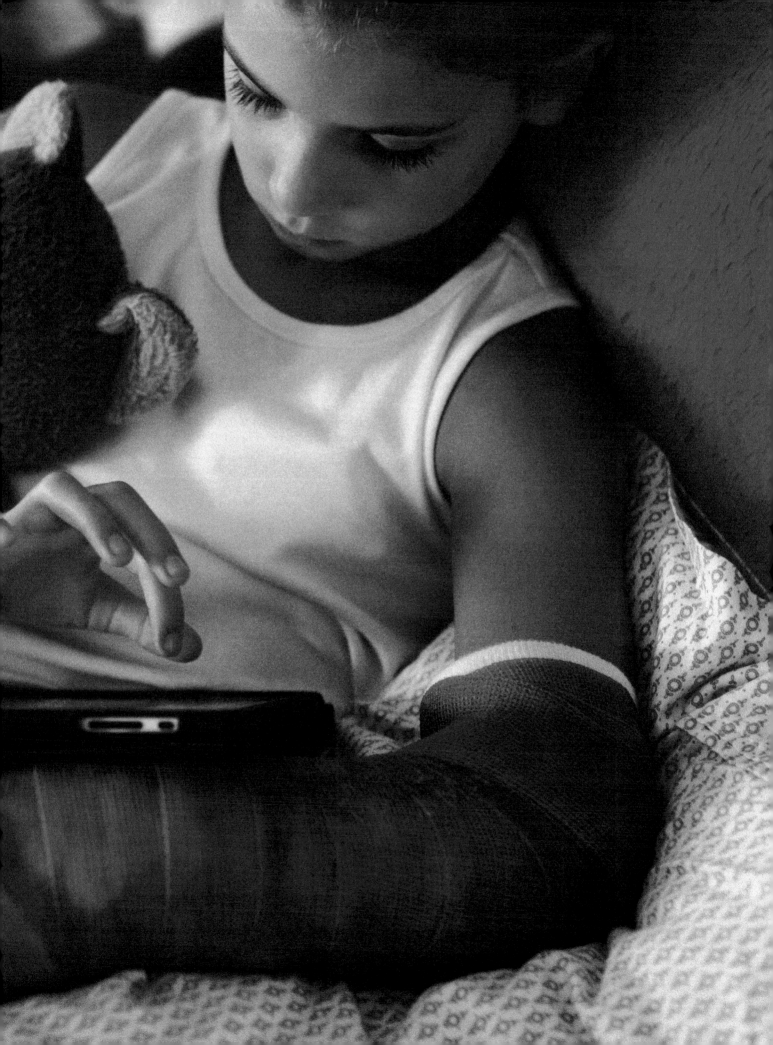

Part 4

Chapters

54 Nutrition in childhood

Figure 54.1 Nutritional assessment.

> Questions are directed here to the child in terms of a subjective and objective assessment, but could be directed to parents or legal guardians

Subjective data

Practical questions for assessment of children's nutritional status

- What foods do you like? Include preferences including snacks, patterns, and times of meals
- What foods don't you like? Include any allergies or diet restrictions
- What do you use to eat? Include any equipment
- When do you prefer to eat and drink? Include times and preference
- Does the child need any help? Include anyone who helps and following any observations of chewing and swallowing
- Does the child get tired? Note any fatigue or longer time taken over feeding

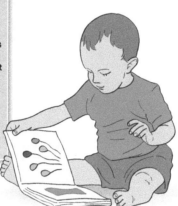

Objective data

Practical questions for assessment of children's nutritional status

- Weight is the most sound indicator of current nutritional status. It should be measured at regular intervals
- Usual approximate body weight is helpful. Use medical notes. Assess any change such as dry skin or tongue
- Height or length is a useful growth parameter and should be plotted on a percentile chart
- As head circumference growth during the first 2 years is very rapid, head circumference is a good indicator of nutritional intake and growth
- Fat distribution or musculoskeletal changes. Triceps skin-folds (TSF) measurements should be performed only by those trained in this method (e.g. dietitian, nutritional care specialist, or medical staff)
- If problems are identified, the physical assessment might include some more in-depth assessments such as mid-arm circumference (MAC). This is made with a tape measure with the arm down in a fully relaxed position, and indicates muscle and fat stores

Figure 54.2 The importance of good nutrition.

Good nutrition gives a child the best start in life and begins at an early stage. Childhood nutrition should be a balance between the vitamins, protein, carbohydrates, and minerals required for healthy growth and development:

- **Bread, cereals, grains, potatoes, pasta, and rice** provide energy, fibre, vitamins, and minerals
- **Fruit and vegetables** provide fibre, vitamins, and minerals, and are a source of antioxidants
- **Meat, fish, poultry, and alternatives**, which include eggs and pulses, provide protein and vitamins and minerals, especially iron. Pulses also contain fibre
- **Milk and dairy foods** such as yoghurt and cheese provide calcium for healthy bones, growth, and teeth, plus vitamins and minerals

Any healthy diet needs to be in association with regular physical exercise. Worryingly, research has found that many children and young people have inadequate intakes of many nutrients, including vitamin A, riboflavin (vitamin B2), zinc, potassium, magnesium, calcium, and iron, particularly once they reach age 12+ and have more control over what they eat

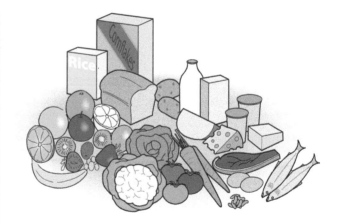

Importance of good nutritional assessment

This chapter focuses on the nursing assessment of children's and young people's nutrition, both when healthy and when ill. Assessment of children's and young people's nutritional status is important in order to plan and evaluate care. Poor nutrition complicates many diseases of childhood and affects both the physical and psychological wellbeing of children and young people.

In order to facilitate a good understanding of nutrition, Figure 54.1 contains a list of questions nurses could use when assessing children and young people. It is crucial that the nurse has a good knowledge and understanding of 'normal' development.

Nutrition in the under-5s

Healthy young children have a high energy requirement because of their rapid growth and increasing activity. As the young child becomes more independent and adept at holding a spoon or drinking from a beaker, this is the time to introduce variety. As they have small stomachs, it is advisable to offer small, frequent meals. To help prevent dental caries there should be restriction of sugary snacks such as fizzy drinks and sweets.

Although obesity is a major problem, children and teenagers still need enough calories to grow and develop into healthy adults. Table 54.1 gives a rough guideline to the daily calorie needs of

Children and Young People's Nursing at a Glance, Second Edition. Edited by Elizabeth Gormley-Fleming and Sheila Roberts.
© 2023 John Wiley & Sons Ltd. Published 2023 by John Wiley & Sons Ltd.

Table 54.1 Calorie intake for children

Age (years)	Calories per day	
	Boys	**Girls**
1–3	1230	1165
4–6	1400	1200
7	1649	1530
8	1745	1625
9	1840	1721
10	2032	1936
11	2200	2150
12	2406	2290
13	2510	2300
14	2629	2342
15	2820	2390
16	2964	2414
17	3083	2462
18	3155	2462

boys and girls at different ages. Children and young people who are very physically active may need more; those who are inactive may need less.

As the child develops, milk is no longer the main source of nutrients, although the under-5s should still drink a pint a day (440 mL). Whole-fat milk is recommended for those over 12 months and can be used until age 5 years to provide plenty of calories, unless the child is overweight or under medical care. Some evidence suggests that semi-skimmed milk (but not skimmed) can be introduced after 2 years of age, but the overall diet must provide enough energy.

The diet must also be high in vitamins and minerals. In particular, a good supply of protein, calcium, iron, and vitamins A and D is required. It is recommended that the pre-school child should progress from the very high-energy diet of infancy (with about 50% of total energy coming from fat) to the diet for a 5-year-old, which should have a much greater emphasis on a lower fat content (but still about 35% of energy from fat).

Diet-related problems

Obesity is less likely in under-5s but is increasing in some countries. Young children should not be put on weight-reduction diets, but a healthy family approach to food and regular physical activity are important in avoiding excessive weight gain and obesity.

Worryingly, iron-deficiency anaemia is common at this age, resulting from high requirements for growth and poor dietary intake, especially in the 'faddy or fussy eater'. It is associated with frequent infections, delayed development, and poor weight gain. Vitamin C present in orange juice can enhance iron absorption from the gut.

Constipation is common in the under-5s and can be prevented by gradually increasing the amount of fibre in the child's diet. Foods high in fibre include vegetables, wholemeal bread, baked beans, and high-fibre white bread. A high fluid intake, not of fizzy drinks, is also important.

Toddler diarrhoea is common and may be linked with too many sugary drinks and fruit juice, especially between meals.

Nutrition in school-aged children

The same principles apply for school-aged children as for the under-5s. The younger school-aged child, 4–6-year-olds, still need smaller and more frequent meals, as they do not have large enough stomachs to cope with adult-sized meals. The requirement for energy remains due to growth and activity, but gradually an 'adult-style' healthy diet should be introduced, reducing high fat content foods and increasing fibre-rich foods.

Diet-related problems

Disorders associated with inadequate nutrition continue to increase, with obesity now a significant health problem of childhood. In the 4–5-year age group, 14.4% of children are obese when they start school, with a further 13.3% classed as overweight. In the 10–11-year age group this rises to 25.5% being obese, with 15.4% classed as overweight. There is a significant link to obesity prevalence among children living in deprived areas. Boys tend to be more obese than girls. In these situations, medical or dietetic referral is required. Nurses can also support any weight loss in encouraging a child to lose weight gradually and increase activity while their height also increases. This may require a healthy lifestyle for the whole family. It should also be noted that the proportion of underweight children increases with school age, the number doubling by year six compared to in reception.

Nutrition in young people aged 12+

It is particularly important that young people over 12 years eat a healthy diet rich in vitamins and minerals. Growth in girls occurs prior to puberty and slows down thereafter, while boys grow following puberty. Young people often have higher requirements for nutrients than adults in order to support growth. For example, 15–18-year-old boys need more thiamin (vitamin B1), niacin (vitamin B3), vitamin B6, calcium, phosphorus, and iron than adult men. Similarly, 15–18-year-old girls need more niacin, calcium, phosphorus, and magnesium than adult women.

The Food Standards Agency has provided guidance on the safe maximum consumption levels for oily fish: boys aged under 16 can have up to four portions of oily fish a week and girls up to two portions. The lower recommendation in girls is because substances found in oily fish can accumulate in the body and high levels may be detrimental to the developing foetus in a later pregnancy.

Diet-related problems

As young people become more independent, have new interests away from family life such as relationships, and have concerns such as career choices and body image, their energy needs are paramount. At the same time, they may tend to develop health-compromising eating behaviours such as skipping meals, fad dieting, overeating, or an eating disorder such as binge eating or anorexia. They need a diet that provides the high energy needed for this stage of life while delivering nutritious and convenient foods that promote long-term health (Figure 54.2). Medical help should be sought in eating disorders.

Key points

- Childhood obesity is a worldwide issue, and the children and young person's nurse is ideally placed to provide education about a healthy lifestyle and eating habits to circumvent longer-term physical and mental health issues.
- A healthy, varied diet should be offered, and portion sizes known to the child and family.
- The introduction of food labelling should be used positively to educate children and young people about good nutrition.
- Behaviour management is key to promoting healthy eating and lifestyles.

55 Breastfeeding

Figure 55.1 Choosing to breastfeed.

The Baby Friendly Initiative in the United Kingdom and Ireland encourages healthcare professionals to promote and support breastfeeding. Children's nurses have a pivotal role in the promotion, protection, and support of breastfeeding.

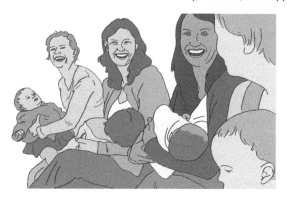

Breastfeeding is a normal way to feed and care for a baby. Breast milk is uniquely designed to provide the best nutrition and protection to meet the baby's needs and its properties can never be reproduced in formula milks. Colostrum is produced in the few first days. It is high in protein, immunoglobulins, vitamins, anti-infective agents, living cells, and minerals – and helps babies to resist infection.

Breast milk is then produced. It is a constantly changing food that adjusts to the age and needs of the baby or child. Protection from infection is provided by iron binding in the baby's gut and maternally derived antibodies.

Children's nurses should actively promote breastfeeding as it offers many health benefits for both baby and mother. These health benefits extend beyond the breastfeeding period and into later life.

Children who do not receive breast milk
- Are more likely to develop ear, nose, and throat infections
- Are more likely to develop gastroenteritis, kidney and chest infections
- Have a greater risk of obesity and of developing diabetes
- Have a higher risk of allergies and eczema
- Have an increased risk of sudden infant death syndrome
- Have a higher risk of necrotizing entercolitis (in the preterm baby)

Breastfeeding babies gain comfort, warmth, and security close to the mother. For the parent, breastfeeding helps protect against breast and ovarian cancer, as well as helping achieve and maintain a healthy post-pregnancy weight

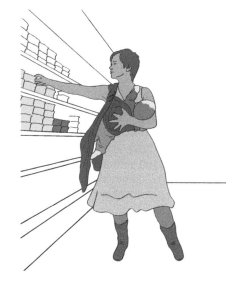

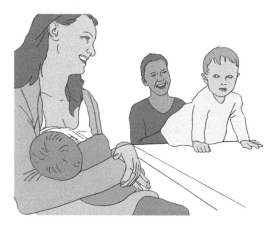

The World Health Organization recommends 6 months, exclusive breastfeeding continued with complementary foods to 2 years of age or older. In the United Kingdom 74% of parents, and 55% of parents in Ireland, initially choose to breastfeed their baby. However, by 6 months these numbers are greatly reduced. Children's nurses can help the parent plan achievable goals in relation to breastfeeding and support them in sustaining breastfeeding

Children and Young People's Nursing at a Glance, Second Edition. Edited by Elizabeth Gormley-Fleming and Sheila Roberts.
© 2023 John Wiley & Sons Ltd. Published 2023 by John Wiley & Sons Ltd.

Figure 55.2 Advice on breastfeeding.

Breastfeeding support

A children's nurse can offer breastfeeding support by:
- Providing consistent and accurate information to families
- Providing reassurance and encouragement to families
- Providing the opportunity for families to discuss issues
- Proving the parent with evidence-based information on how to address any problems that may occur
- Assisting in getting timely assistance from trained peer support, relevant heath professionals, and parent-to-parent support

Initiating breastfeeding

Breastfeeding or expressing milk as soon after delivery as possible will aid in breastmilk production. The breastfeeds should be frequent, effective, exclusive, and on demand. It is advised to avoid giving a breastfed baby formula or use bottles initially, as this may lead to a reduction in milk production

The baby may be unable to feed at the breast due to illness or abnormalities, or if the parent is away from the baby, they may choose to express their breastmilk by hand, hand pump, or electric pump, and it can be delivered by another method. The children's nurse should provide information on how to obtain, clean, and use equipment and on the safe storage and delivery of the expressed milk

Protecting breastfeeding

The children's nurse should be aware of and adhere to the International Code of Marketing of Breastmilk Substitutes (WHO/UNICEF)

Further information for both mothers and health professionals can be found at www.breastfeeding.nhs.uk (UK) and www.breastfeeding.ie (Ireland)

Attachment

It is important that the baby latches on to the breast with a widely open mouth, so that not just the nipple is in the baby's mouth but also the areola and underlying breast tissue. On attaching, the chin should touch the breast first and the baby's head be allowed to tip back slightly so the tongue can reach as much of the breast as possible

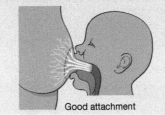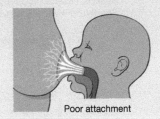

Good attachment — Poor attachment

Positioning

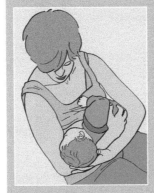

There are many different breastfeeding positions: the cradle hold, underarm hold, laid back, and lying down.

There is no best way, and each parent and baby should try different positions in different circumstances. To facilitate the baby to self-attach and feed well, the principles are always the same: the parent should feel comfortable; the baby needs to be in a position that is close, facing the breast, straight, and supported.

Signs that a baby is breastfeeding well

- Gaining weight after the first 2 weeks
- 1–2 wet nappies in the first 48 hours, then at least 3 from day 3–4, then 5–6 every 24 hours
- Passing meconium by day 2, by day 3 a changing stool that is lighter and easier to clean. From day 4 and for the first few weeks at least three soft or runny yellow stools every day
- At least 8 feeds in a 24-hour period and feeds for 5–30 minutes at most feeds
- Breast and nipples should not be sore
- Baby is content and satisfied after most feeds

The World Health Organization republished its guidance on the implementation of the Baby-Friendly Hospital Initiative (BFHI) in 2018. The aim of this initiative is to help motivate maternity and newborn hospital services worldwide to implement the 10 steps to successful breastfeeding. By putting the BFHI into practice, an integrated systems approach is adopted and organizations are required to fulfil their responsibilities to this initiative (Figures 55.1 and 55.2). The 10 steps are:

1 Hospital policies
2 Staff competencies
3 Antenatal care
4 Care after birth
5 Support mothers with breastfeeding
6 Supplementing
7 Rooming in
8 Responsive feeding
9 Bottles, teats, and pacifiers
10 Discharge

There is substantial evidence to suggest that the 10 steps significantly improve breastfeeding rates.

Key points

- Mothers need support to breastfeed, particularly with latching on and positioning.
- Knowing when the baby is getting enough milk is an important part of education about breastfeeding.
- Evidence-based guidance around the use of donor breastmilk has led to increased usage as safety has improved.

56 Bottle feeding

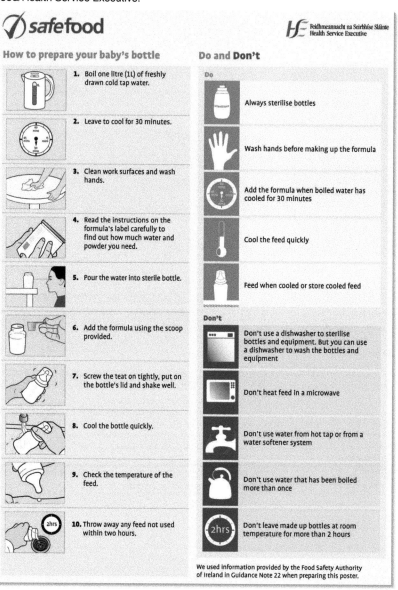

Figure 56.1 Do and don't for safe preparation of a formula feed. Reprinted courtesy of Safefood/Health Service Executive (2018). *Source:* How to prepare your baby's bottle? 2018. Available at www.safefood.net. Reproduced with permission of Safefood/Health Service Executive.

safefood

HSE Feidhmeannacht na Seirbhíse Sláinte
Health Service Executive

How to prepare your baby's bottle

1. Boil one litre (1L) of freshly drawn cold tap water.
2. Leave to cool for 30 minutes.
3. Clean work surfaces and wash hands.
4. Read the instructions on the formula's label carefully to find out how much water and powder you need.
5. Pour the water into sterile bottle.
6. Add the formula using the scoop provided.
7. Screw the teat on tightly, put on the bottle's lid and shake well.
8. Cool the bottle quickly.
9. Check the temperature of the feed.
10. Throw away any feed not used within two hours.

Do and Don't

Do
- Always sterilise bottles
- Wash hands before making up the formula
- Add the formula when boiled water has cooled for 30 minutes
- Cool the feed quickly
- Feed when cooled or store cooled feed

Don't
- Don't use a dishwasher to sterilise bottles and equipment. But you can use a dishwasher to wash the bottles and equipment
- Don't heat feed in a microwave
- Don't use water from hot tap or from a water softener system
- Don't use water that has been boiled more than once
- Don't leave made up bottles at room temperature for more than 2 hours

We used information provided by the Food Safety Authority of Ireland in Guidance Note 22 when preparing this poster.

Balanced nutrition is critical for normal growth and development of an infant. Breastfeeding is the recommended method of infant feeding; however, by choice or necessity, some mothers may formula feed their infant. Formula companies must comply with legislation that governs the production, composition, marketing, and distribution of formula milk. In particular, the composition of formula milk is adjusted by modifying the protein, carbohydrate, and fat content, and adding important vitamins, minerals, and trace elements to increase its similarity to breast milk. Despite such modifications, formula milk continues to differ in the source and amounts of its constituents and does not contain the biologically active ingredients contained in breast milk. The nutritional composition of both breast and formula milk should satisfy the complete nutritional requirements of an infant until the introduction of complementary foods, at around 6 months of age, and continue to contribute to nutritional intake for the first year.

Children and Young People's Nursing at a Glance, Second Edition. Edited by Elizabeth Gormley-Fleming and Sheila Roberts.
© 2023 John Wiley & Sons Ltd. Published 2023 by John Wiley & Sons Ltd.

Types of infant formula

Infant formula milk is commonly made from modified cows' milk, which is dominant in either whey or casein protein. Choosing an infant formula milk is based on the infant's age and nutritional requirements, and in some circumstances the infant's medical condition.

Standard infant formula

First infant formulas should be based on the whey protein in cow's milk as whey is similar, although not identical, to the protein in breast milk. Whey-dominant formulas are suitable from birth to 1 year. Casein-dominant formula is marketed for hungrier infants as it requires more complex digestion and is thought, although not scientifically proven, to provide feelings of increased fullness and satiety. Both whey and casein-dominant formulas have the same calorific and nutritional content, but the casein protein is less similar to the protein found in breast milk. Protein levels in all infant formulas must comply with a lower protein range, closer to that seen in breast milk, to normalize infant weight gain. A range of whey and casein-based formula milks are available for term infants (Table 56.1).

Follow-on formula is suitable for infants from 6 months of age and contains additional protein and minerals for growth and development. Infants do not have to switch from a first infant milk to a follow-on formula, as the introduction of complementary foods generally provides an adequate source of additional nutrients. Daily fluid and feed requirements differ depending on the infant's age, weight, and percentile (Table 56.2).

Specialized infant formula

A range of specialized infant formula milks are available for infants with specific nutritional requirements that cannot be met by standard formula. These specialized formulas should only be used on the advice of a healthcare professional. Some examples of these specialized milks are:

- Pre-term hospital formula milk – Aptamil® Preterm, SMA® Gold Prem 1; Cow & Gate® Nutriprem 1, Cow & Gate® Hydrolysed Nutriprem 1.
- Pre-term post-hospitalization formula milk – Cow & Gate® or SMA® Nutriprem 2, SMA® Gold Prem 2.
- Colic and/or constipation – Cow & Gate® Comfort.
- Lactose intolerant – SMA® LF.
- Regurgitation – pre-thickened feeds.
- Malabsorption or cow's milk allergy – hydrolysed or partially hydrolysed protein formulas.
- Soy-based formula – galactosaemia.

Partial or completely hydrolysed protein formula is recommended for infants with cow's milk allergy, rather than using sheep, goat, or soy-based formula.

Preparing infant formula

Infant formula is available as ready-to-feed (RTF) or powdered infant formula. RTF is a sterile formula that does not require refrigeration and is stored at room temperature. It is ready to feed to the infant and warming the feed is dependent on infant preference. Powdered infant formula is non-sterile and can be contaminated with a number of harmful bacteria, including the *Cronobacter* species and *Salmonella*. It is imperative that strict safety guidelines are followed in the preparation of powdered infant formula to ensure that the prepared feed is not contaminated by harmful bacteria. Key safety statements in relation to the safe preparation of formula feeds are presented in Figure 56.1 and Box 56.1.

> **Box 56.1** Guidelines for safe preparation of powdered infant formula
>
> - Wash hands.
> - Cleanse work surface with warm, soapy water, rinse, and dry.
> - Wash and sterilize all equipment.
> - Check that the powdered infant formula is in date.
> - Check the required volume of water and the number of scoops of formula.
> - Boil 1 L of fresh, cold tap water and allow it to cool for 30 minutes. This ensures the temperature remains greater than 70° C (to kill any bacteria that might be present in the powdered infant formula).
> - Do not use water from the hot tap, bottled/fizzy/spring/filtered/mineral water, or artificially softened water, or water that has been boiled more than once.
> - If boiled tap water is not suitable for drinking, then boiled bottled water with a sodium content of less than 20 mg can be used.
> - Use the measurements on the bottle and pour in the required amount of boiled water.
> - Use the leveller in the pack to level each scoop and add the required number of scoops of formula to the bottle of boiled water. Do not pack the powder into the scoop.
> - Reseal the pack to protect against moisture and bacteria.
> - If the bottle is not for immediate use, place the disc on the neck of the bottle, screw on the collar, and shake until all powder is dissolved. Then cool and store in the back of the fridge at 5 °C or less.
> - If feed is for immediate use, replace the disc with the sterile teat, cover the teat with the bottle cap, and shake until all of the powder is dissolved.
> - Cool the feed to the desired temperature (hold bottle under running cold water or stand it in a container of cold water). Ensure the water does not reach the neck of the bottle.
> - Check the temperature of the feed and use immediately.
> - Throw away any unused feed within two hours.

Table 56.1 Whey- and casein-based formula milks.

	Examples	Protein/g/100 mL	Energy/100 mL
Whey dominant	SMA® Advanced First Infant Milk	1.2 g (whey : casein 100 : 0)	63
	SMA® Pro First Infant Milk	1.24 g (whey : casein 70 : 30)	67
	Aptamil® First Infant Milk	1.3 g (whey : casein 50 : 50)	66
	Aptamil® Profutura First Infant Milk	1.3 g (whey : casein 62 : 38)	66
Casein dominant	Aptamil® Hungry Infant Milk	1.3 g (whey : casein 23 : 77)	66
	Cow & Gate® Hungry Infant Milk	1.3 g (whey : casein 23 : 77)	66
	SMA® Extra Hungry Infant Milk	1.5 g (whey : casein 20 : 80)	68

Table 56.2 Daily fluid and feed requirements.

Age (months)	Approximate number of feeds in 24 hours	Daily fluid intake mL/kg
0–3	6–8 every 3–4 hours	150
4–6	4–6 every 4–6 hours	150
7–9	4 (also having food)	120
10–12	3 (also having food)	110

Key points

- Ensure that the infant formula is correctly prepared and given, and follow all safety guidelines. Safe preparation of infant formula is essential if gastroenteritis is to be avoided.
- Extreme care must be taken when checking the temperature of infant formula.
- All feed volumes should be recorded on the infant's feeding chart in the hospital setting.
- Mothers who choose to formula feed their baby rather than breastfeed must not be judged, but given the same encouragement and support to bond with their baby.

57 Feed calculations

Figure 57.1 Feed calculations for the correct amount of feed required by an infant during a 24-hour period.

The feed requirement should be calculated by using the equation:

Total mL/kg × weight of the infant (kg) = total feed requirement in 24-hour period (mL)

↓

Once the volume required in a 24-hour period has been calculated, this figure can be used to calculate an hourly rate if the infant is on a continuous feed:

Total feed requirement in 24-hour period /24 = hourly rate for continuous feed (mL/h)

↓

The volume can also be used to calculate the total feed required every 3 hours (or whatever frequency necessary for bolus or oral feeds)

Total feed requirement in 24-hour period/8 (for every 3 hours), or /6 (for every 4 hours) = feed required

Calculating the amount of feed required for bolus feeds can be slightly more difficult than calculating for continuous feeds as there is more maths involved. For example, if you wish to feed the infant every 3 hours, you need to be aware that the infant will require 8 feeds in a day as 8 × 3 = 24 hours. Similarly, if you wish to feed the infant every 4 hours, the infant will require 6 feeds in a day as 4 × 6 = 24 hours.

Example: A term baby has been admitted to a children's ward. The baby weighs 3 kg and should have 150 mL/kg/day of feed

How much feed does the baby require in a 24-hour period?

mL × kg – 150 × 3 = 450 mL (total feed requirement in 24-hour period)

↓

The baby is to be fed continuously via a nasogastric pump. What should the hourly rate for continuous feed be?

450 mL (total feed requirement in 24-hour period)/24 = 18.75 mL/h

↓

A couple of days later the baby is improving and requires feeding every 3 hours. How much feed will the baby require every 3 hours?

450 mL (total feed requirement in 24-hour period)/24 (hours in a day) × 3 (hours) = 56.25 mL

↓

The baby's parents request that the baby is fed every 4 hours. How much feed will the baby require every 4 hours?

450 mL (total feed requirement in 24-hour period)/24 (hours in a day) × 4 (hours) = 75 mL

Children and Young People's Nursing at a Glance, Second Edition. Edited by Elizabeth Gormley-Fleming and Sheila Roberts.
© 2023 John Wiley & Sons Ltd. Published 2023 by John Wiley & Sons Ltd.

While it is well documented that breastfeeding is the optimum form of nutrition for infants, sometimes it is not possible for breastfeeding to occur. The reasons for this could be maternal choice, problems with the technique required to breastfeed, the baby not taking enough feed to thrive, or the baby being ill and therefore unable to breastfeed. Some babies are unable to feed orally and will require nutrition via a nasogastric or gastrostomy tube.

The amount of fluid that is required for a term baby who is receiving all of their nutrition from feed varies (Figure 57.1). If the baby is ill then the requirement may be restricted.

The premature infant should receive up to 220 mL/kg, which is dependent upon their gut tolerance and the fluid balance. To achieve an adequate level of nutrition the feed volume of the premature infant should be at least 220 mL/kg, and they should be fed every three to four hours and not on demand to ensure that they are receiving the required nutrients.

The term baby should be fed on demand with 150–200 mL/kg until they have been established on a weaning programme. Infant-led weaning is now widely practised.

The amount of feed that a baby requires will depend on their gut tolerance, whether they have an acute illness, and their current weight. It is normal practice that when a baby is acutely unwell the feed requirement that they receive is reduced to allow their gut to be rested and to give the baby some recuperation time. If the baby is finding it difficult to feed orally, then a nasogastric tube may be passed in the short term to ensure that they receive the required nutritional intake.

It is important that children's nurses understand how to calculate the feed requirement, volume for each feed, and rate of each feed to ensure that the baby receives the optimum amount of nutrition at an appropriate pace.

Key points

- Demand feeding for the full-term baby should be the norm.
- The children's nurse must know how to calculate the feed requirements for the infants in their care. Over- or underfeeding will have an impact on normal growth and development.
- While breastfeeding is recommended and baby-friendly initiatives are promoted, the children's nurse should respect parental choice of feeding methods,

58 Growth charts

Figure 58.1 Measuring head circumferences.

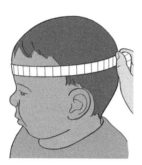

Why. Head circumferences provide information on head anomalies such as hydrocephalus or craniosynostosis, which may require treatment

When and Where. Neonates should have their first head circumference measurement taken after 36 hours, which allows moulding and oedema from birth to settle. After this, children up to 2 years should have their measurement taken on each visit to clinic, doctor, or hospital admission

How. Follow universal precautions at all times. Ensure the child is comfortable and settled to provide accurate measurement. The measuring tape should be placed above the ears and midway between eyebrows and hairline, then around the occipital prominence of the back of the head. This ensures the largest head circumference has been taken

Document. Always document on the correct boy or girl growth chart, the child's healthcare records, and local documentation paperwork

Figure 58.2 Measuring weight.

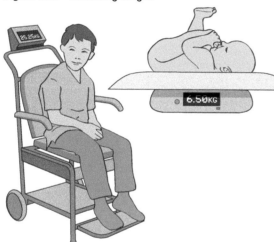

Why. Measuring weight is a useful tool in combination with height to determine the child's BMI. It indicates if the child is under-or overweight for that child's age and gender. Additionally, it provides accurate medication and fluid requirements

When and Where. Weight should be taken in the morning for accuracy and should be taken on each visit to clinic, doctor, or hospital admission

How. Follow universal precautions at all times. For neonates and infants remove all clothing and nappy. Children should wear minimal clothing and remove shoes. Use either baby scales or chair. Ensure scales are zeroed and place or ask the child to sit in the chair with feet on the ledge provided to ensure all weight is evenly spread

Document. Always document on the correct boy or girl growth chart, the child's healthcare records, and local documentation paperwork

Figure 58.3 Measuring height.

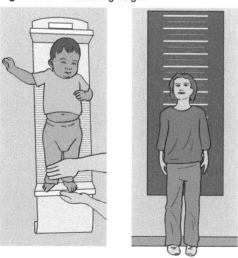

Why. In order to determine if a child is growing at a healthy rate. Measuring height is also a useful tool in combination with height to determine a child's BMI

When and Where. Height should be taken in the morning for accuracy and should be taken on each visit to clinic, doctor, or hospital admission

How. <2 years: the child should lie supine and measurement be taken on a roller mat. >2 years: or a standing height recorder. Feet should remain together and flat on the floor. The body should be straight with the head at 90° and the bottom against the backboard

Document. Always document on the correct boy or girl growth chart, the child's healthcare records, and local documentation paperwork

Children and Young People's Nursing at a Glance, Second Edition. Edited by Elizabeth Gormley-Fleming and Sheila Roberts.
© 2023 John Wiley & Sons Ltd. Published 2023 by John Wiley & Sons Ltd.

Definition

The assessment of a child's growth involves the serial measurement of their length or height and their weight and then comparing these to growth standards. Growth reference standards have been determined from worldwide research on children who were receiving recommended feeding and care. This arrived at the prescriptive standard rather than the descriptive references for growth. Growth charts or percentile charts are used to follow the measurements of a baby or child to ensure they are following a predictable trend. The lines on the chart are called centile lines. These provide a guide to show the expected growth rate over time. Deviation from the expected rate of growth is easily identifiable and can identify children at risk of becoming undernourished or obese.

Background

The World Health Organization (WHO) growth charts are now used throughout the UK for the documentation of children's head circumference (Figure 58.1), weight (Figure 58.2), height/length (Figure 58.3), and body mass index (BMI). The centile measurements are based upon statistics from breastfed children of non-smoking parents. The charts are suitable for all ethnicities. They represent the normal growth a healthy child should follow, providing professionals with a tool to monitor whether a child is growing (or developing through puberty) as expected. The newer charts (Childhood and Puberty Close Monitoring [CPCM] charts), published in June 2013, allow for closer monitoring of children who may be of concern due to growth, nutritional, or puberty problems.

Who can use them?

The centile charts can be used for every baby or child, irrespective of how they are fed. Although the data were collected from breastfed babies to determine the centiles, these do not impact the interpretation of the results. Establishing breastfed babies as the model for normal growth and development has helped raise the profile of breastfeeding from a public and policy perspective.

The charts provide a quick snapshot of how a baby or child is developing according to their weight and height. It is important to discuss with parents the results and if the baby moves from either above or below two centiles of the baseline centile line. This needs to be discussed to find out if there are any causes and how support can be provided, and additional weight measurements need to be taken.

Potential triggers

There are a multitude of reasons that a child may not be growing as anticipated. For instance, a greater than expected increase in head circumference may indicate hydrocephalus. There may also be safeguarding reasons why a child may not follow a centile, for instance in cases of neglect the child may not gain weight as expected. These triggers should not be ignored and a full assessment should be carried out by a qualified healthcare professional.

The following charts are available:
- Early years chart 0–4 years
- Neonatal and Infant Close Monitoring (NICM) chart
- Personal Child Health Record (PCHR) charts – otherwise known as the 'red book'
- UK Down's syndrome chart (DS) 0–18 years
- School-age charts 2–18
- CPCM chart
- BMI chart (https://www.rcpch.ac.uk/resources/growth-charts)

Further information can be found on the RCPCH website.

Key points

- The appropriate chart must be selected for the correct monitoring purpose and the child's age.
- The instructions on the chart must be followed exactly to ensure accurate records.
- Healthcare professionals must remember to date, time, and sign their entries in the documentation.
- Any deviation from expected growth (e.g. sudden increase in head circumference) should be investigated by an appropriate professional.

59 Child development: 0–5 years

Figure 59.1   Fine motor development.

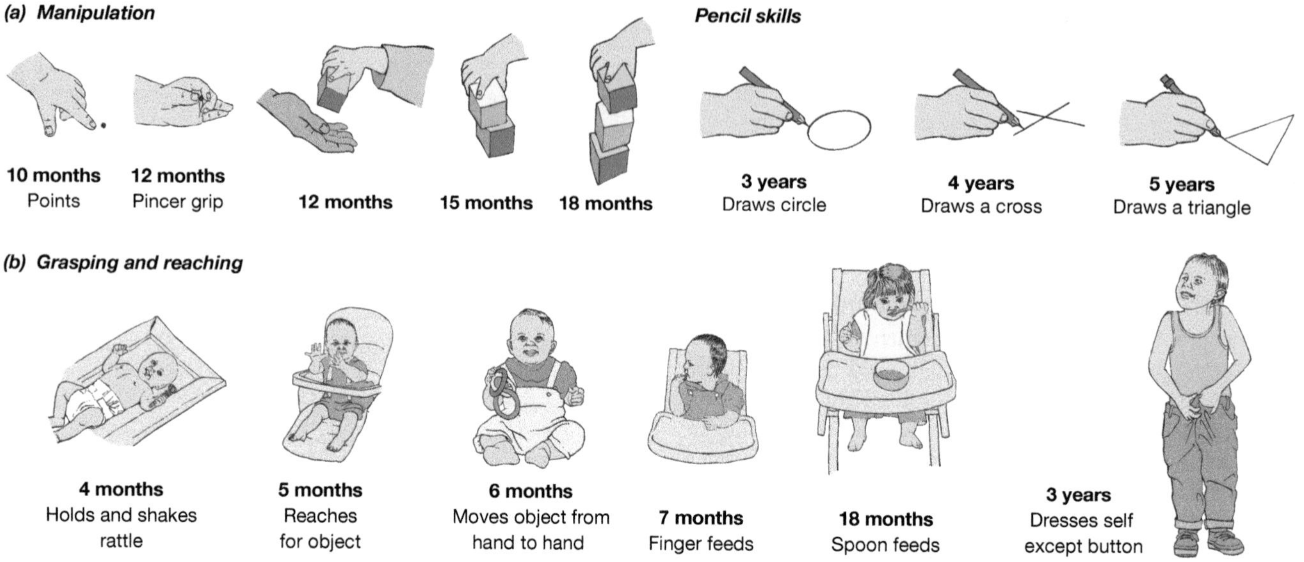

(a) Manipulation

  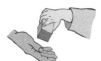 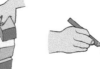

10 months
Points

12 months
Pincer grip

12 months

15 months   **18 months**

Pencil skills

 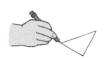

3 years
Draws circle

4 years
Draws a cross

5 years
Draws a triangle

(b) Grasping and reaching

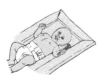   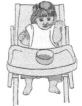 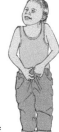

4 months
Holds and shakes
rattle

5 months
Reaches
for object

6 months
Moves object from
hand to hand

7 months
Finger feeds

18 months
Spoon feeds

3 years
Dresses self
except button

Figure 59.2   Speech and language.

3 months Vocalizes	**18 months** 10 words
8 months Dada mama	**24 months** 2 linked words
12 months 2 words with meaning	**3 years** Full sentences

Figure 59.3   Social development.

6 weeks
Smiles

4 months
Laughs

 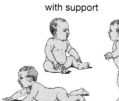

9 months
Plays peek a boo

About 2.5 years
Toilet trained by day

Figure 59.4   Gross motor development.

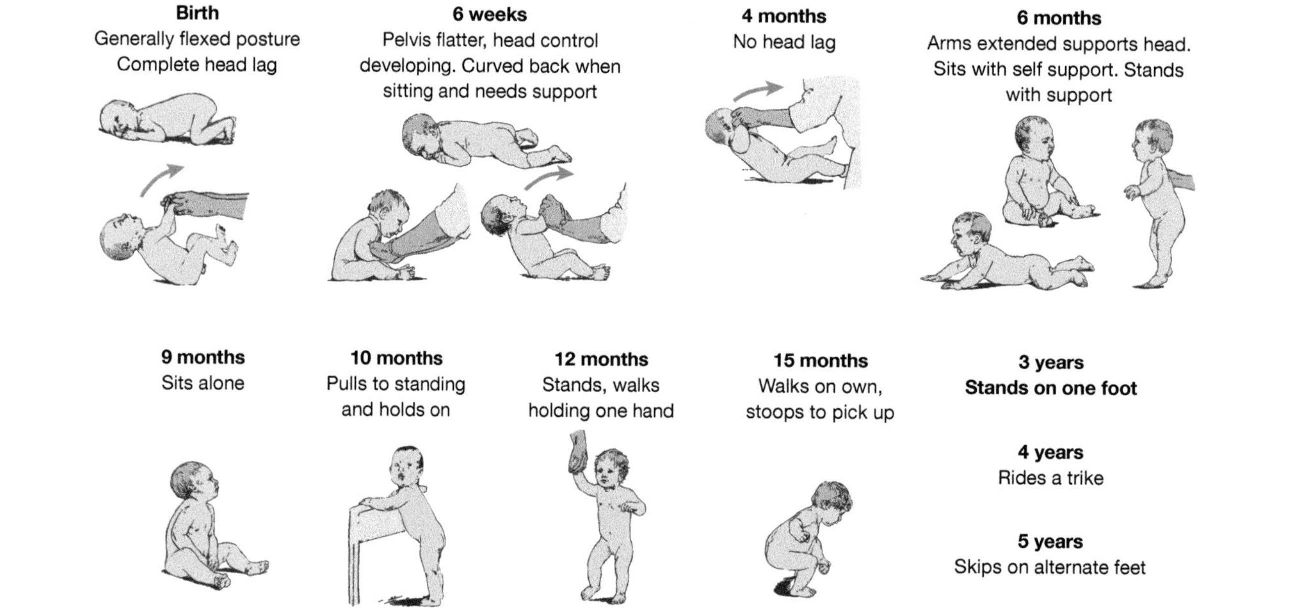

Birth
Generally flexed posture
Complete head lag

6 weeks
Pelvis flatter, head control
developing. Curved back when
sitting and needs support

4 months
No head lag

6 months
Arms extended supports head.
Sits with self support. Stands
with support

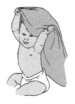 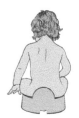

9 months
Sits alone

10 months
Pulls to standing
and holds on

12 months
Stands, walks
holding one hand

15 months
Walks on own,
stoops to pick up

3 years
Stands on one foot

4 years
Rides a trike

5 years
Skips on alternate feet

  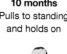   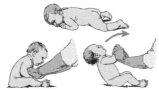

Children and Young People's Nursing at a Glance, Second Edition. Edited by Elizabeth Gormley-Fleming and Sheila Roberts.
© 2023 John Wiley & Sons Ltd. Published 2023 by John Wiley & Sons Ltd.

Growth and development occur throughout the lifespan. Growth is an increase in the size and number of cells, resulting in an increase in the size and weight of the whole, or any of its parts. It occurs in a continuous pattern, the pace varies, and the most rapid growth takes place *in utero*, in the first two years of life, and in adolescence. Growth of the infant is measured by estimating the weight, length, head circumference, and, in some instances, skinfold thickness.

Development is the increase in complexity of the individual, involving structure and function, and the emerging of an individual's capacities through learning, growth, and maturation. Development is measured using developmental scales and follows patterns of development (Table 59.1).

Development is divided into four major areas:
• *Gross motor*: gross motor skills, primitive reflexes, and postural responses.
• *Fine motor*: fine motor skills and vision (Figure 59.1).
• *Communication*: non-verbal communication, speech and language, and hearing (Figure 59.2).
• *Psychological*: emotional, behavioural, social (Figure 59.3).

Factors influencing growth and development include prenatal and birth factors, genetic and chromosomal factors, health status, psychosocial factors including socioeconomic status, intrauterine and postnatal nutrition, and hormonal milieu.

Growth is rapid in the first year of life. Length is increased length by 50%, most of it occurring in the trunk. Weight doubles by the age of 5–6 months and triples by the end of the first year. The posterior fontanelle is usually closed by 2 months. Growth slows during the second year, with toddlers growing approximately 9–12.5 cm/year and gaining 220 g/month, and head circumference increasing 2.5 cm/year. The anterior fontanelle closes between 12 and 18 months. By the age of 2 years, birth weight has quadrupled to an average of 12.3 kg, the child is about half their adult height, and has 20 teeth (Figure 59.4). At 2–3 years, toddlers grow 5–6.5 cm, gain 1.5–2.5 kg, and head circumference has slowed to an increase of approximately 1.3 cm/year. Preschool children grow about 6.5–7.5 cm/year and gain 1.5–2.5 kg, weighing on average 14.5 kg. Not all body systems grow at the same rate. Full maturation is not complete until the end of the second decade.

Development is checked by assessing developmental milestones that children should reach by a certain age, some of which are essential to remember (Tables 59.1–59.3).

Normal infant reflexes

Neonatal behaviour is controlled by reflex. These reach a peak at 4–8 weeks of age and then begin to diminish from about 3 months, except for the protective reflexes that include blink, parachute, cough, swallow, and gag.

Table 59.1 Patterns of development.

Pattern	Path of progression	Examples
Cephalocaudal	From head to toe	Head control precedes the ability to walk
Proximodistal	From the trunk to the tips of the extremities	The neonate can move arms and legs, but cannot pick up objects with fingers
General to specific	From simple tasks to more complex	Progression from crawling to walking to skipping

Table 59.2 Dental development.

Baby teeth	Erupt (months)	Lost (years)
Central incisor	8–12	6–7
Lateral incisor	9–13	7–8
Canine	16–22	10–12
First molar	13–19	9–11
Second molar	25–33	10–12

Table 59.3 Essential developmental milestones.

Age	Milestone
4–6 weeks	Fixes to faces with eyes
	Smiles in response
6–7 months	Sits up unsupported
9 months	Gets to a sitting position
10 months	Pincer grasp
	Waves goodbye
12 months	Walks unsupported
	Two or three words with meaning
18 months	Feeds self with spoon
	Points to things
	Tower of three to four cubes
	Throws a ball without falling
24 months	Sentences of two to three words
	Runs
	Kicks a ball

Key points
• The children's nurse must be knowledgeable about normal growth patterns and expected developmental milestones or 'windows of achievement' in order to undertake a holistic assessment of the child.
• Development is a highly interactive process and outcomes are influenced by the child's environment and family life.
• Monitoring of the child's physical growth can provide an indication of potential risk of undernutrition or obesity.

60 Child development: 5–16 years

Figure 60.1 Child development 5–16 years.

Physical changes are less obvious than at 0–5 years

Children grow taller, change shape, and acquire new skills.
- By 5 years, the child's height and weight are increasing steadily at the rate of 5 cm and 2–3 kg/year
- Boys are on average 2.5 cm taller and 1 kg heavier than girls during early school years; however, by 12 years girls are both taller and heavier than boys

Age 6
Swings by arms, and skips with rope

Age 7
'Walks the plank', uses a bat and ball

Age 8–10
Hopscotch, skipping games

5–7 years
Reorganization of the brain occurs and ability to memorize and reason improves

By 7 years
Growth is nearly complete at 90% of final size. The volume of grey matter increases, continuing to the second decade

Shape of the child's face changes from infancy to adulthood

- Eruption of permanent teeth forces the shape of the jaw to change
- The jaw grows forward and the forehead becomes more prominent
- The head and eyes are extra large in children, and by the age of 8 years the child's head is 90% of its adult size

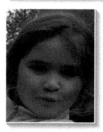
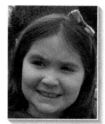
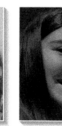

Pubertal growth spurt
- The rate of growth can double
- The final 20–25% of linear growth is achieved; this can be as much as 12.5 cm in a peak year
- Girls gain an average of 5–20 cm in height and 7–25 kg in weight
- Boys gain 10–30 cm in height and 7–30 kg in weight

Raging hormones
Testosterone production in boys rockets to 18x that of childhood and oestrogen 8x in girls

The normal age of menarche varies between 9 and 18 years

Developmental tasks of adolescence
- Leaving biological family
- Achieving a new relationship with parents
- Developing intimate, nurturing, and caring relationships outside family
- Finding a career based on interest and capacity
- Becoming at ease with sexuality
- From dependence to independence… and to interdependence
- Change from concrete to abstract cognitive thinking
- Thinking about thinking
- Making more and more complicated decisions, analysing, and hypothesizing

Figure 60.2 Growth rates for girls and boys.

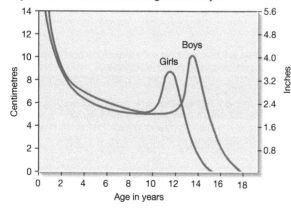
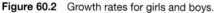

Figure 60.3 Chain of hormonal events in puberty.

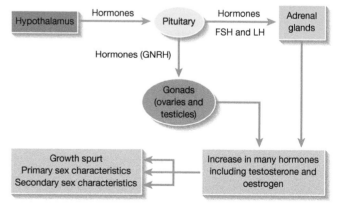

Children and Young People's Nursing at a Glance, Second Edition. Edited by Elizabeth Gormley-Fleming and Sheila Roberts.
© 2023 John Wiley & Sons Ltd. Published 2023 by John Wiley & Sons Ltd.

Figure 60.4 Sequence and range of sexual development in puberty.

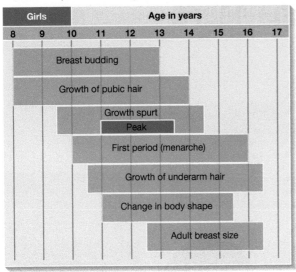

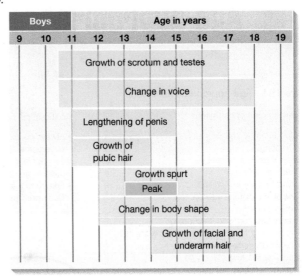

Between 5 years and puberty the physical changes in children are less obvious than at 0–5 years. However, as would be expected, children grow taller, change shape, and acquire new skills. The 5-year-old draws a recognizable person or house, and writes their own name. They can hop, skip, swing, jump, balance, climb, dance, and throw a ball. They also ride a two-wheel bicycle and begin to choose their own friends. They can undress and dress except for laces and ties and perform domestic and dramatic play, alone or with friends. Language in middle childhood continues to develop, in both vocabulary and complexity, with the child now able to correct their own mistakes and understand double meanings. There is an acceptance of rules but not necessarily an understanding of them, and the child has a much better grasp of cause and effect.

Physically, the growth of the trunk and extremities now exceeds that of the head, the centre of gravity lowers, and body proportions become slimmer. Growth hormone stimulates longitudinal growth in a dose-dependent manner and is reflected in limb length. Girls stop growing sooner than boys as a result of epiphyseal unity under the effect of oestrogen secretion. Boys' longer growth is reflected in their greater height and longer arms and legs. The extremities grow first, followed by neck, hip, chest, shoulder, trunk, and depth of chest. Muscle growth follows that of bone and is therefore greater in boys. More fat is deposited in girls on the thighs, hips, and buttocks, giving a smoother, more rounded body contour. In the cardiovascular system the systolic blood pressure rises at an accelerated rate during puberty; pulse rate decreases; blood volume, haemoglobin, and red blood cells rise more in boys than in girls; and by adulthood women have 1 million fewer red cells per mL than men. The size and capacity of the respiratory system increase, rate decreases, and boys are able to take in more air at one breath because of their larger chest and shoulder size. This growth is reflected in peak flow rate, with normal ranges increasing from 150 L/min at 5 years to 240 L/min at 10 years and 400 L/min at 15 years. Oestrogen causes the skin of the female to develop a soft, smooth, and thicker texture. The sebaceous glands are particularly active and the eccrine and apocrine sweat glands become fully functional. Body hair takes on the characteristic distribution patterns and the texture changes. The lymphoid system including the tonsils and adenoids decreases in size, improving asthma in some teens, and children start to lose their deciduous teeth. Permanent teeth appear at about the rate of four per year between the ages of 7 and 14 years (Figure 60.1).

Adolescence is a time of continued brain growth. There is no actual increase in number of neurons, but growth of the myelin sheath continues until at least puberty, thus enabling faster neural processing that corresponds with the development of cognitive abilities. The more mature the brain, the more the prefrontal cortex works as a mechanism that enables a serious 'second thought' as decisions are made. This ability expresses itself in self-control and judgement. Younger teens may respond with less maturity because their brains are less mature. In early childhood and again at the onset of puberty, the prefrontal cortex fires up with new growth and millions of new neuro-connections are made, yet, after each growth spurt, the brain prunes away unused or unneeded connections. The connections that remain are more efficient, more powerful, and stronger. Research suggests that growth and changes in the prefrontal cortex continue well into the teen years.

During the pubertal growth spurt the rate of growth may double. The final 20–25% of linear growth is achieved; this can be as much as 12.5 cm in a peak year. Girls gain an average of 5–20 cm in height and 7–25 kg in weight. Boys gain 10–30 cm in height and 7–30 kg in weight (Figure 60.2).

The biological changes of puberty, which are considered to begin in adolescence, are universal, but their expression, timing, and extent show enormous variety depending on sex genes and nutrition. Puberty is triggered by a chain of hormonal effects controlled by the anterior pituitary in response to a stimulus from the hypothalamus (Figure 60.3).

During puberty, sexual development can be seen to occur in a set sequence, with variations in timing between individuals (Figure 60.4).

There are features of adolescent development that occur universally: the onset of puberty causes biological changes; the emergence of more advanced cognitive abilities is seen in cognitive changes and developing self-image; intimacy and relations with others demonstrate emotional changes; and finally the transition into new roles in society exemplifies social changes.

Key points

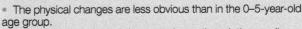

- The physical changes are less obvious than in the 0–5-year-old age group.
- Brain growth during adolescence is continued, the myelin sheath growth continues, and this enhances cognitive ability.
- Sexual development occurs in a set sequence with some variation in timing for individuals.

61 Age-appropriate behaviours

Figure 61.1 Age-appropriate behaviour.

Determinants of behaviour

- Chronological age
- Parenting
- Developmental progress
- Prematurity
- Overall health and wellbeing
- Social and cultural environment
- Socialization
- Family structure and functioning
- Presence of illnesses or conditions in the child
- The child's global development
- Social functioning
- Impact of school and peers

Issues to consider

- Child's social and cultural circumstances
- Parenting behaviours and competence
- Parental reports of behaviour
- Where the child has a specific illness or condition impacting upon growth and development
- Children with learning disabilities
- Children with mental health problems
- Any history of abuse
- Bullying
- Substance misuse
- Influence of peer groups and antisocial behaviours

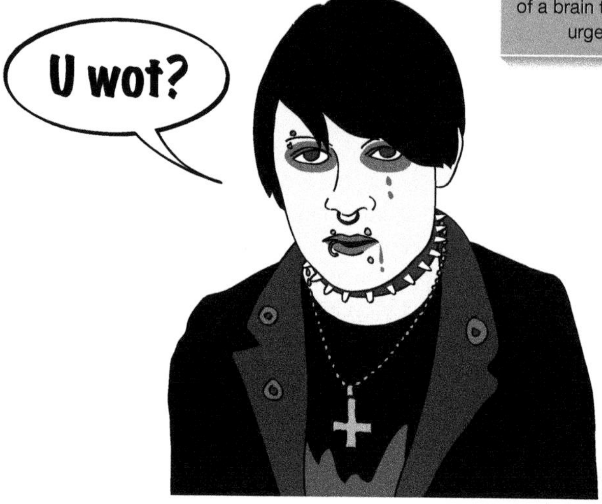

Observation and record keeping

- Always consider the need to record growth, development, events, and behaviours
- Be open and honest about issues when the need arises
- Adhere to the Nursing and Midwifery Council Code principles on record keeping and referral

Warning!

Any sudden and unexplained behavioural change in children could be due to the presence of a brain tumour and so needs urgent assessment

U wot?

Age-appropriate sexual behaviours TRAFFIC LIGHT SYSTEM		Example
RED	Outside healthy and safe behaviours for age. In need of immediate protection and support from professionals – GP, social worker, health visitor	Birth – 5 years: persistent touching of genitals 5-9 years: persistent masturbation, possibly in front of others 9-12 years: sending nudes or sexually provocative images via social media 13-18 years: compulsive masturbation, exposing genitals, sexual harassment
AMBER	Area of concern. Has potential to become unsafe and outside health behaviour if they persist. Requires a response from relevant protective adult with close monitoring	Birth – 5 years: pulling other children's clothing down 5-9 years: questions about sexual activity, engaging in mutual masturbation 9-12 years: behavioural changes, provocative dressing, bullying involving sexual aggression, sharing contact details with online acquaintances 13-18 years: sexual preoccupation, preoccupation with online chatting, sexual aggression
GREEN	Natural and expected behaviour. It does not mean that these behaviours should continue, but they should provide an opportunity for discussion and education	Birth – 5 years: body stroking and holding genitals 5-9 years: masturbation to self-soothe, increased curiosity about adult sexuality 9-12 years: use of sexualised language, having a boyfriend/girlfriend 13-18 years: sexually explicit conversations with peers. Flirting, interest in erotica, sexual activity, consenting oral sex

Assessing the development and behaviours of children encompasses a wide range of approaches measuring growth, cognitive ability, educational performance, and social maturation, and also in specific circumstances such as behaviours in children with disorders (Figure 61.1). These methods help us to understand whether children are developing, evidenced through their behaviours, as well as identifying when they are not and the possible reasons for this. It is only through knowledge of what is appropriate at a certain age or level of development that nurses, and others, are able to identify delays. While it is possible to assess, measure, and monitor development, children are individual in terms of their growth, self, health, and wellbeing, all of which are influenced by their circumstances, culture, family, and socialization. Changes in technology, availability of information, and education also impact upon development and are issues to consider. Ultimately, children follow similar patterns of growth and development, some variance being deemed acceptable. However, absent, delayed, or inappropriate behaviours are issues of concern and need to be identified, assessed, and addressed appropriately.

Growth

Growth of children generally follows a similar pattern, which is reflective of bone and neuromuscular development; this is the same on both sides of the body. Such growth and development can be assessed using age- and sex-appropriate growth charts that plot weight, height, head circumference, and body mass index. These are based on averages for children of similar ages and stages of development, and so allow the practitioner to ascertain any abnormalities or deviations, particularly in behaviour.

Development

Biological growth is the foundation for the child's overall development. However, as they age, so do their abilities, skills, and communication. These can be understood with reference to assessing the following factors.

Physical development

While growth continues, the child develops the psycho-motor skills necessary to function, which in turns supports their physical and non-verbal behaviour.

Cognitive development

Cognitive development includes aspects of personality, reasoning, and concepts of self. The ways in which the child behaves clearly reflect all of the above and are particularly influenced by the relationships they have with carers.

Language development

Language acquisition is a crucial aspect of children's functioning and behaviour. Not only does it reflect their development, it is a part of how others perceive a child's behaviour.

Social development

Children learn social behaviours through observing others (predominantly parents and peers) and by conditioning (e.g. rewards). Role models are critically important for social learning and it is with reference to these that children develop their own behaviours. Poor or dysfunctional role models may thus lead to the child developing and displaying inappropriate behaviours.

Age-inappropriate behaviours

There are a wide range of circumstances, conditions, and illnesses that can result in age-inappropriate behaviour, impede appropriate behaviour, or influence overall development.

Peer influence

Peers are a powerful influence on behaviour and can be valuable in developing a sense of esteem, group ownership, and appropriate social behaviour. Equally, the shared behaviours of the group may be perceived as inappropriate and potentially antisocial.

Drug- and alcohol-mediated behaviour

There is an increasing concern about young people's access to and use of alcohol and illegal drugs. Consumption of these may be linked to intrafamilial issues such as parental use, co-presence of family/parental discord and dysfunction, as well as child abuse. Peer groups are also a powerful influence on children participating in taking alcohol or drugs. Both substances impact on behaviour, often leading to disruption, antisocial incidents, criminal acts, self-harming, and suicide, in addition to the impact on their physiology.

Child criminal exploitation

Children and young people can be coerced into storing and transporting drugs to suburban areas and towns for payment by gangs. These are highly organized and sophisticated networks of criminals who will use children and young people to take the majority of risks and to undertake criminal activities from which they will distance themselves. There are other forms of criminal exploitation too, such as sexual exploitation, gang and knife crime, and trafficking.

Hospitalization

Children with chronic illness often attend hospital and are exposed to adult behaviour, medical language, and environments that may impact on their development. As children develop, they may be perceived as being manipulative, 'knowing too much', and adult-like in their behaviours.

Sexualized behaviour

Sexual behaviour and relationships are often difficult issues for young people and their parents to contend with. Nonetheless, some children display behaviours such as showing body parts, inappropriate touching, kissing, and use of sexual language. When these occur, particularly at younger ages, it can be suggestive of child sexual abuse, access to pornography, or mental health problems.

Learning disabilities

The many conditions that lead to learning disabilities mean that children may display a wide range of behaviours that could be considered age inappropriate. These can be linked to the child's intellectual disability.

Mental health conditions

While mental health conditions will not cause age-inappropriate behaviour, they may impact on the child's overall development. In such cases the child may 'act out' or display behaviours that are considered not to be consistent with the norm.

Key points

- Children's and young people's nurses must be knowledgeable about the stages of physical growth, development, and behaviours across the lifespan.
- Assessment tools such as HEADSSS (see Chapters 1 and 11) may be useful in ascertaining the behaviours of the young person.
- All physical measurements should be plotted on an age- and sex-appropriate percentile chart.

62 Common behavioural problems of childhood

Figure 62.1 Behaviour problems and strategies.

The crying baby

- Wet or dirty nappy
- Too hot or too cold
- Hungry
- Wind
- Colic
- Environmental stress
- Reflux oesophagitis
- Teething

If sudden severe crying, consider:
- Any acute illness
- Otitis media
- Intussusception
- Strangulated inguinal hernia

Temper tantrums

- Normal, peak at 18–36 months
- Screaming
- Hitting
- Biting
- Breath-holding attacks

Strategies that may help
- Avoid precipitants such as hunger and tiredness
- Divert the tantrum by distraction
- Stay calm to teach control
- Reward good behaviour
- Try to ignore bad behaviour until calm
- Use time out

Sleeping problems

- Difficulty getting to sleep
- Waking during the night
- Sleeping in parents' bed
- Nightmares and night terrors

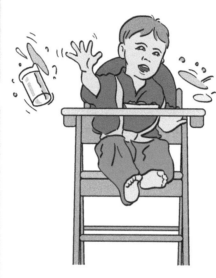

Eating problems in toddlers

- Food refusal
- Fussy eating – only eating a limited variety of foods
- Overeating
- Battles over eating and mealtimes
- Snacking
- Excessive drinking of juice

Unwanted habits

- Thumb sucking
- Nail biting
- Masturbation
- Head banging
- Hair pulling
- Bedwetting
- Encopresis (passing faeces in inappropriate places)

Aggressive behaviour

- Temper tantrums
- Hitting and biting other children
- Destroying toys
- Destroying furniture
- Commoner in boys and in larger families
- May reflect aggression within family
- Requires calm, consistent approach
- Avoid countering with aggression
- Use time out and star charts

Box 62.1 What you need from your evaluation.

History

- Ask what is troubling the parents most – is it the child or other stresses in their lives, such as tiredness, problems at work, or marital problems?
- What are the triggers for difficult or unwanted behaviour? Does it occur when the child is hungry or tired, or at any particular time of day?
- Colic tends to occur in the evenings; tantrums may be more common if the child is tired
- Does the behaviour happen consistently in all settings or is it specific to one place, e.g. the toddler may behave well at nursery but show difficult behaviour at home?
- Does the behaviour differ with each parent?
- How do the parents deal with the behaviour – do they get angry or aggressive, are they consistent, do they use bribery, or do they give in to the toddler eventually?
- What strategies have the parents already tried to deal with the situation?
- Is there any serious risk of harm? Some behaviour, such as encopresis or deliberate self-harm, may reflect serious emotional upset. Most toddlers who are faddy eaters are growing well and do not suffer any long-term nutritional problems
- Babies with colic are usually less than 3 months old, go red in the face with a tense abdomen, and draw up their legs. The episodes start abruptly and end with the passage of flatus or faeces

Examination

- The history usually contributes more than a physical examination
- If the parents are concerned about sudden-onset or severe crying in a baby, it is important to exclude serious infection such as meningitis or urinary tract infection, intussusception, hernias, and otitis media

Management

- In most cases the parents can be reassured that the behaviour is very common, often normal, and that with time and common sense it can be controlled
- With tantrums it can be helpful to use the ABC approach:
  - **A** What antecedents were there? What happened to trigger the episode?
  - **B** What was the behaviour? Could it be modified, diverted, or stopped?
  - **C** What were the consequences of the behaviour? Was the child told off, shouted at, or given a cuddle?
- Generally, it is best to reward good behaviour (catch the child being good) and ignore bad behaviour. Star charts can be very useful: the child gets a star for good behaviour (staying in bed, etc.) and then a reward after several stars
- Parents should try hard not to be angry or aggressive as this may reinforce attention-seeking behaviour

Children and Young People's Nursing at a Glance, Second Edition. Edited by Elizabeth Gormley-Fleming and Sheila Roberts.
© 2023 John Wiley & Sons Ltd. Published 2023 by John Wiley & Sons Ltd.

Common emotional and behavioural problems

These problems are seen so often that many would regard them as normal, although in a small minority of children the behaviour is so disruptive that it causes major family upset. GPs, paediatricians, and health visitors should be comfortable giving basic guidance on behaviour management to help parents through what can be a stressful, exasperating, and exhausting phase of their child's development (Figure 62.1 and Box 62.1).

Crying babies and colic

Crying is a normal physiological behaviour and is usually periodic and related to discomfort, stress, or temperament. However, it may indicate a serious problem, particularly if the onset is sudden. In most instances it is just a case of ensuring that the baby is well fed, warm but not too hot, has a clean nappy, comfortable clothes, and a calm and peaceful environment. A persistently crying baby can be very stressful for inexperienced parents. It is important that they recognize when they are no longer coping and are offered support. On average a baby between 6 and 8 weeks old will cry for 2–3 hours per day.

Excessive crying is a term used to describe periodic crying affecting infants in the first three months of life. It was previously referred to as infantile colic, a term that is somewhat outdated but may still be used by parents. The crying is paroxysmal, and may be associated with hunger, swallowed air, or discomfort from overfeeding or tiredness. It often occurs in the evenings. Crying can last for several hours, with a flushed face, distended and tense abdomen, and drawn-up legs. In between attacks the child is happy and well.

Excessive crying is associated with certain high-risk factors such as maternal depression or abusive head trauma. A sudden onset of irritability and crying in the young baby is a notable concern.

It is important to consider more serious pathology such as intussusception, infection, non-immunoglobulin (Ig)E cow milk or soy protein allergy, lactose overload, or gastroesophageal reflux. Excessive crying is managed by excluding medical causes, parental education and reassurance, and assessing the emotional status of the parents. Screening for postnatal depression should take place, as excessive crying is linked to higher rates of postnatal depression.

Feeding problems

Weaning is a crucial period in a child's life and a period of significant change. Baby-led weaning is a popular alternative approach to spoon feeding. Baby-led weaning promotes self-feeding in infants from the age of 6 months onwards. The child is in control of the weaning process. Food preferences, eating behaviours, and body weight are all influenced during this period.

Toddler eating habits can be unpredictable – eating large amounts at one meal and sometimes hardly anything at the next. At this age, mealtimes can easily become a battle and it is important that they are kept relaxed and the child is not pressurized into eating. Small portions that the child can finish work best, and second portions can be given if wanted. Eating together as a family encourages the child to eat in a social context.

Sleeping problems

Babies and children differ in the amount of sleep they need and parents vary in how they tolerate their child waking at night. In most cases sleeping 'difficulties' are really just habits that have developed through lack of a clear bedtime routine. Difficulty sleeping may also reflect conflict in the family or anxieties, for example about starting school or fear of dying. Successfully tackling sleeping problems requires determination, support, and reassurance.

- *Refusal to settle at night*: Difficulty settling may develop if babies are only put to bed once they are asleep. A clear bedtime routine is important for older children, for example a bath, a story, and a drink.
- *Waking during the night*: This often causes a lot of stress as the parents become exhausted. It is important to reassure the child, then put them back to bed quietly. Sometimes a technique of 'controlled crying' can be helpful – the child is left to cry for a few minutes, then reassured and left again, this time for longer. Taking the child into the parents' bed is understandable, but usually stores up problems for later when it is difficult to break the habit.
- *Nightmares*: The child wakes as the result of a bad dream, quickly becomes lucid, and can usually remember the content. The child should be reassured and returned to sleep. If particularly severe or persistent, nightmares may reflect stresses and may need psychological help.
- *Night terrors*: Night terrors occur in the preschool years. The child wakes up confused, disorientated, and frightened and may not recognize their parent. They take several minutes to become orientated and the dream content cannot be recalled. These episodes should not be confused with epilepsy. They are short-lived and just require reassurance, especially for the parents.

Temper tantrums

Tantrums are very common in the third year of life (the 'terrible twos') and are part of the child learning the boundaries of acceptable behaviour and parental control. They can be extremely challenging, especially when they occur in public.

The key to dealing with toddler tantrums is to try to avoid getting into the situation in the first place. This does not mean giving in to the child's every demand, but ensuring the child does not get overtired or hungry, and setting clear boundaries in a calm, consistent way. It is generally best to ignore the tantrum until the child calms down. If this fails, then 'time out' can be a useful technique. The child is taken to a safe, quiet environment, such as a bedroom, and left for a few minutes (one minute for each year of age is a good guide) until calm. This is usually very effective, as it removes the attention the child desires, and allows the parents time to control their own anger.

Unwanted or aggressive behaviour

Young children often have aggressive outbursts that may involve biting, hitting, or scratching other children. These require consistent, firm management, with use of time out and star charts for good behaviour. It is important not to respond with more aggression, as this sends conflicting messages. If aggressive behaviour is persistent, it is important to explore other tensions or disturbances within the family. In older children, the school may need to be involved.

Unwanted behaviours such as thumb sucking, hair pulling, nail biting, and masturbation are also common in young children. Most can be ignored and resolve with time. Masturbation can usually be prevented by distracting the child or dressing them in clothes that make it more difficult. Older children should not be reprimanded, but informed that the behaviour is not acceptable in public.

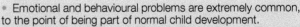

Key points

- Emotional and behavioural problems are extremely common, to the point of being part of normal child development.
- Parents need to be encouraged that they can manage most behaviour with a clear strategy.
- A calm, confident, consistent approach to the child's behaviour is recommended.
- Parents should reward good behaviour and try to minimize attention given to undesirable behaviour.

63 Adolescent development

Figure 63.1 Who am I and how am I?

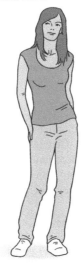

I need services that …

• Treat me with respect and make me feel welcome

• Have staff who are professional, knowledgeable, trustworthy, value me, and know how to help me

• Listen, understand me, appreciate my concerns, and enable me to make informed choices

• Will not be shocked by my behaviour or lifestyle and can signpost me to other services if I need them

• Are accessible at times and locations that are suitable to me

• I can trust to treat what I say in confidence unless I am at risk of harm

• Develop and improve in response to my feedback

Figure 63.2 Adolescent brain development.

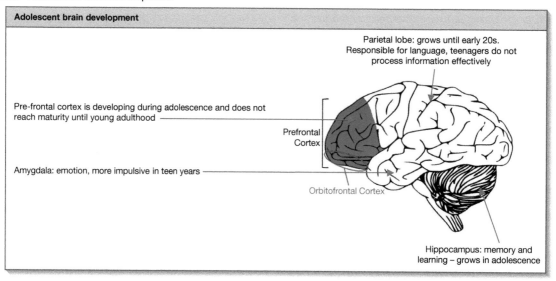

Adolescent brain development

Parietal lobe: grows until early 20s. Responsible for language, teenagers do not process information effectively

Pre-frontal cortex is developing during adolescence and does not reach maturity until young adulthood

Prefrontal Cortex

Amygdala: emotion, more impulsive in teen years

Orbitofrontal Cortex

Hippocampus: memory and learning – grows in adolescence

Brain development: Age 10 – 18 years

Limbic system intensifies during puberty
Rapid emotional, cognitive, rational, and social growth
Risk-taking behaviour

Brain development: Age 18 – 25 years
Pre-frontal cortex continues to develop – controls impulses
Executive functions – ability to consider consequences
Greater control over actions
Less risk-taking behaviour and more balanced judgements

Risk-taking behaviour is a normal part of adolescent development. *Source:* Alex from the Rock / Adobe Stock.

Children and Young People's Nursing at a Glance, Second Edition. Edited by Elizabeth Gormley-Fleming and Sheila Roberts.
© 2023 John Wiley & Sons Ltd. Published 2023 by John Wiley & Sons Ltd.

Adolescence is a period of development that presents the individual with numerous challenges as they progress through the transition from childhood to young adulthood. Growth and maturation make new behaviours possible, provide opportunities for intellectual development and learning, but also present hurdles and challenges to be overcome as new relationships develop and new experiences are encountered. These changes are important to young people because they determine experience, impact on how others view and respond to them, and influence the ways in which they see themselves. They also determine the path from education to the world of work and financial independence.

Physical development

The teenage years mean rapid physical change for both boys and girls. Teenagers experience a growth spurt of several inches a years for several years. Individual differences will be widespread because of factors such as sex and genetic inheritance. Physical changes involve the skeletal and nervous systems, leading to changes in shape and proportion, for example significant changes to hands and feet, arms and legs, and trunk. Strengthening of bones continues and is associated with thickening muscle fibres in boys and increased fat deposits in the breasts and hips in girls. Puberty also results in the development of sex characteristics, which further differentiate the sexes. Hormonal upheaval may also affect teenage time-keeping and sleep patterns; the sleep hormone melatonin, for example, is released at about 10 p.m. in adults, but not until 1 a.m. in teenagers.

Brain development and changes in cognition (thinking)

The cerebral cortex of the brain governs learning and is concerned with increasingly complex thought, perception, language and memory, reflexivity, and empathy as connections between neural pathways are made in response to repeated experiences. These form the 'hard wiring' of the brain and nervous system, a process that will be most successful with repeated positive learning experiences and less effective during periods of stress or inconsistency. Significant periods in the hard wiring of the brain have recently been shown to occur at around the age of 2 years and during the early teens when the synaptic connections are pruned and reorganized (Figure 63.1). During early and mid-adolescence, young people may rely on more primitive areas of the brain, leading to increased impulsivity and risk taking. Gradually, increased myelinization of the new connections in the frontal cortex leads to an ability to transmit messages more effectively, hold in mind more multidimensional concepts, and think in a more strategic manner. These science-based understandings based on modern imaging techniques are consistent with the ideas of the cognitive developmental psychologist Jean Piaget (1951), who saw early adolescence as a period characterized by new ways of thinking as the young person moves from thought processes based on concrete reasoning to more abstract thinking. This means that teenagers are likely to be more reflective in their thinking, and more concerned with ethical and philosophical dilemmas such as their place in society, moral issues, altruism, politics, and the meaning of life.

Identity

Erik Erikson (1950) saw acceptance of both self and society as a task that is especially important between the onset of puberty and young adulthood. He saw this period of development as characterized by an 'identity crisis' when young people struggle to resolve a sense of confusion to establish a consistent sense of themselves, trying out numerous roles to gain a sense of personal integrity and bringing together experiences, values, and aspirations to answer the question 'Who am I?' The young person may discover their place in society or feel they stand outside society. An important aspect of this is maintaining a sense of being true to oneself while at the same time balancing this with the need to conform to the expectations of peers, culture, and wider society. Later, this will lead to the young person becoming less self-absorbed and being able to overcome a sense of isolation to develop an intimate relationship with another person. Erikson's 'storm and stress' view of adolescence has been challenged by other researchers, who argue that the majority of teenagers will go through a relatively smooth transition from childhood to young adulthood.

Changing social relationships

Urie Bronfenbrenner (1979) developed an ecological systems theory to demonstrate that no child or young person will develop in isolation. All young people will be influenced by the sociocultural context within which they live and develop; their family, community, and social institutions; culture and media, generation, and political environment. Most important for young people will be their decreasing dependence on parents and the increasing influence of peers, who may provide a source of friendship, mutual support, and positive learning experiences, but who also may encourage negative health behaviours in more vulnerable young people such as smoking, experimentation with drugs and alcohol, pressure to engage in sexual experimentation, or offending and violent gang culture.

Young people as service users

Young people may access health services from numerous agencies for a variety of reasons (Figure 63.2): access to health information, treatment for health problems, or access to specific services such as stopping smoking, help with drug and alcohol misuse, or contraception and sexual health services. Most young people will treat services with respect, but some may initially present challenging behaviour in order to test out whether they can confidently trust the service provider not to be judgmental or shocked by their concerns. All young people have the right to be treated with dignity and respect and receive services that are accessible, welcoming, and responsive to their needs and concerns, as well as that safeguard their wellbeing. Professionals and practitioners working in these services will need to demonstrate appropriate attitudes and values. They will also need to know about other services that could be additional sources of support for young people in challenging social circumstances.

Key points

- Adolescent development presents unique challenges that will cumulate in the transition to adulthood.
- Brain development continues during adolescence with increased myelination in the frontal cortex, leading to increased ability to think strategically and to be reflective.
- Healthcare professionals need to understand the unique needs of the adolescent and be able to demonstrate the correct attitudes and values to meet those needs.

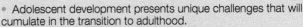

64 Child health promotion

Figure 64.1 What is health promotion?

'Health promotion is the process of enabling people to increase control over, and to improve, their health.'

Health promotion embraces the concept of empowerment, both at an individual and collective level, thus enabling others to make their own decisions and equipping them with resources to determine their health circumstances.

Scenario

Each year a number of children visit their local accident and emergency departments following falls from their bikes. Many sustain head injuries as a direct consequence of not wearing a cycle helmet

There are five key health promotion approaches that can be drawn on to try to remedy this situation :
• Medical
• Behavioural
• Educational
• Client-centred
• Societal change

Figure 64.2 Approaches to health promotion.

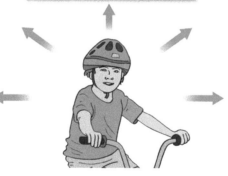

Medical

This approach requires the target population to comply with preventative medical measures. There may be an expectation that medical advice is followed in terms of cycle helmet wearing as this has the potential to reduce head injuries. There could also be an expectation that parents will have ensured that their children have had their immunizations, thus reducing the likelihood of a tetanus infection in the advent of a cycle fall

Behavioural

This approach aims to promote behaviour that reduces the risk of ill-health. The type of healthy behaviours that are expected are normally identified by the professional. Therefore, cycle helmet wearing may be promoted within a school environment; alternatively, a children's nurse may choose to opportunistically promote this to children and their families when they are in the accident and emergency department

Educational

This approach provides people with information, enabling them to make informed decisions. Ideally, children, young people, and families should be given information about the wearing of cycle helmets as well as the opportunity to ask questions. Developmentally appropriate resources should be used to enhance the child's understanding. Individuals are encouraged to make their own decisions based on the knowledge that they have gained

Societal change

This approach modifies the environment, both physically and socially, to make healthier choices the easier ones. Therefore, if it became usual practice, and socially accepted, that everyone wore a cycle helmet, it may make it easier for children and young people to comply

Client-centred

This approach enables children, young people, and families to identify their own health needs. Therefore, unless concerns about cycle helmet wearing are expressed, this would not automatically be addressed by the children's nurse

Figure 64.3 Promoting health to children.

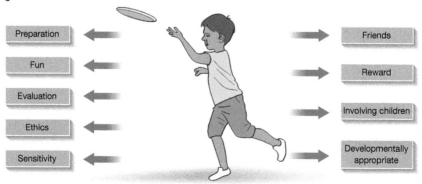

Preparation

Fun

Evaluation

Ethics

Sensitivity

Friends

Reward

Involving children

Developmentally appropriate

Children and Young People's Nursing at a Glance, Second Edition. Edited by Elizabeth Gormley-Fleming and Sheila Roberts.
© 2023 John Wiley & Sons Ltd. Published 2023 by John Wiley & Sons Ltd.

What is child health promotion?

The World Health Organization suggests that 'Health in childhood determines health throughout life and into the next generation . . . Ill health or harmful lifestyle choices in childhood can lead to ill health throughout life, which creates health, financial and social burdens for countries today and tomorrow' (Figure 64.1).

This quote illustrates just how important the promotion of children's health is. Child health promotion focuses upon the enhancement of children's and young people's overall health and wellbeing. There are various approaches that may be considered when promoting health with children (Figure 64.2).

Do children's nurses need to promote health?

Within the Nursing and Midwifery Council's (NMC) standards of proficiency for registered nurses, it clearly indicates that nurses play a key role in improving and maintaining the health and wellbeing of the people they work with. In addition, the Making Every Contact Count (MECC) initiative is now nationally established in the UK. This programme advocates that every healthcare professional supports patients to facilitate healthier choices; there is a clear emphasis placed upon the role of nurses and it is suggested that all nurses, in any context, can make every contact count in order to positively influence the health of their client group. In terms of children's nursing, it may be advising a parent about areas such as children's immunization, sleep requirements, diet, or dental hygiene; alternatively, it may be referring an adolescent who smokes to a Stop Smoking Service.

Involving children

The need to listen to a child or young person's voice and involve them in a range of issues has grown in acceptance and it is now widely established that the views and experiences of children should be taken into account wherever possible. Health promotion is no different and it is essential that children and young people be fully engaged in the promotion of their health from an early age (Figure 64.3).

Engaging with children requires tremendous skill and expertise and there are a range of factors that should be taken into account:
- *Planning*: The child and the nurse need to be clear about the aim of the health promotion initiative. Planning and organization are fundamental if success is to be achieved.
- *Developmental stage*: Considering the child or young person's cognitive developmental stage is crucial. If they do not understand the approach taken, or if the strategy is perceived to be too 'babyish', there will be a lack of engagement. Similarly, physical capability and ability need to be assessed to ensure that appropriate strategies are utilized.
- *Fun*: We all enjoy having fun, so being able to portray a serious health message in an enjoyable and creative manner can be a good way to engage children (particularly those at the primary-school age) and enable them to remember the key issues. For example, a strategy to enhance handwashing may involve educating children about 'germs' and how they are spread. Children could be asked to dip their hands into bright paint, representative of germs, and then use soap and water to remove it. The remains of the paint on the children's hands after washing serve as a demonstration of how germs can then be spread to other areas, such as food.

- *Rewards*: Young children in particular enjoy a reward system (e.g. a certificate or sticker) if they successfully complete a game, for example. However, the older age range are also responsive as long as the 'prize' is age appropriate – wrist bands and pens that reinforce the health message are frequently well received.
- *Friends*: It is widely recognized that children and young people of all ages enjoy spending time with their friends, so health promotion activities that enable this are more likely to be engaging.
- *Sensitivity*: The time and context of any health promotion activity need to be considered. For example, while a child is recovering from an acute illness and family members may well be experiencing increased stress levels, it may not be appropriate to discuss sensitive issues such as a child's excess weight. Perhaps discussion or referral to other health professionals may be more appropriate.

Ethics

Health promotion also presents some ethical challenges. The aim of health promotion is to do good, but sometimes there can be negative outcomes. For example, a children's nurse could advise a teenage girl to reduce her weight as she has a high body mass index, which would be perceived as being in the girl's best interests. However, if the girl started smoking because she had heard that this is a good appetite suppressant, there could be negative consequences. This is one reason why the evaluation of any health promoting activity is so important.

Evaluation

Evaluation is a key aspect of health promotion; in other words, has it worked? Does anything need to be changed for the future? This can be difficult to assess, but it is still important that evaluation is objectively considered. It can include simple strategies such as the children's nurse's reflection on the activity, or feedback from whoever the activity was aimed at.

Where is health promoted to children?

In summary, everywhere. All health professionals have a responsibility to be involved in the promotion of children's health, whether this is in an acute or primary care setting. Schools have been recognized as a key environment in which health can be promoted. However, emphasis has traditionally been upon the promotion of specific health needs around areas such as diet, sexual health, or drug and alcohol abuse, rather than fostering a more holistic and engaging health promotion approach. There is now a recognized need to develop strategies to redress this balance. One way could be the organization of a health promotion 'market', facilitated by health professionals, which exposes children and young people to a range of health promotion initiatives.

Key points

Child health promotion:
- Is the responsibility of all health professionals, including children's nurses.
- Should involve families – in particular parents – as well as the children and young people themselves.
- Must be carefully planned and be appropriate for the development stage and needs of the children or young people.
- Should be evaluated.
- Is complex, but everyone needs to rise to the challenge.

65 Immunity and immunization

Figure 65.1 Immunization.

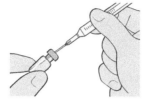

Aims of immunization

- Prevention of infectious diseases and their associated complications
- Prevention of outbreaks of disease
- Eradication of infectious diseases worldwide

Role of the nurse

Nurses are major contributors to immunization programmes. They regularly administer vaccines for childhood immunization programmes (see Chapter 66), annual influenza vaccination campaigns, and travel vaccine schedules

Nursing and Midwifery Council (NMC) Code of Conduct

Nurses have professional accountability when they undertake immunizations. This means that in order to administer immunizations safely and effectively, they have a responsibility to work within their competence and keep their knowledge and skills up to date

When working within the boundaries of their competence nurses ensure that no action or omission is detrimental to patients

Figure 65.2 Safe administration of vaccinations.

Patient Group Direction (PGD)

PGDs are legal written instructions for the supply and administration of vaccines to patients for whom no individual prescription exists

They are used for groups of patients whose requirements and characteristics are consistent

- Patients must meet specific inclusion and exclusion criteria stated in the PGD
- Nurses must be individually named and have signed the PGD to be eligible to use it

Consent

- Consent must be obtained before giving any vaccine to a patient
- There is no legal requirement that this must be in writing, but a consent form can be a record of the information provided about the process, benefits, and risks of immunization as well as the decision
- It is good practice to check the person still consents at each immunization episode

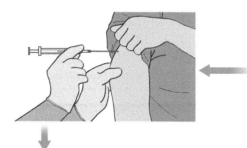

Contraindications

Vaccines should not be given when a patient has had an anaphylactic reaction to a preceding dose

Live vaccines may be temporarily contraindicated in patients who are pregnant or immunosuppressed

Vaccines may be postponed when a patient is acutely unwell or has a febrile illness. This is to prevent wrongly attributing new or worsening symptoms to the vaccine

Adverse events following immunization

Common adverse events include:
- Pain, swelling, or redness at the injection site
- Fever, malaise, headache
- Fainting and panic attacks

Anaphylactic reactions are extremely rare. Typically, onset is rapid and unpredictable with cardiovascular collapse, bronchospasm, and angioedema. Anaphylaxis is treated using intramuscular adrenaline

Documentation and record keeping

Accurate documentation is essential in order to monitor an individual's vaccine status as well as record what action or care was taken

It is best practice to document the vaccine name, dose, batch number, and expiry date as well as the site of administration

Dealing with anxious people

Some people can be anxious about injections. Maternal anxiety can make children nervous. Teenagers can be nervous due to peer influence. To alleviate anxiety nurses should:

- Use a calm, reassuring approach
- Use distraction techniques to divert attention from the procedure
- Prepare the vaccine out of sight of the patient
- Explain the procedure fully

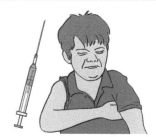

Immunity

Immunity is the ability of the body to protect itself from infectious disease. There are two types of immunity: innate and acquired.

Innate immunity

Innate immunity is present from birth and is a non-specific first line of defence. Innate immunity includes:

- Physical barriers such as intact skin and mucous membranes.
- Chemical barriers such as saliva and gastric acid.
- Phagocytic cells such as macrophages in the mucosa.

Acquired immunity

Acquired immunity is specific to a single organism or group of closely related organisms and is acquired through an active or a passive mechanism. Acquired immunity can be active or passive.

Active immunity is usually long-lasting and can be acquired through exposure to the natural disease or by vaccination. The body responds by producing antibodies and T lymphocytes to act against the infection. Vaccination provides immunity without the risk from the disease and its complications.

Passive immunity provides temporary protection to an individual by the transfer of antibodies. For example:

- Across the placenta from mother to child.
- Transfusion of blood or blood products containing immunoglobulins.

How immunizations work

Immunization is a safe and effective way of preventing infectious disease (Figure 65.1). Vaccines are administered to an individual to provide protection by triggering active immunity and providing immunological memory. This prepares the immune system to respond quickly when exposed to natural infection in the future, therefore preventing or reducing the severity of the disease. Vaccines are generally made from inactivated (killed) or attenuated (weakened) live organisms, or from their component parts or the toxins they produce.

Inactivated vaccines

Inactivated vaccines may require two or more injections to produce sufficient primary antibody response. Reinforcing doses are often given to provide longer-term protection. Inactivated vaccines cannot cause the infectious disease they are intended to prevent.

Attenuated vaccines

Live attenuated vaccines induce the same immune response as natural infection and usually provide a long-lasting antibody response after one or two doses. They do not usually cause the disease itself in healthy individuals.

Population immunity

The main aim of immunization is to protect the individual. People who have been vaccinated are less likely to be a source of infection to others, so reducing the risk of exposure to unvaccinated individuals. This means vaccination programmes can also benefit those who cannot be immunized. This is called population or herd immunity.

Safe immunization

Nurses must have received additional training to be authorized to administer immunizations (Figure 65.2). They must be competent in all aspects of immunization, including contraindications and the recognition and treatment of anaphylaxis. In order to maintain patient safety and remain current on immunization policy and practice, NHS Trusts require nurses to receive regular update courses in immunization and resuscitation.

Safe storage of vaccines

The success of immunization programmes depends on vaccine potency. Vaccines are sensitive to heat, cold, and light. Exposure to these conditions irreversibly reduces the effectiveness of vaccines and puts patients at risk. This can lead to litigation issues if ineffective vaccines are administered. The cold chain is the system used for storing and transporting vaccines within the safe temperature range of 2–8 °C and protected from light. Dedicated fridges are used, temperature is monitored daily, and stockpiling is avoided to enable air to circulate and maintain a constant temperature.

Reporting adverse events

Vaccines are tested for quality, safety, and efficacy before being licensed for routine use. Although adverse effects are identified prior to licensing, careful monitoring is required. The Yellow Card Scheme is a voluntary process for reporting suspected adverse reactions. The scheme is important in the early identification of safety concerns. Vaccine safety is kept under constant review by a committee of experts who carefully review new evidence and make recommendations.

Immunization controversies

Immunization has caused controversy since it was first discovered by Edward Jenner over 200 years ago. False beliefs tend to flourish where there is limited understanding of the evidence. Dissemination of misleading and contradictory information has been facilitated in recent times by the internet and social media. Reporting in the media may give equal weight to both sides of an argument, without giving due emphasis to a robust research base. This can result in a reduction in vaccine uptake and a resurgence of the disease.

One such controversy was that surrounding measles, mumps, and rubella (MMR) vaccination. The findings of this research linked MMR to autism and gastrointestinal problems. The research was seriously flawed and the findings have since been withdrawn. Because of the research, many parents opted not to vaccinate their children and as a result there has since been an increase in the number of cases of measles, predominantly in those who were unvaccinated. Measles is associated with serious complications, including meningitis, pneumonia, and hepatitis. MMR coverage for population immunity had not been achieved and the subsequent impact saw a resurgence of children who contracted measles. Similar controversies with the arrival of the SAR COV-2 vaccination programme have occurred and these have had significant media attention too.

In order to inform practice and be able to respond to patients' concerns, nurses need to know where to find reliable information about current issues and have the skills to critically appraise research.

Key points

- Immunity is either innate or acquired and the children's nurse needs to be able to understand and explain these concepts.
- The children's nurse will have to receive additional training to be permitted to administer vaccinations.
- The children's nurse must be able to identify evidence-based information on vaccination in order to support families and young people to make informed choices about receiving vaccinations.

66 Childhood immunizations

Figure 66.1 Immunization programme from birth to 18 years of age.

Age	Vaccine
8, 12, and 16 weeks	6 in 1 (diphtheria, tetanus, pertussis, polio, Haemophilus influenzae type B (Hib), and hepatitis B
12 weeks and 1 year	Pneumococcal
8, 16 weeks, and 1 year	Meningococcal group B
8 and 12 weeks	Rotavirus
One year	Haemophilus influenzae type B (Hib) and meningococcal group C
One year and 3 years and 4 months	Mumps, measles, and rubella
3 years and 4 months	Diphtheria, tetanus, pertussis, polio
12 – 13 years	Human papillomavirus (HPV)
14 years	Meningococcal group A, C, W, and Y
Eligible groups	Influenza
5 years plus	Covid-19

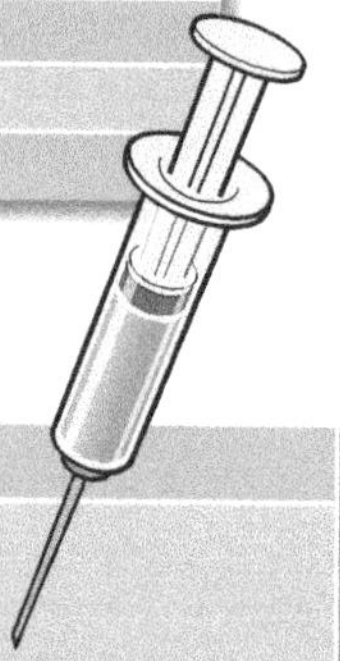

Immunizations should not be delayed because of:

- Minor infections (coughs and colds) without pyrexia
- Family history of bad reactions to immunizations
- The infant or child having had the illness (e.g. mumps)
- Prematurity
- Cerebral palsy
- Contact with an infectious disease
- Has asthma, hay fever, or eczema
- The infant or child is on antibiotics, an inhaler, or using steroid creams
- Breastfeeding
- Jaundice
- Underweight
- Being above the recommended age of immunization
- History of febrile convulsions or allergies

Immunizations are:

- Safe
- Free
- Very unlikely to cause allergic reactions
- Protection against some life-threatening illnesses

Healthcare professionals have a responsibility to:

- Promote immunization
- Reassure parents and carers
- Support parents and carers in their decision-making
- Offer advice on pain control

Immunization saves lives
Be wise – immunize

Figure 66.2 (a) Oral administration of vaccine. (b) Vaccine administration in lower limb. (c) Site for vaccine administration in upper limb.

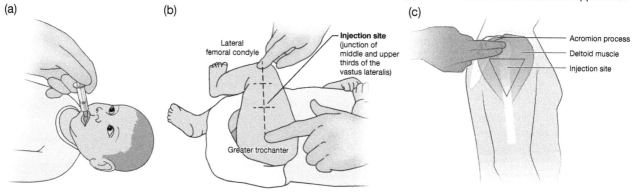

(a)

(b)

Lateral femoral condyle

Injection site (junction of middle and upper thirds of the vastus lateralis)

Greater trochanter

(c)

Acromion process

Deltoid muscle

Injection site

Children and Young People's Nursing at a Glance, Second Edition. Edited by Elizabeth Gormley-Fleming and Sheila Roberts.
© 2023 John Wiley & Sons Ltd. Published 2023 by John Wiley & Sons Ltd.

There are many decisions parents and carers have to make about their infants and children, and immunizations are often an area that parents worry about, particularly with media hype and the misguided research on the adverse effects of immunizations on some children.

The benefits of immunizations outweigh the risks to the infant or child. Healthcare professionals sharing information and reassuring parents and carers is paramount if we are to continue to ensure that some diseases do not return.

Smallpox was officially declared wiped out in 1980, and polio is heading towards eradication. Immunizations have saved more lives and prevented more serious diseases than any advance in recent medical history. There will be more potentially life-saving immunizations in the coming years, as there are more than 150 new immunizations currently being tested.

Immunizations given at 2, 3, and 4 months

By about 2 months of age, the baby's natural immunity gained from the mother begins to diminish and so that is why the immunization programme starts at 2 months. Three doses of the 6-in-1 vaccine are required to ensure the child is protected against these infections. The 6-in-1 vaccine protects the infant against diphtheria, hepatitis B, tetanus, pertussis, polio, and haemophilus influenza type B.

Babies will receive an oral vaccine against rotavirus infection. This is administered as two doses, 4 weeks apart. The first dose is given at 8 weeks and the second at 12 weeks.

Meningitis B vaccine is administered to babies as part of their routine vaccination programme at 8 and 12 weeks of age.

The infant is also given pneumococcal conjugate vaccine (PCV) at 12 weeks of age.

Immunizations given at 12–13 months

A booster of meningitis B is given at 12 months of age. The child will receive their first dose of a combined C and haemophilus influenza type B (Hib/Men C). They can have a second dose of PCV along with the first vaccine for measles, mumps, and rubella (MMR).

Immunizations given at 3 years 4 months or soon after

A booster of MMR is given, along with a pre-school booster of 4 : 1 diphtheria, tetanus, pertussis, and polio (DTaP/IPV).

Immunizations given to all children aged 12–13 years

Human papillomavirus immunization was commenced in 2008 to try to reduce the numbers of cervical cancer, some mouth and throat cancers, and some cancers in the anal and genital area. It also helps protect against genital warts. Initially this vaccine was solely administered to girls, but the vaccine programme was extended to boys aged 12–13 years born after 1 September 2006. The immunization is given via two single injections over a period of two years. The first dose is administered when the child is 12–13 years and the second dose 6–24 months after the first.

Immunizations given to teenagers aged 13–18 years

A booster of diphtheria, tetanus, and polio (3-in-1 teenage booster) is given to all young people at the age of 14 years. MenACWY (a single injection that protects against the four strains of meningococcal bacteria, A, C, W, and Y) is administered at the same time as the 3-in-1 teenage booster.

Other immunizations available

Immunosuppressed children may be offered varicella immunization between the ages of 1 and 12 years in 1 single dose. A child over 13 years will be given two doses 4–8 weeks apart.

BCG tuberculosis immunization is given to infants at birth if they are born in an area of the country where there is a high number of cases, or if there is a high chance of coming into contact with the disease.

Influenza immunization is offered to children who have certain medical conditions or who are immunosuppressed, once a year from 6 months of age.

The Covid-19 vaccination programme includes children and young people, who are receiving two doses of the vaccine (Figure 66.1).

Common problems

The 6-in-1 injection may cause redness and swelling at the site for a few days (Figure 66.2), and mild fever may last up to 10 days after the immunization.

The pneumococcal immunization causes redness and inflammation in 1 in 7 infants. Mild symptoms of irritability, raised temperature, and digestive disturbances can occur.

The meningitis C vaccine can cause swelling and redness to the site. In toddlers, disturbed sleep and mild fever can occur, whereas older children may complain of headaches.

MMR can cause cold symptoms, fever, or swollen salivary glands for a few days up to three weeks after the immunization. Rash and loss of appetite can also occur.

Treatment

All the common problems are manageable and minor. Paracetamol for pain and discomfort according to prescription advice is recommended, along with frequent fluids and rest.

When not to immunize

Immunization should be postponed if a child has a pyrexia (above 38 °C).

If a child has had a bad reaction to a previous immunization, they may require assessment first, and future doses may be given in a hospital setting.

Only children who have had a confirmed anaphylactic reaction to an immunization will be advised not to have further doses.

Key points
- Immunizations are safe.
- Allergic responses are very rare.
- The benefits outweigh the risks.
- Immunization across the globe has saved millions of lives.

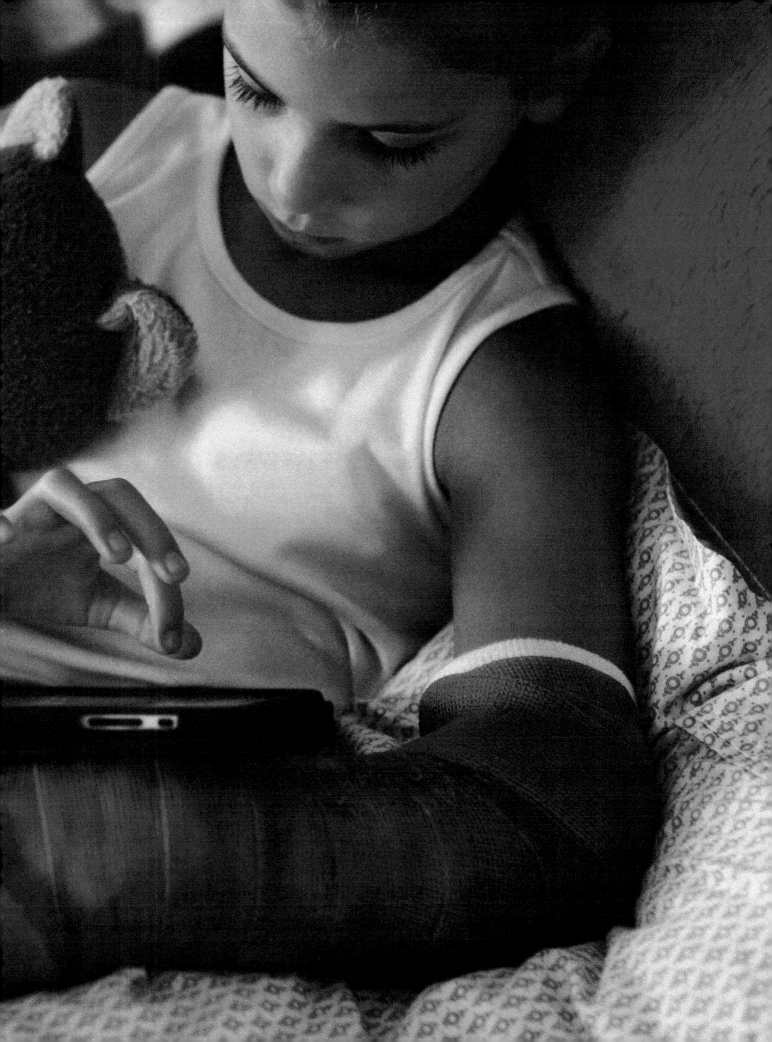

Part 5

Chapters

67 Child and young person health policies

Figure 67.1 Key words of importance in child health policies.

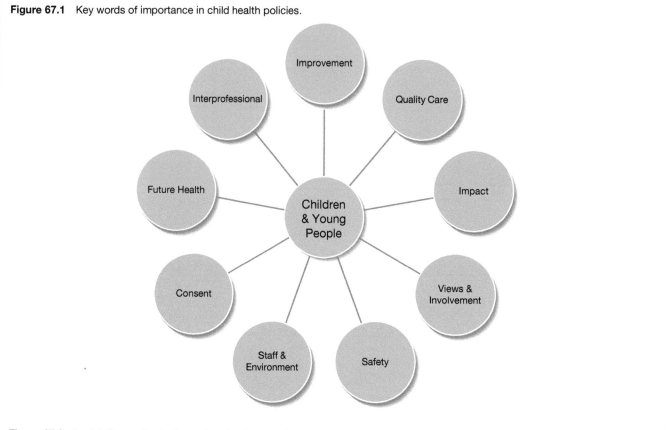

Figure 67.2 Legislation underpinning policy development in practices for nursing children and young people.

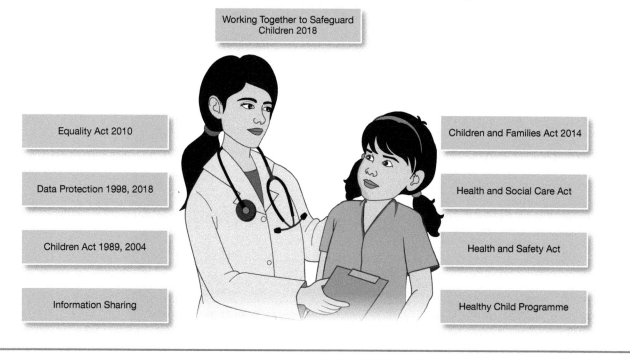

Child health policies aim to maintain or improve the health of children and young people (Figure 67.1). Within the UK, health inequalities remain prevalent, impacting upon the life experiences and opportunities of every child. Investment in these, alongside other measures to challenge child poverty, will influence opportunities and safety for future generations.

Historically, landmark policies have provided a variety of key messages such as the impact of hospitalization upon child development; the importance of promoting the health and ensuring the safety and protection of children in a range of settings; along with recognizing the importance of involving young people in their care (Figure 67.2). The policies have also promoted the need to have paediatric health and social care facilities and staff specifically trained in caring for children, young people, and their families.

Examples of historical and current policies include:
• Platt Report (HMSO 1959): a report looking at the welfare of children in hospital, which made recommendations to hospital authorities in regard to children's welfare.
• Court Report (HMSO 1976): *Fit for the Future* made further recommendations for caring for children, including the need for community paediatricians.
• Children Act (HMSO 1989): Key points include that children's welfare is paramount, and that families are best placed to care for children.
• Welfare of Children and Young People in Hospital (HMSO 1991): key points include the advice to have two Registered Sick Children's Nurses on duty 24 hours a day in all children's departments or wards.
• Allitt Inquiry/Clothier Report (DOH 1994): in light of the Beverly Allitt tragedy, recommendations were made to ensure the safety of children, including an increase in the number of trained children's nurses.
• Kennedy Report into Bristol Children's Heart Surgery (DOH 2001): children must be cared for in an appropriate, safe environment and by competent staff appropriately trained in caring for children.
• Redfern Report into Liverpool Children's Hospital (DOH 2001): the body parts enquiry recommended a tightening of consent to ensure everyone is appropriately informed prior to making a decision.
• Seeking Consent: Working with Children (DOH 2001): this focused on issues that arise when seeking consent from children and their parents.
• Laming Report into the Death of Victoria Climbie (DOH 2003): the report stressed the need for multi-agency working in safeguarding children.
• Children Act (DOH 2004): this established a Children's Commissioner to raise awareness of the views of children and young people and to promote cooperation between services for the benefit of children and young people.
• National Service Framework for CYP and Maternity Services (DoH 2004): set standards for children and young people across health and social care in England.
• You're Welcome: Quality Criteria for Young People Friendly Health Services (DoH 2005/2011): these set out principles that will help health services (including non-NHS provision) become young people friendly.
• Report from the Children and Young People's Health Outcomes Forum (2012): offers advice on how to improve children and young people's health outcomes.
• The Healthy Child Programme (PHE 2009): a national evidence-based universal programme for children aged 0–19.
• Special Educational Needs and Disability (SEND) code of practice: 0–25 years (DforEd and DoHSC 2014): legal requirements and statutory guidance for health and education when caring for children with special educational needs.
• Children and Families Act (UK) (2014): this aims to improve services for key groups of vulnerable children and support families in balancing home and work life.
• All Our Health (PHE 2015): aimed at preventing illness, protecting health, and promoting wellbeing.
• Building the Right Support (NHS England 2015): a national plan to develop community services for people with learning disabilities.
• Healthy Children: Transforming Child Health Information (NHS England 2016): a vision for supporting parents and professionals in providing high-quality care.
• These Are Our Children (DoH 2017): recommendations for improvement in care for children and young people with learning disabilities.
• Child Health in 2030 in England: comparisons with Other Wealthy Countries (RCPCH 2018): recommendations for the future health of children and young people.

This chapter provides a glimpse into government policy in the UK, which is vast and ever evolving. Health policy has been proactive in championing the specific needs of children and young people within society, but embedding the recommendations can be challenging. Regulation and coordination of the range of services and agencies that children and young people come into contact with are complex. The children's nurse has a key role in disseminating, promoting, and collaborating in interprofessional working with children and their families to ensure the best health outcomes for children and young people.

It is imperative that children's nurses keep up to date with evolving policies through professional updating (as part of professional regulation and through employers, e.g. local health organizations and trusts will have clinical governance procedures for implementing and developing national and local policy). Children's nurses have a responsibility to keep abreast of evolving evidence-based guidelines specifically for children and young people, such as NICE Guidance. Staying up to date with policies locally can be achieved by accessing managers and local intranet sites, as well as clinical governance teams. However, government policy relating to healthcare more often relates to the NHS as a whole and seeks to address changes to service provision for the entire population. Children's nurses therefore also have a key role in advocating for the specific rights of children and young people in relation to generic policy recommendations.

The children's nurse is a gatekeeper who can influence and contribute to policy development, since there is still much work to be done to ensure equality of opportunity. Furthermore, it is important to understand that there are implications in adhering to and following policy when working in any one of the four countries that make up the UK. Government policy, instigated from the Department of Health, may be adopted for use within Wales, Scotland, or Ireland, or each country may choose to adapt its own policy (e.g. in child safeguarding).

Key points
• Policies are ever evolving and there is a responsibility to keep up to date.
• Children's nurses should take every opportunity to influence child health policies.
• Adherence to policies is paramount to ensure safe and effective care for all.

68 Children's rights in society and healthcare

Figure 68.1 Children's rights.

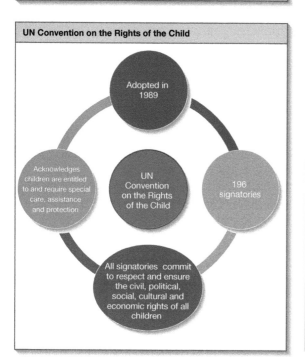

Healthcare rights include the:

What are my healthcare rights?

Right to be protected and be safe in hospital

Right to have the best available care for me

Right to have my parents present

Right to play, education, rest, activities

Right to coordinated healthcare

Right to be treated with respect

Right to be fully informed

UN Convention on the Rights of the Child

Adopted in 1989

Acknowledges children are entitled to and require special care, assistance and protection

UN Convention on the Rights of the Child

196 signatories

All signatories commit to respect and ensure the civil, political, social, cultural and economic rights of all children

European Association of Children in Hospital Charter

Article 1: Children shall be admitted to hospital only if the care they require cannot be equally well provided at home or on a day basis.

Article 2: Children in hospital shall have the right to have their parents or parent substitute with them at all times.

Article 3: Accommodation should be offered to all parents and they should be helped and encouraged to stay. Parents should not need to incur additional costs or suffer loss of income. In order to share in the care of their child, parents should be kept informed about ward routine and their active participation encouraged.

Article 4: Children and parents shall have the right to be informed in a manner appropriate to age and understanding. Steps should be taken to mitigate physical and emotional stress.

Article 5: (5.1) Children and parents have the right to informed participation in all decisions involving their healthcare. (5.2) Every child shall be protected from unnecessary medical treatment and investigation.

Article 6: (6.1) Children shall be cared for together with children who have the same developmental needs and shall not be admitted to adult wards. (6.2) There should be no age restrictions for visitors to children in hospital.

Article 7: Children shall have full opportunity for play, recreation and education suited to their age and condition and shall be in an environment designed, furnished, staffed and equipped to meet their needs.

Article 8: Children shall be cared for by staff whose training and skills enable them to respond to the physical, emotional and developmental needs of children and families.

Article 9: Continuity of care should be ensured by the team caring for children.

Article 10: Children shall be treated with tact and understanding and their privacy shall be respected at all times.

Legislation that impacts on children's rights

UN Convention on the Rights of the Child
Human Rights Act 1998
Children Act 1989 & 2004
Children and Young Persons Act 2008
Children and Social Work Act 2017
Data Protection Act 1998, 2018
Mental Health Act 1983
Child Poverty Act 2010
Serious Crime Act 2015
Sexual Offences Act 2003
Education Act 2002
Borders, Citizenship and Immigration Act 2009
Mental Health Units (Use of Force) Act 2018
Case Law

Children's rights in society

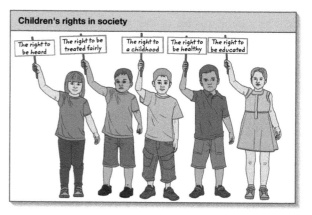

The right to be heard

The right to be treated fairly

The right to a childhood

The right to be healthy

The right to be educated

Children and Young People's Nursing at a Glance, Second Edition. Edited by Elizabeth Gormley-Fleming and Sheila Roberts.
© 2023 John Wiley & Sons Ltd. Published 2023 by John Wiley & Sons Ltd.

All children and young people have rights to be supported with their health and wellbeing (Figure 68.1). These rights are articulated in the United Nations Convention on the Rights of the Child. The UK government has committed to the UN Convention 1989 and this came into force in January 1992. Its primary aim is to provide a comprehensive set of principles and standards to guide and inform planning and practice for children and young people up to 18 years of age. It places clear obligations on practitioners and government leaders to develop policy and practice in accordance with the human rights of children.

What are children's rights?

- A set of entitlements for all children, of whatever age, of whatever background.
- Justifiable claims that require action or non-action from others.
- Rights require positive or negative duties from others, so in the child's case this will be parents, educators, healthcare professionals, and policymakers.

Moral rights

Generally moral rights can be translated into legal rights if there is some recognition of their importance by the rest of society and consequently the imposition of correlative legal duties on others regarding the fulfilment of those rights. For example, the exclusion of a child from school may be considered a violation of their moral right.

Legislative context

A number of changes to English law have enabled children's rights to be upheld in accordance with the UN Convention on the Rights of the Child: for example, the duty of local authorities to protect children, age-appropriate hospital wards (mental health), equality protection, strategy to reduce socio-economic disadvantage, child sexual exploitation recognition, and regulation of the use of force in mental health units.

Significant changes such as Frasier and Gillick competence acknowledged that children and young people have the capacity to be involved in decisions about their health. These are now well understood and applied in the healthcare setting.

However, there are still gaps in the provision of legislation to protect children's rights in all areas of their lives. For example, parents can still hit their child in England based on an 1860 court case, if it would be considered 'reasonable' to do so. However, other nations in the UK have approved legislation that bans smacking. The UK also imprisons more children than any other country in Europe. Parental powers have been progressively modified by legislation.

Children as holders of rights

The child is no longer seen as a passive consumer of services and should now be an active participant. They should not be excluded from conversations or processes where information about them is discussed or shared. Respecting children's right to be heard, for example, does not necessarily mean that their request should prevail, but it does mean that their views and opinions can be considered in decisions that will impact on their lives.

Research involving children and young people has developed, with this group now being recognized as active participants. It has been shown that young children can give powerful testimony about their lives, and about their likes and dislikes.

Conflicting rights

The children and young person's nurse need to be aware that rights can conflict and consider their role in managing situations like the following:

- A child's right to life may conflict with their parent's right to impose their religious practices on their child.
- A child's right to information may conflict with their parent's rights to protect their child, e.g. if they refuse to allow a child to know the child is dying.
- A child's right to confidentiality may conflict with their parent's perceived right to information about the child if they seek contraceptive advice while underage.

Promoting children's rights and welfare in healthcare

The best interest of the child should always be a primary consideration in the broad provision of healthcare services. However, this may require others to advocate on the child's behalf. The children and young person's nurse may assume this position and advocate on behalf of the child.

Healthcare staff have a duty of care to the child and a legal responsibility to protect their rights, interests, and wishes in the healthcare setting. The European Association for Children in Hospital (EACH) charter identifies 10 articles (rights) that are applicable to all children in hospital regardless of age, disability, illness, or background.

All children and young people should feel that their rights are promoted and protected in healthcare and in society in general. It is an integral requirement that children's and young person's nurses understand and act in accordance with the legislative frameworks in practice to promote and protect children's rights. They also need to challenge discriminatory practices and understand their professional responsibility and obligations to the child and the family.

Key points

- All children and young people should be able to have information about their rights in healthcare and in other aspects of their lives.
- Children and young people are active participants in all decisions that affect them.
- Children's and young person's nurses need to be conversant with the rights of the child and current legislative frameworks that impact on healthcare practice.
- The best interest of the child will always remain paramount in any decision-making process.

The NHS change model

Figure 69.1 The NHS Change Model.

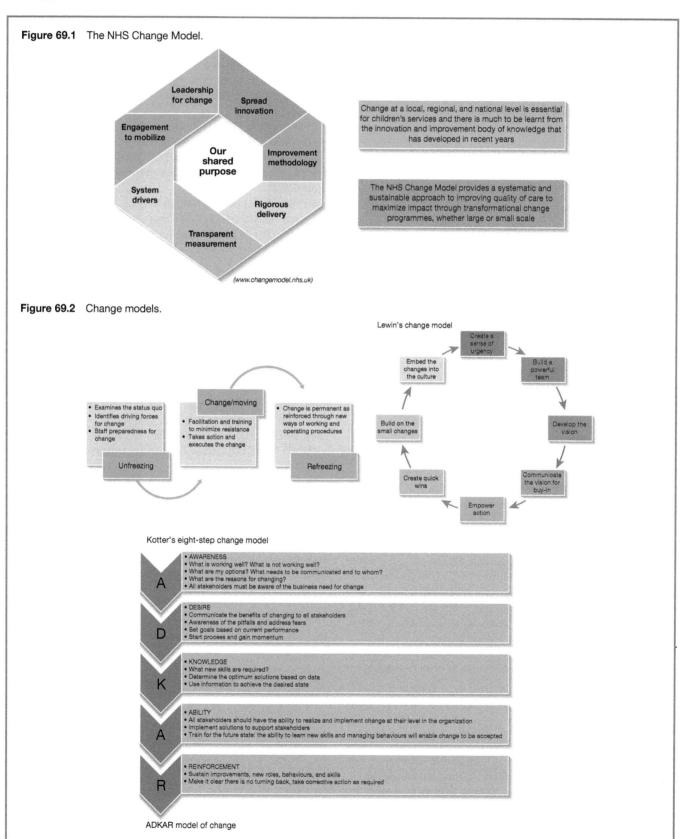

Leadership for change

Spread innovation

Engagement to mobilize

Our shared purpose

Improvement methodology

System drivers

Rigorous delivery

Transparent measurement

Change at a local, regional, and national level is essential for children's services and there is much to be learnt from the innovation and improvement body of knowledge that has developed in recent years

The NHS Change Model provides a systematic and sustainable approach to improving quality of care to maximize impact through transformational change programmes, whether large or small scale

(www.changemodel.nhs.uk)

Figure 69.2 Change models.

Lewin's change model

- Examines the status quo
- Identifies driving forces for change
- Staff preparedness for change

Unfreezing

Change/moving
- Facilitation and training to minimize resistance
- Takes action and executes the change

Change is permanent as reinforced through new ways of working and operating procedures

Refreezing

Create a sense of urgency

Build a powerful team

Embed the changes into the culture

Develop the vision

Build on the small changes

Communicate the vision for buy-in

Create quick wins

Empower action

Kotter's eight-step change model

A • AWARENESS
- What is working well? What is not working well?
- What are my options? What needs to be communicated and to whom?
- What are the reasons for changing?
- All stakeholders must be aware of the business need for change

D • DESIRE
- Communicate the benefits of changing to all stakeholders
- Awareness of the pitfalls and address fears
- Set goals based on current performance
- Start process and gain momentum

K • KNOWLEDGE
- What new skills are required?
- Determine the optimum solutions based on data
- Use information to achieve the desired state

A • ABILITY
- All stakeholders should have the ability to realize and implement change at their level in the organization
- Implement solutions to support stakeholders
- Train for the future state: the ability to learn new skills and managing behaviours will enable change to be accepted

R • REINFORCEMENT
- Sustain improvements, new roles, behaviours, and skills
- Make it clear there is no turning back, take corrective action as required

ADKAR model of change

Children and Young People's Nursing at a Glance, Second Edition. Edited by Elizabeth Gormley-Fleming and Sheila Roberts.
© 2023 John Wiley & Sons Ltd. Published 2023 by John Wiley & Sons Ltd.

Around 21% of the population of England and Wales are under 18. While NHS England states that providing a good start in life and enabling children to be physically and emotionally healthy is critical in ensuring they reach their full potential and lead fulfilled, productive adult lives, the Royal College of Paediatrics and Child Health states that this population group still does not have the priority and focus required at governmental level to secure equitable healthy futures. Sustained advocacy and action are thus required to improve the health of babies, children, and young people.

The Child Mortality and Social Deprivation Report (2021) finds a clear association between the risk of child death and the level of deprivation (for all categories except cancer). Specifically, it states that over a fifth of all child deaths might have been avoided if children living in the most deprived areas had the same mortality risk as those living in the least deprived, which translates to over 700 fewer children dying per year in England. Of the 700 cases of children's deaths reviewed between 2019 and 2020, 243 related to difficulties in accessing services, lack of access to interpreting services, poor communication between agencies, and the lack of a coordinated response to increasing vulnerability.

The establishment of Integrated Care Systems (ICS) across England offers opportunities across healthcare, local authorities, and education to redefine models of care that are shaped around need rather than demand. The ICS approach should include embedding co-production with children, young people, and their families as part of service redesign, along with the use of technology, data, and analytics to underpin the necessary improvement in health that is required.

Change at a local, regional, and national level is clearly essential in meeting the ambitions of the NHS Long Term Plan in which babies, children, and young people have a profile. There is much we can learn from the innovation and improvement in the body of knowledge that have developed in recent years. The NHS Change Model (Figure 69.1) provides a systematic and sustainable approach to improving quality of care to maximize impact through transformational change programmes whether large or small scale. It utilizes improvement science methodology to improve health systems.

The model brings together collective improvement in knowledge and experience from across the NHS into eight key components. Through applying all eight components, effective change can be achieved. The approach is able to fit each unique context as a way of making sense at every level of 'how and why' to deliver improvement, to consistently make a bigger difference, whether it be reducing emergency admissions, transforming services as a result of user engagement, or introducing new processes such as SBAR (Situation, Background, Assessment, and Recommendation) to enhance communication.

• Central to successful change is the agreement of a *shared purpose*. Clarity of focus is essential so that the intent of the change programme is clear to all.

• Evidence suggests that the *leadership* style and philosophy that are most likely to deliver change generate a commitment to a shared purpose through collaboration. Role modelling of leadership behaviours, skills, and attributes and setting a high ambition for performance ensure a connection to values and empower others to commit to action. By doing these things, the scale and pace of improvement are maximized.

• Change cannot be achieved in isolation. *Engagement* of the multidisciplinary team, complemented by engagement of children, young people, and families, as well as education and voluntary organizations, is essential if we are to collaboratively make services better. True co-production in improvement of services must be the ultimate aim. Mobilization enables all stakeholders to build relationships quickly, focusing on creating 'urgency' for change from which to organize resources through developing 'commitments' to each other and to the common goal.

• When we want to change something, even if it is just something small, conditions need to be right if the change is going to both work as we wanted it to and also stay changed for the future. A range of models exist to enable change to be managed (Figure 69.2). Key to these is whether the broad conditions for change, the *system drivers*, can be lined up to support what we are trying to do. These drivers might take the form of incentives for change such as commissioning for quality and innovation payments, or specific standards to be achieved if penalties are to be avoided. Aligning these drivers with the quality improvement intent and thereby making the best use of them is crucial.

• Using an evidence-based *improvement methodology* ensures that the change will be delivered in a planned, proven way. There is a range of methodologies available to support different kinds of change, such as Plan, Do, Study, Act (PDSA) cycles. With the use of effective evidence-based improvement methodologies, the adoption and systematic spread of change are more effective and delivery of leadership goals and the overall success of a change effort are more likely to be assured

• Evidence suggests that an effective approach for the *rigorous delivery* of change and the monitoring of progress towards planned objectives are essential to making that change a reality. A project management approach will increase the likelihood that changes will deliver the planned benefits, because accountabilities are shared and clear, and the scale and pace of improvement are enhanced. A rigorous approach requires discipline and focus.

• *Transparent measurement* of the outcomes of change is crucial to provide evidence that the change is happening, and the desired results are being achieved. Using appropriate measurement techniques ensures that remedial action can be taken to mitigate risk, unforeseen consequences can be dealt with promptly, and, importantly, success can be celebrated.

• We need to accelerate the speed and extent of the *spread and adoption of innovation*, locally, regionally, and nationally, in order to improve the quality of care.

Use of the NHS Change Model provides a framework and supports a culture that values quality improvement to ensure we consistently improve outcomes for and with babies, children, young people, and their families.

Key points

• Quality care is paramount when considering change at local or national level.
• Change needs to include the multidisciplinary team alongside children, young people, and their families.
• Evaluation or measurement of the change is key to ensuring goals are being met.

70 Nursing and midwifery council standards for pre-registration nurse education

Figure 70.1 Five pillars as set out in the standards framework for nursing and midwifery education.

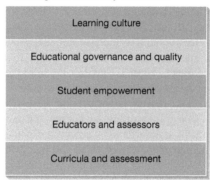

- Learning culture
- Educational governance and quality
- Student empowerment
- Educators and assessors
- Curricula and assessment

Figure 70.2 Roles to support student supervision and assessment.

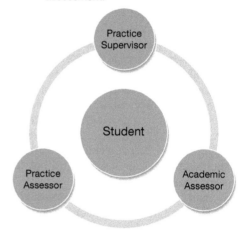

Practice Supervisor

Student

Practice Assessor

Academic Assessor

Figure 70.3 Students' journey through the pre-registration nursing programme standards.

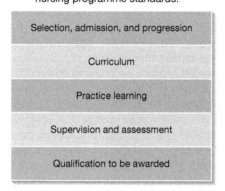

- Selection, admission, and progression
- Curriculum
- Practice learning
- Supervision and assessment
- Qualification to be awarded

Figure 70.4 Expectations at the point of registration.

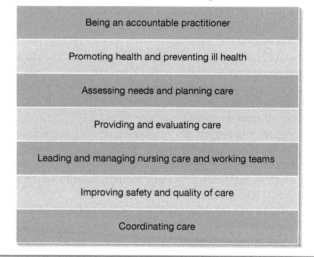

- Being an accountable practitioner
- Promoting health and preventing ill health
- Assessing needs and planning care
- Providing and evaluating care
- Leading and managing nursing care and working teams
- Improving safety and quality of care
- Coordinating care

The Nursing and Midwifery Council (NMC) introduced the current education standards in 2018 to reflect the changing needs of service users and the requirements for contemporary nursing practice. This education framework seeks to provide a single set of education and training standards and requirements.

These standards raised the ambition and expectations of nurses and midwives at the point of registration. New ways of working and embracing technology to equip the nurses of the future are embraced in these standards. The standard framework will provide nurses with the knowledge and skills required to deliver evidence-based, excellent care across a range of settings.

The standards framework ensures that all education institutions and practice placement partners put the safety and wellbeing of people first. There is a continued focus on partnership working between Approved Education Institutions (AEIs) and practice placement partners. The overall responsibility and accountability for the management of the quality of education remains with the AEI in partnership with practice placement partners. The practice placement providers are responsible for ensuring learning opportunities for student nurses, nursing associates, and midwives.

The design principles for the education framework seek to achieve consistent, proportionate, regulatory standards that embed public protection, equality, and the potential for collaboration with others.

These are outcome-based standards that are measurable and assessable. The standards grant AEIs and their practice placement partners more autonomy in respect of a number of areas, including entry criteria, progression, and simulation. AEIs have the autonomy to be creative and innovative in their design and delivery of curricula.

There are three parts to the NMC standards that are used in conjunction with the standards of proficiency for nursing. As a collective, the three sets of standards specify the knowledge and skills that all registered nurses must be able to demonstrate when caring for a diverse range of patients, across all care settings throughout the life span.

• *Part 1: Standards framework for nursing and midwifery education.* This provides information on the overall standards for nursing and midwifery programmes. Universities will work with their local partners in providing evidence to the NMC regarding achievement of these.

• *Part 2: Standards for student supervision and assessment* (SSSA). This outlines the SSSA, which will be explored in this chapter. The responsibilities attached to each role are outlined, including preparation and ongoing support.

• *Part 3: Programme standards.* This refers to the specific programme standards that reflect the processes and policies underpinning the student journey from recruitment to registration, and will need to reflect a collaborative partnership approach.

The standards framework for nursing and midwifery education applies to all AEIs and their practice learning partners. It is arranged in five pillars: learning culture, educational governance and quality, student learning and empowerment, educators and assessors, and curricula and assessment (Figure 70.1). These pillars are the underpinning for all NMC-approved programmes. Each pillar has a number of standards and requirements. The NMC will use these standards to assess the effectiveness of the AEIs and their practice learning partners in all learning environments.

Standards for student supervision and assessment

The SSSA saw a shift from the role of the mentor to the introduction of three new roles: practice supervisor, practice assessor, and academic assessor (Figure 70.2). The standards set out the expectations for all three roles. There are three specific aspects to the SSSA:

• Effective practice learning.
• Supervision of students.
• Assessment of students and confirmation of proficiency.

The process of effective student supervision and assessment is one of partnership between the AEI and practice placement provider, with the overall aim of upholding public protection. Students in practice learning must be supported to learn in a positive learning environment in order to enhance their personal and professional development and become resilient, critical thinkers and decision makers who have the skills to analyse and reflect in order to continually improve their practice. To do this, they need to be supported to learn, hence supernumerary status is essential while still being considered part of the nursing team.

The NMC code of conduct states that all nurses, nursing associates, and midwives have a duty to support students' and colleagues' learning to help them develop their professional competence and confidence. This means that all nurses and midwives can undertake the role of supervisor if it is within their scope of practice.

The SSSA does not mandate specific training for these roles, but there is an expectation that suitable preparation and training will be provided to enable all to undertake their roles effectively. The separation out of the supervision and assessment roles will ensure greater objectivity, fairness, and transparency of assessment. This shared decision making should result in a more consistent and

Table 70.1   Roles of practice supervisors, practice assessors, and academic assessors

Role	Requirements and responsibilities
Practice supervisor	Is a registered nurse, midwife, or registered health or social care professional
	Can support learning in line with their scope of practice
	Has current knowledge and experience of the area in which they are providing support, supervision, and feedback
	Has been appropriately prepared and receives ongoing support to reflect and develop
	Identifies and ensures learning opportunities are available and facilitated
	Contributes to the student's record of achievement by periodically recording relevant observations of conduct, proficiency, and achievement
	Contributes to assessment to inform decisions and records regular feedback
	Has sufficient opportunities to engage with practice assessors and academic assessors
Practice assessor	Is a registered nurse or midwife
	Must be appropriately prepared and must maintain current knowledge and expertise
	Is able to conduct assessments that are informed by feedback from practice supervisors
	Is able to make and record objective decisions, utilizing records, observations, student reflection, and other resources
	Observes the student periodically
	Gathers and coordinates feedback from practice supervisors and other relevant people
	Plans communication with academic assessors at relevant points in the student's journey
Academic assessor	Is a registered nurse or midwife
	Collates and confirms student achievement of proficiencies and programme outcomes in the academic environment
	Makes and records objective, evidence-based decisions on conduct, proficiency, and achievement, and recommendations for progression drawing on student records and other resources
	Is appropriately prepared and maintains current knowledge and expertise
	Works in partnership with the practice assessor to evaluate and recommend the student for progression in each part of the programme
	A different academic assessor is required for each part of the programme
	Must understand the student's learning and their achievement in practice
	Enables scheduled communication with all parties

objective assessment process. Each role has clearly delineated responsibilities, as outlined in Table 70.1.

Programme standards

This set of standards is specific to each approved programme. The student journey in the standards for pre-registration nursing programmes is considered under five headings (Figure 70.3). For pre-registration nursing these standards set out the legal requirements, entry requirements, assessment requirements, recognition of prior learning, length of programme, and information about the award that is offered on successful completion of the programme. Providers of pre-registration nurse education programmes (AEIs) must structure their curricula around the published proficiencies and assess students against these proficiencies to ensure they are able to provide evidence-based, safe, and effective care.

Standards of proficiency for registered nurses

The proficiencies for registered nurses specify the knowledge and skills that a registered nurse must be able to demonstrate when caring for all people across the life span in all care settings. The standards of proficiency for registered nurses are presented as seven platforms (Figure 70.4) and two annexes. Annex A focuses on communication and relationship management. Annex B identifies the nursing procedures that registered nurses need to be able to demonstrate if they are to practise safely. The annexes provide a description of what all registered nurses should be able to demonstrate at the point of registration in order to deliver safe, effective care.

Key points

- The standards of proficiency apply to all nurses irrespective of their field of practice.
- There is increased focus on public health and supporting lifestyle choices.
- An evidence-based, person-centred approach to physical and mental healthcare is important.
- Communication and relationship management and nursing procedures (Annexes A and B) apply to all nurses irrespective of field of practice, but the level of knowledge and expertise required will vary depending in the chosen field of practice.
- Whole-body systems assessment, including skills to support this e.g. chest auscultation, is now included in pre-registration education.
- Nurse must be prepared to deliver care at home or near home settings.
- There is a focus on nurses having the skills to take an increased leadership and management role in the delivery of care.
- Pharmacokinetics and prescribing theory are included in the proficiencies.
- Improvement methodologies such as audit, health economics, and political awareness are included in pre-registration curricula.
- The proficiencies set out the standards nurses must achieve and reflect public expectations of all registered nurses.
- The theory : practice split remains at 50 : 50, so 2300 hours of theory and 2300 hours of practice.

Part 6

Chapters

71 Pain assessment

Figure 71.1 Factors affecting a child's behaviour when in pain.

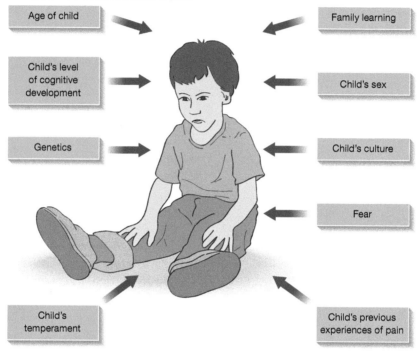

Age of child

Child's level of cognitive development

Genetics

Child's temperament

Family learning

Child's sex

Child's culture

Fear

Child's previous experiences of pain

Figure 71.2 Pain assessment tool.

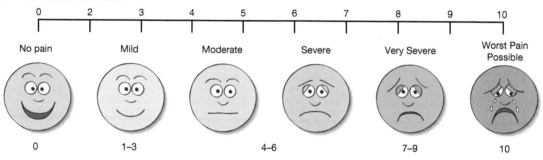

| 0 | 2 | 3 | 4 | 5 | 6 | 7 | 8 | 9 | 10 |

No pain — 0
Mild — 1–3
Moderate — 4–6
Severe
Very Severe — 7–9
Worst Pain Possible — 10

Box 71.1 Key steps in pain assessment.

- Record a pain history
- Assess the child's pain using a developmentally appropriate pain assessment tool
- Reassess pain having allowed time for pain-relieving interventions to work

Box 71.2 Three approaches to assessing pain.

- *Self-report:* what the child says
- *Behavioural:* how the child behaves
- *Physiological indicators:* how the child's body reacts

Box 71.3 Self-report tools.

These should be used with children who are:
- Old enough to understand and use self-report scale (e.g. 5 years and older)
- Not overtly distressed
- Not cognitively impaired

Box 71.4 Some of the more commonly used and well-validated pain assessment tools.

For non-verbal children
Revised FLACC
Children's Hospital of Eastern Ontario Pain Scale (CHEOPS)
COMFORT Scale

For verbal children
Faces Pain Scale-Revised (FPS-R)
Wong-Baker FACES Pain Scale
Oucher
Numerical rating scale

Children and Young People's Nursing at a Glance, Second Edition. Edited by Elizabeth Gormley-Fleming and Sheila Roberts.
© 2023 John Wiley & Sons Ltd. Published 2023 by John Wiley & Sons Ltd.

Pain is the most frequent symptom experienced by children in hospital. Pain assessment is the first step in the effective management of pain. The children's and young person's nurse is in a unique position to assess and manage the child's pain, as they have the most contact with the child in comparison to other healthcare professionals. To treat pain effectively, ongoing assessment of the presence and severity of pain and the child's response to treatment is essential. However, pain assessment poses many challenges in children because of the subjective nature of pain, as well as developmental and language limitations. Pain assessment is a multidimensional observational assessment based on the experience of the child (Box 71.1). It is complex and is founded on observation of the child, understanding the context and significance of their pain, and then the formation of clinical judgements about what is required to treat their pain.

In addition, not all children behave in the same way when in pain, so the factors identified in Figure 71.1 need considering when carrying out a pain assessment.

Self-report tools

A range of self-reporting pain assessment tools are available for use (Box 71.2). Self-reporting is the gold standard, as it is what the child says their pain is. Some of the most commonly used pain assessment tools are listed in Boxes 71.3 and 71.4.

Faces pain scales

Faces pain scales are the most popular self-report tool (Figure 71.2). The design of faces scales is intended to enable a child to provide a representation of their pain intensity. Faces scales are popular with children, but they need to be explained carefully to the child. It is important to note that faces pain scales are not designed to be used as observational scales; they should only be used as a self-report tool. Faces pain scales can be used by most children aged 5 years and over.

Numerical rating scale/visual analogue

When using a numerical scale, the child is asked to rate their pain from 0 to 10 (or 0 to 5). Very little research has explored the use of numerical pain rating scales in paediatrics, but there is some evidence to support their use with children aged 8 years and older.

Behavioural cues

There are a number of behavioural cues that can be used to assess whether a child is in pain:

- Changed behaviour
- Irritability
- Flat affect
- Unusual posture
- Screaming
- Reluctance to move
- Aggressiveness
- Disturbed sleep pattern
- Increased clinging
- Unusual quietness
- Loss of appetite
- Restlessness
- Whimpering
- Sobbing
- Lying 'scared stiff'
- Lethargic

How these cues are displayed varies from child to child and so it is important to involve parents in assessing pain in order to ascertain the child's normal behaviour. A good rule of thumb is that a change in a child's normal behaviour should be considered an indication that they might be in pain.

Behavioural pain assessment tools should be used with infants, toddlers, and pre-verbal, cognitively impaired, and sedated children. If a child is overtly distressed (e.g. due to pain or anxiety), no meaningful self-report can be obtained at that point in time. In this situation the child's pain should be estimated using a behavioural pain assessment tool until the child is less distressed.

Revised FLACC

The r-FLACC is a behavioural pain assessment tool that has good clinical utility. FLACC is an acronym for Facial expression, Leg movement, Activity, Cry, and Consolability. The original version was revised in 2006. FLACC has been validated for postoperative pain in children aged 2 months–8 years, as well as procedural pain in children aged 5–16 years. FLACC is also one of only three scales considered valid and reliable for the assessment of pain in children with cognitive impairment, and has been shown to be a valid and reliable pain measure in the paediatric intensive care unit. However, the scale cannot be used in children who are intubated as 'cries' will not be audible, nor is it suitable for children who are paralysed or have impaired mobility, as this will make it difficult to assess the 'leg movement' category.

Physiological cues

Physiological cues that can be used to assess pain include increase in heart rate and respiratory rate, raised blood pressure, sweating and dilated pupils. On their own, physiological indicators do not constitute a valid clinical pain measure for children. A multidimensional tool that incorporates physiological and behavioural indicators, as well as self-report, is therefore preferred whenever possible. Alterations to vital signs alone may not be a useful or reliable indicator of pain level. If used with a behavioural assessment tool, reliability is increased. However, in the case of the child who is ventilated or sedated, altered physiological signs are a more reliable indicator of pain.

Reassessment of pain

A key component of caring for a child in pain is reassessing their pain at regular intervals. This enables the child's response to pain management interventions to be reviewed. Children should have their pain assessed:

- When they visit an emergency department or an ambulatory clinic.
- On admission to hospital.
- At least once per shift.
- Before, during, and after an invasive procedure.

Following surgery and/or if the patient has a known painful medical condition, pain should be assessed hourly for the first six hours. After this, if the pain is well controlled, it can be assessed less frequently (e.g. every four hours). If the pain is not well controlled, regular assessment should continue.

Key points

- Pain should be assessed using developmental and cognitive-specific tools.
- Reassess pain after all interventions in appropriate time frames so effectiveness can be evaluated.
- Pain assessment should include assessment on movement and at rest.
- Parent/carer involvement is essential when assessing pain level in children with cognitive impairment.

72 Pain management

Figure 72.1 The stages of pain management.

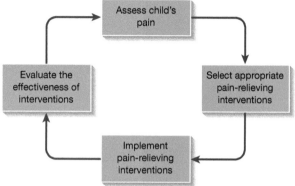

- Assess child's pain
- Select appropriate pain-relieving interventions
- Implement pain-relieving interventions
- Evaluate the effectiveness of interventions

Figure 72.2 The three Ps of pain management.

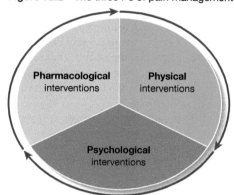

- Pharmacological interventions
- Physical interventions
- Psychological interventions

Figure 72.3 Interventions.

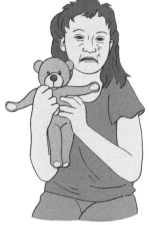

Pharmacological interventions

- Administering prescribed analgesic drugs is the mainstay of acute pain management
- Should adhere to the World Health Organization's two-step ladder
- Multimodal analgesia should be used

Physical and psychological interventions

Interventions that can be used include:
- Acupuncture
- Distraction
- Guided imagery
- Music therapy
- Relaxation

Figure 72.4 The WHO two-step approach to pain management.

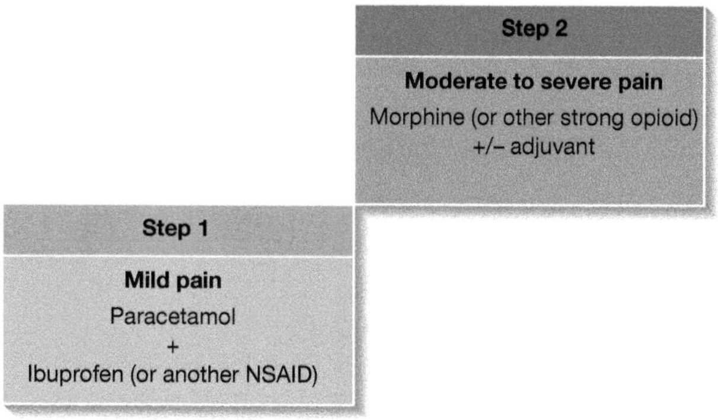

Step 2
Moderate to severe pain
Morphine (or other strong opioid) +/– adjuvant

Step 1
Mild pain
Paracetamol + Ibuprofen (or another NSAID)

Box 72.1 Consequences of unrelieved pain

Physical effects
- Rapid, shallow, splinted breathing, which can lead to hypoxaemia and alkalosis
- Inadequate expansion of lungs and poor cough, which can lead to secretion retention and atelectasis
- Increased heart rate, blood pressure, and myocardial oxygen requirements, which can lead to cardiac morbidity and ischaemia
- Increased stress hormones, which in turn increase the metabolic rate, impede healing, and decrease immune function
- Slowing or stasis of gut and urinary systems, which leads to nausea, vomiting, ileus, and urinary retention
- Muscle tension, spasm, and fatigue, which lead to reluctance to move spontaneously and refusal to ambulate, further delaying recovery

Psychological effects
- Anxiety, fear, distress, feelings of helplessness or hopelessness
- Avoidance of activity, avoidance of future medical procedures
- Sleep disturbances
- Loss of appetite

Other effects
- Prolonged hospital stays
- Increased rates of readmission to hospital
- More outpatient visits

Children and Young People's Nursing at a Glance, Second Edition. Edited by Elizabeth Gormley-Fleming and Sheila Roberts.
© 2023 John Wiley & Sons Ltd. Published 2023 by John Wiley & Sons Ltd.

Why managing pain in children is important

Painful experiences are part of life for every child. Pain has an important purpose, serving as a warning or protective mechanism; people who are unable to feel pain often suffer extensive tissue damage. However, unrelieved pain has a number of undesirable physical and psychological consequences (Box 72.1). When these adverse effects are considered, the need to manage children's pain effectively is clear.

Summary of current guidelines

A review of clinical guidelines relating to the management of pain (Figure 72.1) in children and young people indicates that effective management of pain requires nurses to:

* Take a pain history on admission.
* Assess pain using a validated pain assessment tool.
* Reassess pain following the implementation of pain-relieving interventions.
* Discuss the child's pain management with their parents or carers.
* Involve the child in decisions about their pain management.
* Ensure the child has appropriate analgesic drugs prescribed.
* Administer analgesic drugs as prescribed.
* Use appropriate physical and psychological interventions.
* Prepare the child for painful procedures.
* Use analgesic creams for planned painful procedures.
* Ensure pain assessments are recorded on a flow chart.
* Document the pain-relieving interventions used and their effectiveness in the child's notes.

What does pain management involve?

Pain is a biopsychosocial phenomenon. This means that when managing pain in children pharmacological, physical, and psychological interventions need to be used.

Aims of pain management

The aims of managing acute pain in children (Figure 72.2) are to:

* Rapidly identify pain.
* Prevent pain if possible.
* Control pain by administering analgesic drugs.
* Use multimodal analgesia.
* Monitor to prevent adverse events.
* Address emotional components of pain.
* Continue pain control after discharge from hospital.

Pharmacological interventions

See Figure 72.3.

Non-opioids

Paracetamol

Paracetamol is appropriate for mild pain. It is thought to act by inhibiting prostaglandin synthesis in the brain. Paracetamol has antipyretic activity, but minimal anti-inflammatory effects. Paracetamol can be administered via oral, rectal, or intravenous routes. Due to their immature liver function, newborn babies require reduced doses.

Non-steroidal anti-inflammatory drugs

Non-steroidal anti-inflammatory drugs (NSAIDs), such as ibuprofen and diclofenac, are used for mild to moderate pain. They act by inhibiting the synthesis of prostaglandins via inhibiting the production of COX-1 and COX-2 enzymes. NSAIDs have antipyretic activity as well as anti-inflammatory and analgesic activity. Any easy way of remembering the adverse effects of NSAIDs is by using the acronym SKAB:

* *Stomach*: NSAIDs can cause gastric irritation.
* *Kidneys*: NSAIDs should not be given to people with impaired kidney function.
* *Asthma*: NSAIDs can exacerbate symptoms in some people with asthma.
* *Bleeding*: NSAIDs should not be given to people with impaired platelet function.

Important point: these adverse effects can occur with *all* routes of administration, not just the oral route.

Opioids

Opioids, such as morphine, diamorphine, and fentanyl, are used for treating moderate to severe pain. Adverse effects of opioids include:

* Vomiting
* Constipation
* Respiratory depression
* Bronchoconstriction
* Pruritus (itching)
* Urinary retention

Multimodal analgesia

Multimodal analgesia is the combination of two or more analgesic drugs with different mechanisms of action. This improves children's pain scores and allows for lower doses of analgesic drugs, thus minimizing adverse effects.

World health organization two-step approach to pain management

The World Health Organization (WHO) analgesic ladder offers a two-step strategy for treating pain and recommends that analgesic drugs are given according to pain severity. Analgesic drugs should be given around the clock to start with and then as needed to keep the child pain free (Figure 72.4).

Addiction

Addiction is a psychological dependence on drugs. Many healthcare professionals worry that patients will become addicted to opioids. However, in reality this rarely happens. If children are on opioids for more than a few days they may become tolerant to the drug and need an increased dose to keep them pain free – this does not mean they are addicted. Likewise, if a child is on opioids for more than three days or so they are likely to experience withdrawal symptoms if the drug is stopped abruptly. Again, this does not mean the child is addicted to the drug, but rather that a weaning protocol needs to be implemented.

Physical and psychological interventions

Several physical and psychological interventions can be used to enhance the effectiveness of the analgesic drugs administered. Some of the interventions used most often for the child in acute pain are outlined in Figure 72.3. The clinician needs to choose an intervention that is appropriate for the age and development of the child.

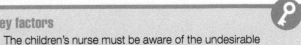

Key factors

* The children's nurse must be aware of the undesirable consequences of pain for the child or young person and seek to avoid these.
* Managing pain in children requires pharmacological, physical, and psychological interventions.
* Multimodal analgesia is known to improve children's and young people's pain scores.

73 Preoperative assessment and preparation

Figure 73.1 Preadmission preparation.

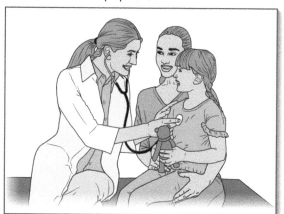

The child and family will need:
- physical assessment
- preadmission screening
- fasting instructions
- risk assessment and management of identified risk
- information to give informed consent
- information to manage all expectations
- opportunity to ask questions

World Health Organization Surgical Safety Checklist

SIGN IN – before the induction of anaesthetic
TIME OUT – before the start of surgical intervention
SIGN OUT – before any member of the team leaves theatre

Advice and activities for parent to do at home to prepare their child for hospital

- Be honest with your child and tell them as much as you can about going into hospital
- Answer questions truthfully
- Use words that they will understand
- Read them age-appropriate books about going to hospital
- Visit the hospital's website so they can see the facilities
- Access other child-appropriate websites or specialist we sites
- If you need any additional support such as an interpreter, request this in advance of attending the hospital
- Label and remember to bring all items of importance to your child – cuddly toys, religious items, mobility aids, clothing, and medicines
- If the child is unwell within three days of admission or has come into contact with infectious diseases such as chicken pox, do inform the ward/day unit

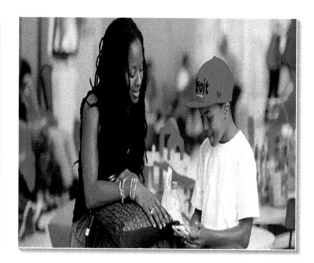

Figure 73.2 Preoperative checklist.

	Yes	No	N/A	Theatre
Identity band present				
Clinical observations and weight recorded				
Loose teeth/fillings/caps/crowns/braces				
Fasting: time of last food, time of last fluids				
Bath/shower; passed urine				
Prosthetics: aids, jewellery, nail varnish removed, body piercings				
Local anaesthetic applied: Ametop Emla (please circle)				
Allergies				
Premedication given				
Consent form signed				
Medicine prescription record included				
Investigation records; blood results				
Discharge letter attached				
Seen by Dr Seen by anaesthetist				
Signed:	Ward nurse		Date	
Signed:	Theatre		Date	

Children and Young People's Nursing at a Glance, Second Edition. Edited by Elizabeth Gormley-Fleming and Sheila Roberts.
© 2023 John Wiley & Sons Ltd. Published 2023 by John Wiley & Sons Ltd.

Preadmission clinic

Preadmission clinics are nurse-led clinics that aim to prepare patients for admission to hospital for elective surgery (Figure 73.1). Children and young people are assessed in relation to their medical fitness for the procedure. These clinics also provide information about the planned surgery, deal with any concerns the child and family may have, and provide post-surgery and discharge information. All the necessary tests or investigations may be carried out at this appointment. Preoperative testing for SARS-CoV-2 should be undertaken in accordance with public health guidance. All necessary precautions and consistent information about precautions and hand washing should be provide to the parents and to the child prior to being admitted to hospital for their surgery. Following attendance at the preadmission/assessment clinic, the child and family will receive confirmation of their date of admission.

Hospital admission

The child/young person and their family are usually admitted on the day of their surgery. Restrictions on the number of family members in attendance at the hospital may be in place, but the needs of the child should be considered as unique, parents permitted to attend, and local adjustments made to accommodate this. Admission processes and associated documentation are completed, including a comprehensive assessment of the child's and family's needs and preoperative procedures such as patient identity, vital signs, weight, and any relevant investigations indicated by the surgical team.

Effects of hospitalization

Hospitalization can be a daunting experience for children and their families. Children need to gain knowledge and understanding of why they are in hospital and what is likely to happen during their stay. A warm welcome and a friendly approach can do much to reduce anxiety, alongside developing a sound therapeutic relationship.

Informed consent

Informed written consent is a legal requirement and good practice in both elective and emergency procedures. Children should be involved in this process whether or not they are of an age to consent (16 years), alongside parents or carers. Information pertaining to the benefits, risks, and complications of the procedure needs to be discussed by the surgeon and family to ensure informed consent has been achieved.

Patient safety and risk management

Many factors contribute to the safety of the patient in the preoperative period, including patient identification, potential risks to safety (i.e. allergy status, prosthetics, loose teeth, laboratory reports, or other investigation results) (Figure 73.2). Indication of the site of surgery should also be observable, checking the child has voided urine, and skin and nail preparation has occurred. Pre-medications or local anaesthetics may be prescribed and administered prior to surgery.

Fasting guidelines

In order to ensure that the child's safety is maintained in the preoperative period, it is vital to ensure that the required fasting times are adhered to: six hours for solid foods, four hours for breastfeeds, and two hours for clear fluids. Explanations must be given to the child and parents of what clear fluid means, for example. It must also be clear that chewing gum is not permitted. This minimizes the risk of the child aspirating stomach contents during the anaesthetic procedure. Parents should be advised to provide food and drink until the stated fasting time to ensure the child remains well hydrated and nourished. This may involve waking the child in the night to give them a drink. If the child has a prolonged period of fasting or an underlying medical disorder, it may be necessary for them to receive intravenous replacement fluids. If the child requires regular oral medication during the fasting period for a pre-existing condition, then this should be discussed with the anaesthetist. Normally it is advised that regular medication is continued unless specified otherwise.

Key points

• Preoperative assessment provides a level of assurance about the medical fitness of a child for surgery and gives an opportunity for the child and parents to gain information about the surgery and post-procedural care.
• All investigations should be completed at this time if delays on the day of surgery are to be avoided.
• It is imperative that preoperative fasting requirements are understood by the child and parents prior to them leaving the hospital/telephone call.
• The parents and child should always have an opportunity to ask questions and be aware of all possible outcomes.

74 Postoperative care

Box 74.1 Phases of postoperative care.

Immediate phase (recovery unit)	Intermediate phase (children's ward)	Discharge phase
Airway – will require equipment (artificial airway) and positioning to maintain patency of airway; observe for vomitus/secretions in the airway; suctioning equipment	Nurse child beside oxygen and suction – aim to maintain airway independently	Child is able to maintain airway independently or airway patency is as prior to admission
Breathing – close observation of the child's breathing pattern and supportive care in the form of oxygen is administered	Observe effort, rate, depth, and rhythm closely in the initial period after return to ward; be aware of the effects of opioids	Breathing pattern should have returned to within normal limits for the patient
Circulation – assessment of perfusion – centrally and peripherally, capillary refill time, manual heart rate/pulse to assess strength, rate, and rhythm	Continue to monitor, as in the immediate phase – observe colour of child's lips and nail beds	Normal perfusion and circulatory performance is achieved
Clinical observations – monitored very closely in the recovery room, respiratory rate, heart rate/pulse, blood pressure, temperature, oxygen saturation levels, level of consciousness	As per ward policy or guideline; however, continues to be monitored closely (i.e. half-hourly to hourly), physiological data recorded as per early warning systems or ward policy	These should have returned to within normal limits for the individual, parents advised re observation of child's recovery from surgery (i.e. temperature checking)
Wound management – close observation of wound sites, dressings, or drains for signs of primary haemorrhage	Wound assessed for any sign of oozing, swelling, bleeding, and/or pain at site – record findings. Ensure any dressings remain in situ. Ensure surgeon speaks to child and parents prior to discharge	Written and verbal advice given regarding care of wound in home, any dressings, suture removal, and analgesia. Referral to local community children's nursing team may be necessary
Pain management – can be patient or nurse controlled, commenced in perioperative period, need to monitor effectiveness, need for additional analgesics	Accurate assessment of the degree and severity of child's pain using an age-appropriate pain scoring tool is vital, in order to measure and effectively control pain	Pain management strategies discussed with parents prior to discharge. Advice re safe storage of medications in the home
Fluid replacement – consider prolonged fasting times, theatre time, postoperative instructions, may be necessary for the child to have intravenous (IV) fluid therapy	Record the site of child's IV cannula, closely monitor for potential complications, reintroduction of oral fluid intake and discontinuation of IV replacement therapies	Ensure IV cannula is removed prior to discharge, noting condition of site and removal in the patient's notes
Nutrition – introduction of clear oral fluids, when child fully alert, as per surgeon's instructions, small amounts initially	Offer light diet – toast or ice cream – when child feels ready to eat	Child should be tolerant of a light diet prior to discharge
Mobilizing – recovery position initially until regains consciousness, change of position if this is restricted postoperatively, bed rest until return to ward area	Gentle mobilization as tolerated or as condition permits	Able to mobilize gently
Elimination – monitor postoperative elimination; observe for possible urinary retention, postoperative nausea and vomiting (PONV) – record frequency, amount and nature	Monitor and record intake and output chart, noting any signs of dehydration or urine retention. Manage any episodes of PONV	Ensure child has passed urine prior to discharge. Child is not experiencing any PONV
Complications – numerous potential problems, most common – hypoventilation, primary haemorrhage, nausea and vomiting	Raised body temperature, risk of shock, respiratory depression, intermediate haemorrhage, nausea and vomiting, signs of wound infection	Wound dehiscence, advice regarding how to manage any possible complications (e.g. secondary haemorrhage following discharge)
Psychological care – communicate with the child – what is happening, parental presence in recovery room	Parents and child kept fully informed and included in all aspects of postoperative care and decisions	Parents happy to take child home and have necessary information and support to continue care at home
Discharge planning – when fit for return to ward, child and family discharged in line with hospital criteria	Ongoing communication with child and family regarding potential discharge date and time and resources to support discharge	Health education and promotion opportunities – restricted activities, importance of nutrition in healing, supplies, and letter for general practitioner. Contact numbers for ward to parents

Figure 74.1 Stages of wound healing.

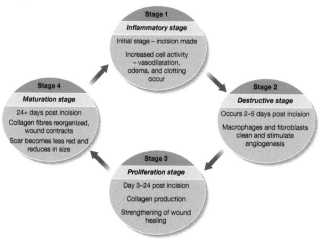

Stage 1
Inflammatory stage
Initial stage – incision made
Increased cell activity – vasodilatation, odema, and clotting occur

Stage 2
Destructive stage
Occurs 2–5 days post incision
Macrophages and fibroblasts clean and stimulate angiogenesis

Stage 3
Proliferation stage
Day 3–24 post incision
Collagen production
Strengthening of wound healing

Stage 4
Maturation stage
24+ days post incision
Collagen fibres reorganized, wound contracts
Scar becomes less red and reduces in size

Children and Young People's Nursing at a Glance, Second Edition. Edited by Elizabeth Gormley-Fleming and Sheila Roberts.
© 2023 John Wiley & Sons Ltd. Published 2023 by John Wiley & Sons Ltd.

Postoperative handover

Following the immediate recovery period and once the child is stable, they need to return to their ward or day-care unit (Box 74.1). The care of the child is handed over to ward staff. The SBAR format should be used (Situation, Background, Assessment, Recommendation) and the nurse should ensure that the following details are included:

- Details of the anaesthetic, including medication administered in theatre, dose, and time.
- Operation performed.
- Specific postoperative instructions and management plan.
- Oxygen therapy administered and prescribed. Time airway adjunct rejected.
- Level of consciousness and rousability.
- Current PEWS (Paediatric Early Warning Score) – this should be repeated by the nurse receiving handover before leaving the recovery room.
- Intravenous fluids or blood products received in theatre and in recovery along with instructions for continuation of intravenous fluids.
- Analgesia administered in theatre and in recovery, with effect. Current pain score should be recorded. Prescription chart should be checked that adequate analgesia is prescribed.
- Any postoperative nausea or vomiting and any treatment given.
- Wound site should be checked and strike-through noted on dressings.
- Drains and catheters should be checked for output and at their insertion sites.
- Neurovascular or neurological observations (if required) should be checked before leaving recovery area.

The ward nurse collecting the child from the recovery area should have oxygen with oxygen tubing and correct-size mask available and other monitoring equipment that may be indicated.

Community perspective

Transition from hospital to home can be a complex and lengthy process in the case of major surgery or trauma. It may require discharge planning from the point of admission, by making practical plans with the child and parent in relation to identifying needs post surgery and resources required, aiming to avoid a failed discharge or readmission for the child and family. However, children who have day surgery may also require community care. The early identification of needs and initiation of effective communication pathways between the hospital and the community children's nurse, health visitor, and other appropriate members of the multidisciplinary team should achieve a timely and successful discharge. Additional resources or those with expertise such as the tissue viability nurse may become involved with patients and families who experience issues with wound healing or choice of dressings (Figure 74.1).

The importance of adhering to and completing treatment regimes following discharge should be emphasized and supported by community nursing teams until the child and family no longer require the input of such services. Infection prevention and control are a key aspect of ongoing care for the child and family, ensuring that all personnel involved in care delivery, whether in the hospital or community, are aware of effective hand hygiene and maintain good standards of hygiene around wounds until effective wound healing is complete.

Key points

- The children and young person's nurse is responsible and accountable for determining the frequency of observations based on the clinical need of the child or young person in the postoperative period.
- Discharge after day-case surgery should focus on a safe and effective discharge process and this will require early preparation for discharge.
- Safety-netting advice for parents and carers must be provided if the family are to feel secure on discharge.

75 Pressure area care

Figure 75.1 Development of pressure ulcers.

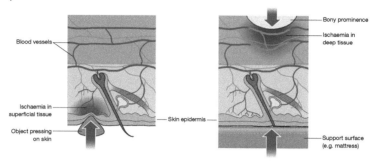

Figure 75.2 Some common sites for pressure ulcers. CPAP, continuous positive airway pressure; ECG, electrocardiogram; IV, intravenous.

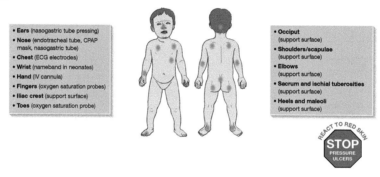

- **Ears** (nasogastric tube pressing)
- **Nose** (endotracheal tube, CPAP mask, nasogastric tube)
- **Chest** (ECG electrodes)
- **Wrist** (nameband in neonates)
- **Hand** (IV cannula)
- **Fingers** (oxygen saturation probes)
- **Iliac crest** (support surface)
- **Toes** (oxygen saturation probe)

- **Occiput** (support surface)
- **Shoulders/scapulae** (support surface)
- **Elbows** (support surface)
- **Sacrum and ischial tuberosities** (support surface)
- **Heels and maleoli** (support surface)

REACT TO RED SKIN
STOP PRESSURE ULCERS

Figure 75.3 Grade of pressure ulcers.

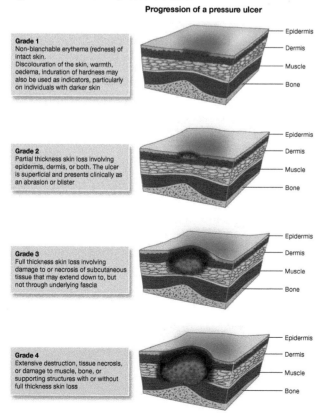

Progression of a pressure ulcer

Grade 1
Non-blanchable erythema (redness) of intact skin.
Discolouration of the skin, warmth, oedema, induration of hardness may also be used as indicators, particularly on individuals with darker skin

Epidermis
Dermis
Muscle
Bone

Grade 2
Partial thickness skin loss involving epidermis, dermis, or both. The ulcer is superficial and presents clinically as an abrasion or blister

Epidermis
Dermis
Muscle
Bone

Grade 3
Full thickness skin loss involving damage to or necrosis of subcutaneous tissue that may extend down to, but not through underlying fascia

Epidermis
Dermis
Muscle
Bone

Grade 4
Extensive destruction, tissue necrosis, or damage to muscle, bone, or supporting structures with or without full thickness skin loss

Epidermis
Dermis
Muscle
Bone

Figure 75.4 Think SSKIN when assessing a child who is at risk of pressure ulcers.

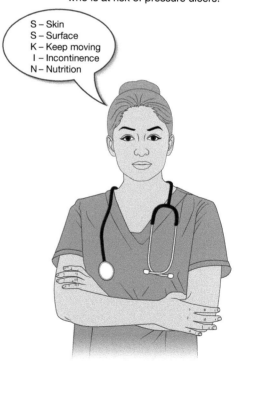

S – Skin
S – Surface
K – Keep moving
I – Incontinence
N – Nutrition

Children and Young People's Nursing at a Glance, Second Edition. Edited by Elizabeth Gormley-Fleming and Sheila Roberts.
© 2023 John Wiley & Sons Ltd. Published 2023 by John Wiley & Sons Ltd.

A pressure ulcer is an area of damage to the skin caused by the external pressure of the support surface or objects pressing on the skin and underlying tissues, with enough pressure to reduce blood flow and for a long enough time to cause tissue ischaemia (Figure 75.1). In this case, pressure damage starts at the skin and may progress to deeper ulceration if pressure is not relieved. This can be seen initially as redness of the skin that does not blanch on light finger pressure (grade 1 pressure ulcer). Pressure injury and ulcers are generally preventable and avoidable. Prevention of the pressure injury is the aim.

Children with certain conditions are at increased risk of injury from pressure and these include children with spina bifida, those with neurological impairment that restricts their movement, and those who need to wear prosthesis or orthosis. Children who are malnourished, or have a weakened immune system, or are critically ill all have an increased risk of developing pressure ulcers.

Pressure damage may also start in deep tissues at a bony prominence (Figure 75.2). If a child is lying in one position for a long period of time, tissues are compressed between the support surface and the bony prominence. The support surface may distribute skin pressure, but internal pressure will be concentrated at the bone. In this case, the ischaemia starts where the bone is pressing on muscle, and tissue damage progresses towards the skin. This may be first seen as swelling, heat, and discoloration over the area of ischaemia. Both deep and superficial pressure ulcers can be very painful.

About half of pressure ulcers seen in children appear to be related to objects (such as medical devices) pressing or rubbing on the child's skin. All areas where devices may press or rub on the child's skin must be inspected frequently and, if possible, a cushioning layer should be placed between the device and the child's skin. Children with reduced mobility must have their position changed and skin inspected frequently. Sitting in wet or damp clothing/nappies for long periods may cause skin damage. Crumpled bed linen or clothing with thick seams may also lead to undue pressure on the child's skin.

Grade of pressure ulcers

Pressure ulcers are graded according to the amount of skin damage that occurs, ranging from grade 1 to grade 4 (Figure 75.3).

This is useful when describing any lesions in patient records and planning treatment and nursing care. Grade 1 pressure ulcers usually heal without complications if the source of the localized pressure is removed. Moisture lesions (such as nappy rash) should not be confused with pressure ulcers.

- *Grade 1*: intact skin with non-blanchable redness of a localized area, usually over a bony prominence. The skin may be discoloured, warm to touch, and some oedema, induration, or hardness may also be present, particularly or dark skin.
- *Grade 2*: partial thickness. Loss of epidermis or dermis or both, presenting as a shallow open ulcer with a red/pink wound bed, without slough. The ulcer is superficial. May also present as an intact, open, or ruptured serum-filled blister.
- *Grade 3*: full-thickness tissue loss. Subcutaneous fat may be visible, but bone, tendon, or muscle is not exposed. Slough may be present, but does not obscure the depth of tissue loss. May include undermining and tunnelling.

- *Grade 4*: full-thickness skin loss with exposed bone, tendon, or muscle. Extensive destruction. Slough or eschar may be present on some parts of the wound bed. Often includes undermining and tunnelling.

Prevention of pressure ulcers

Evidence-based guidelines recommend that all children who need nursing care or who have reduced mobility should have an initial pressure ulcer risk assessment documented. Children deemed to be at risk should have skin assessment and preventative action recorded in their care plan (Figure 75.4). This plan may include the following:

- Positioning in bed or chair.
- Use of slide sheets/hoists to move and transfer child.
- Use of absorbent bedsheets.
- Prophylactic use of barrier film for children in nappies or pads.
- Nutritional assessment.
- Use of continuous low-pressure or alternating-pressure mattresses/cushions.
- Frequent inspection of at-risk areas of skin.

Pressure ulcer risk assessment should be repeated whenever a child's condition changes.

Care at home

Parents may need advice for discharge, as pressure injuries often take a long time to heal or may have the potential to occur in certain conditions, such as when wearing a cast or prosthetic, or lack of immobility post surgery. They can be painful and add to the existing health problems that the child has. Parents need to be told about the following:

- *Observing* the child's skin regularly, particularly high-risk areas, and looking for blisters, bruising, scratches, cracks, or changes in skin colour. Particular attention should be paid to areas that are moist, such as the groin and buttocks. If the child has a cast, then look for increased pain or discomfort.
- *Positioning*: encourage child to change position at least every two hours and to be as active as possible. No dragging the skin when changing position and make sure bed line is wrinkle free where possible.
- *Nutrition*: a balanced diet with good fluid intake is necessary for wound healing and maintaining healthy skin.
- *Pressure-relieving devices*: parents should know where to access and how to use them. An occupational therapist may need to be involved.
- *How to seek help* and to have a low threshold for seeking help if they have any concerns.

Key points

- Prevention of pressure ulcers is always better than having to treat one.
- All pressure ulcers, irrespective of grade, should be reported as an incident in accordance with local policy.
- The children's nurse should adjust the child's care plan according to the child's need following comprehensive pressure area risk assessment. Risk assessment should be repeated in accordance with the child's changing condition.

76 Managing fluid balance

Figure 76.1 Common causes of fluid imbalance.

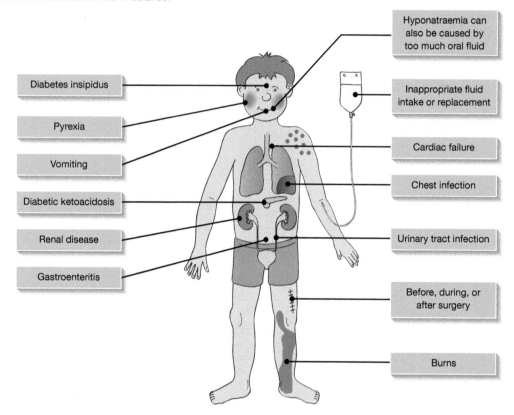

- Diabetes insipidus
- Pyrexia
- Vomiting
- Diabetic ketoacidosis
- Renal disease
- Gastroenteritis

- Hyponatraemia can also be caused by too much oral fluid
- Inappropriate fluid intake or replacement
- Cardiac failure
- Chest infection
- Urinary tract infection
- Before, during, or after surgery
- Burns

Box 76.1 What you need from your evaluation. AVPU, Alert, Verbal, Pain, Unresponsive.

History

- How long has the child been unwell?
- Any history of vomiting or diarrhoea or recent gastroenteritis in the family?
- Has the child been pyrexic?
- In an infant or young child: have the nappies been wet?
- In an older child: is the child passing urine?
- Is the child able to tolerate any oral fluids?
- How much and what type of fluids have been offered?

Key observations/investigations

- Temperature, pulse, respirations, blood pressure, AVPU
- Capillary refill time
- Weight
- Urinalysis
- Blood glucose
- Glasgow coma scale
- Blood for urea and electrolytes
- Blood gas analysis in the ill child

Assessing the child: signs and symptoms of dehydration

- Pallor
- Sunken eyes
- Sunken fontanelle
- Dry skin/mucous membranes
- Presence of lethargy or irritability
- Reduced urinary output
- Weight loss
- Increased capillary refill time (>2 seconds)
- Cool, mottled extremities
- Decreased tissue turgor
- Increased pulse and reduced blood pressure
- Dehydration may be mild, moderate, or severe

Assessing the child: signs and symptoms of over-hydration

- Altered urinary output
- Generalized or peripheral oedema
- Cerebral oedema: altered consciousness or seizure activity
- Weight gain

Distribution of body fluids

The percentage of body weight made up by fluid varies with age, as does its distribution within the body. The percentage of total body water decreases with age, with infants and young children having 75–80% of their body weight composed of fluid. Fluids are contained within a number of compartments in the body. Intracellular fluid (ICF) is contained within the cells. Extracellular fluid (ECF), contained outside the cells, is further subdivided into three types: interstitial fluid that surrounds the cell (e.g. that found in cartilage or connective tissue); intravascular fluid, found within the blood vessels; and transcellular fluid, found in body cavities (e.g. cerebrospinal or intestinal fluid). Body fluids and associated electrolytes are in constant motion around the body by diffusion, osmosis, and active transport in order to achieve a state of homeostasis. Thus, the body works continuously to distribute fluid and achieve optimal fluid balance.

Mechanisms of fluid balance

The kidneys have a vital role in fluid balance by filtering plasma fluid during the formation of urine. There are three additional key mechanisms that control fluid balance in the body: thirst, antidiuretic hormone, and the renin–angiotensin–aldosterone system. When these systems are unable to maintain homeostasis, fluid moves unregulated between compartments; this can result in a fluid and electrolyte imbalance. See Figure 76.1 for some common causes of fluid and electrolyte imbalance.

Management of the child with fluid imbalance

As with any aspect of children's nursing, a child- and family-centred approach is essential. Careful and appropriate information sharing, involving the child and family, open communication, negotiation, and thorough preparation, including play and distraction techniques, will help to reduce anxiety. Ongoing monitoring and assessment of the child, together with the multidisciplinary team, and adherence to local policies are key aspects of ensuring safe and effective care. Appropriate measuring, recording, and reporting of all intake and output in the fluid balance chart and documentation in the nursing notes are also vital. Some children (e.g. those with meningitis or electrolyte disturbance) may need fluid restriction, while those in specialist areas may have very individual requirements. Communication with the medical team is paramount. Key considerations in the management of a child with fluid imbalance are outlined in Box 76.1.

Oral fluid requirements

Oral fluids are the preferred option for maintaining fluid balance in children where possible. If the child has a history of vomiting, an oral rehydration solution (ORS), such as Dioralyte™ (Sanofi, Reading, UK), given orally or via a nasogastric tube, may be recommended. Parents have a key role in encouraging ORS intake

Table 76.1 Intravenous fluid calculations (https://www.nice.org.uk/guidance/ng29/evidence/full-guideline-pdf-2188636813).

Fluid requirements	Per day (mL/kg)
For the first 10 kg	100
For the second 10 kg	50
For each kg over 20 kg	20

For example:
- 6 kg infant would require 6 × 100 mL = 600 mL/day
- 18 kg child would need 1000 + 400 = 1400 mL/day
- 25 kg child would need 1000 + 500 + 100 = 1600 mL/day

NB Maximum daily amounts should be specified in local policies.

(as opposed to water or other oral fluids) in small but frequent amounts. However, many children who are ill require intravenous (IV) fluid therapy. Oral requirements for neonates vary according to hospital policies. As a general rule, by 5 days old onwards, 150 mL/kg/day body weight is required.

Intravenous fluid requirements

The choice of the IV fluid will be governed by local policy and the individual assessment of the child. If shock is present, a rapid bolus of appropriate IV fluid can be given initially, in accordance with local policy. The fluid deficit, based on the estimated percentage of dehydration, may also be calculated and is normally replaced by sodium chloride 0.9% over the next 48 hours. This should take account of any boluses given. Large volumes of IV medication and ongoing losses should also be taken into consideration when calculating IV fluid requirements. Maintenance fluids are calculated by the formula in Table 76.1. This formula is applicable to infants and children over 28 days of age. For neonates under 28 days, see NICE guidance (https://www.nice.org.uk/guidance/ng29/resources/intravenous-fluid-therapy-in-children-and-young-people-in-hospital-pdf-1837340295109).

Ongoing monitoring and assessment of the child, accurate recording, reporting, and evaluation are key aspects of the children's nurse's role as a member of the multidisciplinary team.

Key points
- Accurate calculation of fluid requirements and knowledge of suitable fluid therapy are vital.
- Assessing and managing fluid imbalance are an important part of the nurse's role.
- Ongoing monitoring of the child and accurate documentation are key.
- Optimal multidisciplinary working is essential.
- Children's nurses must maintain competence through regular training updates and adhere strictly to local policy

Acknowledgements. The authors would like to thank Dr Damien Armstrong for his assistance in the preparation of this chapter.

77 Administering medication

Figure 77.1 Medication procedure.

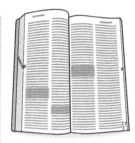
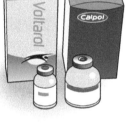
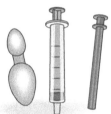

1 Before you make a start

- Familiarize yourself with your local medicines policy and procedures
- Be aware of NMC Code of Conduct (2018)
- Understand why your patient has been prescribed this medication, check the care plans as well as dose, possible adverse effects, contraindications, and special precautions
- Check prescription charts regularly. Omission is the second most common reason for medication error
- Gather together the prescription chart, keys, and second registered nurse to act as checker if required
- Wash your hands

2 Check prescription chart

- Has the correct patient identification. Full name, NHS number, and/or hospital number if required by local policy
- Has a completed and signed confirmation of allergy status on the front of the chart
- Provides a clear, legible prescription of medication to be administered. If this appears ambiguous it is safer to request that the prescription chart is rewritten. Prescriptions should include date of prescription, the generic drug name, route, dosage, date and time to be administered, and the prescriber's printed name and signature
- Remember all checks should be completed independently

3 Preparing the medicine

- With the second checker, select the correct medication and check that it is within the expiry date. Consider formula/spoon/oral syringe preference for children
- Check that the dose prescribed is correct for the age and weight of the patient using a reference source (e.g. British National Formulary for Children (BNFC))
- Independently calculate the volume of liquid or number of tablets required. Compare answers. Recalculate if you disagree
- Measure the dose required. Both practitioners should witness all stages of the process and confirm the amount prepared. Both nurses should undertake final bedside checks together

4 Administering the medicine

- Check that the patient's name, date of birth, and NHS number on the nameband correlate with these details on the prescription chart
- If possible, ask the patient/parent to tell you their name and date of birth
- Check the allergy section on the prescription chart for contraindications to administration
- Explain purpose of the medication to the patient/family and gain consent for administration
- The patient/family/non-registered nurse/play specialist may wish to be involved in the administration procedure. Remember this must always be performed under the supervision of a registered nurse who remains accountable for any delegation of this task

5 Closing the intervention

- After administering the medication both nurses should sign the prescription chart to evidence that the medication has been given
- Offer the patient a drink, particularly if the medicine has an unpleasant taste
- Record reasons for non-administration of the drug on the prescription chart and in the nursing documentation
- Make the patient comfortable. Offer bravery rewards if appropriate. Ask whether there are any further interventions required. Inform the patient and/or family when you will be returning
- Dispose of equipment safely with clean spacers as required. Wash your hands
- Observe patient for adverse effects

Figure 77.2 Medication never events.

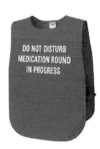

- Mis-selection of strong potassium solution
- Administration of medication by the wrong route
- Overdose of insulin due to abbreviations or incorrect dose
- Overdose of methotrexate for non-cancer treatment
- Mis-selection of high-strength midazeolam during conscious sedation

Box 77.1 The 10 'rights' of safe medication administration.

1. Right Patient
2. Right Medication
3. Right Dosage
4. Right Route
5. Right Time
6. Right Documentation
7. Right Education
8. Right to Refuse
9. Right Assessment
10. Right Evaluation

Children and Young People's Nursing at a Glance, Second Edition. Edited by Elizabeth Gormley-Fleming and Sheila Roberts.
© 2023 John Wiley & Sons Ltd. Published 2023 by John Wiley & Sons Ltd.

Contemporary issues

The administration of medicines to children and young people is very common. However, this is a complex procedure, not least because of the intricate weight-related calculations, the frequent inability of the patient to identify or advocate for themselves, and the widespread use of unlicensed medications in this patient group (Figure 77.1). The Nursing and Midwifery Council (NMC) Code of Conduct (2018) identifies the standards that all children's and young people's nurses must adhere to. The four themes are all relevant to medication administration:

- Prioritise people
- Practise effectively
- Preserve safety
- Promote professionalism and trust

Section 18 in Preserve safety focuses specifically on the role of the nurse in medication administration. The NMC Future Nurse: Standards of Proficiency for Registered Nurses identifies the procedural competencies required for best practice and evidence-based medication administration.

Although the use of medications that are not licenced for use in neonates, children, and young people has traditionally been common, this practice has recently been deemed unacceptable. Work is currently underway with the pharmaceutical industry to develop medicines that are safe and suitable for administration to neonates, children, and young people.

Involving the child, young person, and family

The admission process for children and young people should assess and record details of the child or young person's prescribed medication, together with their preferences for when this is usually taken and how all medications are usually given (e.g. tablet, syrup, spoon, oral syringe). Many children's hospitals operate parent administration procedures that maintain home routine, facilitate integrated family and healthcare partnership working, and help to protect against medication errors. The role of the children's nurse in this process is to provide support to families, but remain mindful of their legal and professional requirements to ascertain that medication has been administered as recorded.

As children and young people are reliant upon parental understanding of medicine regimes for their wellbeing, they are particularly vulnerable. The children's nurse therefore has a key role in explaining the rationale for dose, frequency, specific instructions, and adverse effects of medication to children, young people, and their parents and carers. Where hospital leaflets are unavailable, www.medicinesforchildren.org.uk is a valuable resource.

Medicine errors and safety

Medication errors continue to be the most frequent adverse incident reported. A medication error is an act or an omission in care that could contribute to unintended consequences. Medication errors or mistakes are classed as preventable events. The term 'near-miss' is used to describe a situation where a patient has been exposed to a situation and this has not resulted in harm or injury. There are a number of medication-related 'never' events (Figure 77.2). Some 10% of errors affect the 0–4-year age group. Medication errors can occur at any stage in the process:

- Prescription
- Transcription
- Dispensing
- Administration
- Monitoring the patient's condition

The most common error is incorrect dose, followed by omitted doses and incorrect frequency. The actual number of incidents and the harm they cause are unknown, as reporting is not yet mandatory. It is widely acknowledged that although these events are preventable, healthcare providers will never achieve a position of zero medication incidents. The true extent of the issue is unknown, as errors in medication administration in the home are largely unreported. What is important is that children's nurses learn from these events and review their practices in line with best evidence and local policy.

All medication errors including near misses must be reported using the UK-based incident reporting system. The duty of candour is a statutory duty that requires all nurses to be open and transparent when errors are made. If a nurse makes a mistake when administering medication to a child, they should do the following:

- Tell the child and parents as soon as possible that a mistake has been made.
- Apologize to the child and to the parents.
- Advise on any new treatment/intervention required in the immediate time period.
- Explain fully any long- and short-term effects as a result of the error.

Safe medication administration continues to be an area of focus and a number of initiatives have been implemented, such as removing distractions when calculating and dispensing medication; protected drug rounds with the nurse responsible clearly visible and wearing a red apron labelled with 'Do not disturb, Drug round in progress', and the use of automated dispensing cabinets. However, a simple strategy for reducing medication errors is to follow the 10 'rights' (Box 77.1). If there is any doubt at any stage in the process, the children's nurse should always seek advice from the prescriber, senior colleagues, or pharmacist rather than proceed and potentially harm a child.

Calculation formula

Familiarity with common drug calculation formulae is important and practice will lead to confidence development.

$$Dose = \frac{What\ you\ want}{What\ you\ have} \times Amount\ it\ is\ in$$

For example: you need to administer 60 mg paracetamol, which comes as a 120 mg in 5 mL preparation:

$$Dose = \frac{60}{120} \times 5 = \frac{1}{2} \times 5 = \frac{5}{2} = 2.5 mL$$

Units of measurement

$$1\ gram(g) = 1000\ milligrams(mg)$$
$$1\ milligram(mg) = 1000\ micrograms(\mu g)$$
$$1\ microgram(\mu g) = 1000\ nanograms(ng)$$
$$1\ litre(L) = 1000\ millilitres(mL).$$

Calculating intravenous fluid rates

$$Rate = \frac{Volume}{Time}$$

Example: 500 mL over four hours:

$$Rate = \frac{500}{4} = 125\ mL/hour$$

Key points

- Medication administration errors occur frequently in children's nursing practice so safe practice is key.
- The health literacy of parents is an important factor in managing medication administration in the community.
- The children's nurse must follow local policy in the administration of medication and be competent in this procedure and able to administer medication to a variety of routes safely.

78 Drug calculations

Box 78.1 Fractions

A useful resource when undertaking drug calculations is to learn common fractions expressed as a decimal. This is helpful when calculating dosages from ampules.

1/2 = 0.5	1/4 = 0.25	1/5 = 0.2
	2/4 = 0.5	2/5 = 0.4
	3/4 = 0.75	3/5 = 0.6
		4/5 = 0.8

Worked Example
If you require half of a 1 mL ampule you will require 0.5 mL

Box 78.2 Dividing and multiplying by 10, 100, and 1000

Many drug doses and stock strengths are given in multiples of 10. A useful skill is to be able to recognize when a dose is a multiple of 10 or 100 and to understand their relationship.

$10\,mg = 10 \times 1\,mg$
$100\,mg = 10 \times 10\,mg$
$20\,mg = 10 \times 2\,mg$
$50\,mg = 10 \times 5\,mg$
$1000\,mg = 10 \times 100\,mg$

Box 78.3 The metric system

To undertake drug calculations it is imperative to understand the units of measurement used in the prescribing and administration of drugs. The units are expressed using the Système Internationale within the standard metric system of weights and measures.

Units	Abbreviations	Conversions
Kilogram	kg	1 kg = 1000 g
Gram	g	1 g = 1000 mg
Milligram	mg	1 mg = 1000 µg
Microgram	µg	NA
Litre	L	1 L = 1000 mL
Millilitre	mL	NA

NA, not applicable.

Box 78.4 Proportions

Many calculations that are undertaken on a children's ward are based on weight and volume. This is because a dosage weight of drug has been dissolved in a volume of liquid. For example, an elixir that contains the dose strength of 125 mg in 5 mL means that in every 5 mL of liquid will be 125 mg of the drug.

Strength of the medicine 125 mg in 5 mL
If you halve the dose 62.5 mg in 2.5 mL
If you double the dose 250 mg in 10 mL

Box 78.5 Formula method

This method requires relevant numbers to be inserted into an equation, which once solved provides the necessary volume of liquid or number of tablets that need to be administered.

$$\frac{What\ you\ want\,(prescription)}{What\ you\ have\ got\,(stock\ strength)} \times What\ it\ is\ in\,(volume)$$
$$= Volume\ to\ be\ administered$$

$$\frac{What\ you\ want\,(prescription)}{What\ you\ have\ got\,(stock\ strength)}$$
$$= Number\ of\ tablets\ to\ be\ administered$$

Worked Examples
You need to administer 120 mg of paracetamol. The dose strength available is 120 mg of paracetamol in 5 mL

$$\frac{120}{120} \times 5 = 5\,mL$$

You need to administer 25 mg of prednisolone. This is available in 5 mg tablets

$$\frac{25}{5} = 5\ tablets$$

Numeracy

It is vital that paediatric nurses have sound numeracy skills to assist them within a range of healthcare activities. One such activity is drug calculation and administration (Boxes 78.1 and 78.2). Poor numeracy skills may lead to medication errors. The causes of medication errors are varied; however, nurses' poor mathematical skills are a leading cause of patient safety incidents.

Nursing and midwifery council

To ensure that nurses are equipped with a high level of numeracy skills, the Nursing and Midwifery Council (NMC) has established key competencies within the Standards Framework for Nursing and Midwifery Education that must be met to enable students to be allowed to progress onto the professional register, along with providing standards for registered nurses. However, long-term numerical fears, potentially stemming from school days, cause many qualified nurses to not feel confident in their numerical competence; regular revision and skills acquisition within the work place are beneficial to all concerned.

Skills

There are several resources that could provide assistance to nurses in utilizing a multifaceted approach to drug calculations (Box 78.3). These include being regularly exposed to drug calculations within their area, having basic numeracy knowledge and opportunities to practise that knowledge, possessing calculator skills, and being proficient in the effective use of equipment such as syringes.

Estimation

Being able to estimate the answer that you are seeking is essential in drug calculations (Box 78.4). Many medication errors occur because the practitioner has not thought through what a sensible answer or dose would be. A moment taken to approximate the calculation will prevent serious errors, such as a misplaced decimal point. Simple strategies such as 'would I swallow that many tablets' can help.

Using a calculator

Paediatric nurses should be able to undertake non-complex drug calculations without the use of a calculator. A calculator provides an answer to the equation that is keyed in; if the equation is incorrect, it is easy to generate the wrong answer. However, it would be acceptable to calculate the dose you need and then check the answer using a calculator. For more complex drug calculations, it may be necessary to use a calculator, although you should estimate the correct answer to ensure your calculation is correct.

Checking the dose

Before you administer a drug to a child, you must be sure that the prescribed dose is correct. While errors may be made by prescribers as well as those who administer the prescription, accountability sits with both. The majority of medicines can be administered by a single healthcare professional. However, there may be instances when a second checker is required, for example for intravenous medication. It is important that nurses check the relevant organizational policy as to who can administer medications and when a second checker is required. Double checking should involve each nurse independently undertaking the calculation and then both checking the answer together. There are some academics who believe that double checking may increase the risk of error, as each becomes complacent and relies on the other to spot an error. Therefore, it is imperative that nurses undertake the calculation independently before doing it jointly.

Recommendations for practice

Medication administration incidents are most frequently due to the wrong dose, delayed or omitted medication, or the wrong medication being administered, with the most frequently cited error being calculation error (Box 78.5). Universities and healthcare organizations must ensure that they implement routine and regular assessment of numeracy skills through education programmes and as part of their continuing professional development programmes. The implementation of such strategies should lead to an increased awareness and knowledge of the importance of numeracy and accuracy of drug calculations, leading to improved quality of care for patients and a reduced risk of medication errors.

Key points
- Understand your professional responsibility and accountability.
- Understand units of measurement.
- Possess sound knowledge of calculation formulae.
- Estimate the required volume/number of tablets.
- Double check when appropriate.
- Universities and employers should demonstrate yearly assessment of practitioners' numeracy skills.

79 Enteral and nasogastric feeding

Figure 79.1 Enteral feeding routes.

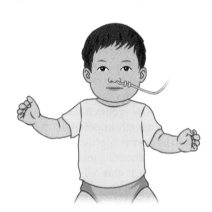

Nasogastric tube

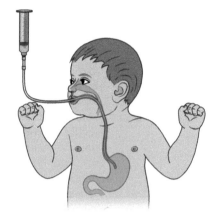

Orogastric feeding

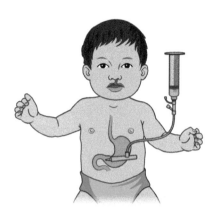

Gastrostomy feeding

Figure 79.2 Troubleshooting nasogastric tube placement.

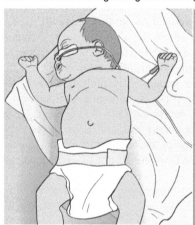

- The position of the tube should always be checked prior to administering any medication or feed
- Confirming tube position can sometimes be difficult
- Some medication such as H2 receptor blocking agents can alter the pH readings
- It can also be difficult to assess the pH of the stomach contents in children who are receiving continuous feeds
- Tips to try and check correct position:
  - ask the child to have a small drink if possible and safe to do so
  - reposition the tube to try to increase the amount of aspirate collected
  - reposition the child on their left side as this can increase the aspirate obtained
  - inject 10–20 mL air into the tube and then aspirate
- If no aspirate can be obtained then it may be necessary to confirm the position of the tube using X-ray. Local guidelines should always be followed in these cases

Box 79.1 Administering a bolus feed.

- Collect equipment and feed:
  - use correct personal protection equipment (PPE)
  - syringes
  - feed checked for correct child and expiry date
  - pH paper
  - water for flushing tube
- Wash hands and put on PPE
- Check tube position
- Check amount of feed to be delivered
- Attach syringe to nasogastric tube
- Administer feed slowly using gravity
- Flush nasogastric tube with water or air
- Dispose of all equipment following local policy
- Document actions

Box 79.2 Administering a continuous feed.

- Collect equipment and feed:
  - use correct PPE
  - syringes
  - feed checked for correct child and expiry date
  - pH paper
  - giving set
  - pump
- Wash hands and put on PPE
- Check tube position
- Check amount of feed to be delivered
- Prime giving set and place in pump
- Set hourly rate and volume to be administered on pump following local guidelines
- Dispose of all equipment following local policy
- Document actions

Box 79.3 Administering medication.

- Collect equipment and medication
- Check medication following local guidelines
- Wash hands and put on PPE
- Check tube position
- Administer each medication, flushing with water between each one
- Flush tube at finish
- Document actions

Children and Young People's Nursing at a Glance, Second Edition. Edited by Elizabeth Gormley-Fleming and Sheila Roberts.
© 2023 John Wiley & Sons Ltd. Published 2023 by John Wiley & Sons Ltd.

Enteral feeding

Enteral feeding is used when a child or young person is unable to maintain their own nutritional intake. The main reasons for using enteral feeding are as follows:

- Children who are unable to feed orally because they have a swallowing problem.
- Children who are unable to feed orally because they have breathing difficulties that are compromising their feeding.
- Children who are unable to maintain an optimal nutritional intake because they need a high-calorie diet or supplementation of their nutritional intake.

Enteral feeding can be short or long term and the chosen route for enteral feeding will be determined by its duration. It is important that children, young people, and their carers are involved in the decision to start enteral feeding and all the options are explained to them. Prior to commencing enteral feeding the child will require a full physical and nutritional assessment. Decisions should be taken utilizing the expertise of the multidisciplinary team, including the involvement of community healthcare practitioners if the child is to be discharged home with enteral feeding in place.

There are different routes by which children can be fed enterally (Figure 79.1):

- Nasogastric (NG)
- Orogastric (OG)
- Nasojejunal (NJ)
- Gastrostomy

Nasogastric feeding

NG feeding is the most common form of enteral feeding. Different types of NG tube are available and the choice of which type to use will be dependent on the duration of the feeding. Tubes for short-term use are made from polyvinylchloride (PVC) and can be left in place for 3–10 days; they can also be used for OG feeding. Tubes for long-term use are made of polyurethane and usually have a guide wire to assist insertion. These tubes can remain in place for up to 6 weeks, but the individual manufacturer's guidelines should be followed. Before insertion of the NG tube an explanation of the procedure should be provided to the child and their carers and informed consent obtained.

Inserting a nasogastric tube

The first step in NG tube insertion is to determine the size of tube required. This is usually decided by the size of the child's nostril. It is important that the NG tube does not obstruct the nostril so that the child can breathe around the tube. The most commonly used sizes are 6 Fr and 8 Fr. The appropriate length of tube should also be chosen, again dependent on the size of the child. The procedure for inserting the tube is as follows:

- Prepare child and family.
- Collect all the equipment required:
  ○ Correct size of tube.
  ○ pH paper.
  ○ Appropriate size of syringe (usually 20 mL).
  ○ Tape to secure the tube.
  ○ Sterile water to flush the tube once the position has been established.
  ○ A drink with a straw or dummy for the child to suck on if appropriate.
- Wash hands and put on personal protective equipment.
- Open the tube and check it is intact and suitable to use.

- Measure the tube using the NEX measurement (nose, ear, xiphisternum).
- If necessary lubricate the end of the tube with sterile water.
- Pass the tube gently into the child's nostril, advancing it along the nasopharynx into the oral pharynx. If any resistance is met or the child starts coughing or having difficulty breathing, the tube should be withdrawn.
- Once the measured length has been reached, the tube should be temporarily secured and tested using the pH paper.
- An aspirate pH of 5.5 or less indicates the tube is in the correct position.
- Once the correct position has been confirmed, the tube should be secured ensuring the child's skin is protected if necessary. Size of tube and date of insertion should be recorded in the child's records.

Orogastric feeding

OG feeding is not a common choice, but it may be used for some groups of children where it is not possible to pass an NG tube. These may be children (usually infants) who are for example receiving continuous positive airway pressure (CPAP) non-invasive ventilation, who have a congenital abnormality, or children admitted to the accident and emergency department with a suspected basal skull fracture. The procedure for passing an OG tube is similar to that for an NG tube. The key differences are:

- The tube is passed through the mouth.
- The measurement is from the xiphisternum to the lips.
- Care must be taken when securing the OG tube not to damage the lips or gums.

Nasojejunal feeding

NJ feeding is also not a common choice, but may be used when the child is unable to tolerate or absorb feeds via their stomach or in cases of severe vomiting or reflux. The NJ tube is passed beyond the stomach, through the pylorus, and into the jejunum. Initial position confirmation by X-ray is required followed by checking for signs of displacement. Aspirate is not required prior to feeding.

Gastrostomy feeding

Gastrostomy tubes provide a more long-term enteral feeding solution for children who are unable to maintain their nutritional status by oral feeding. A gastrostomy tube is inserted surgically by making an incision and placing the tube directly into the stomach through the abdominal wall. The tube is then held in place either by an internal flange or by a balloon. The type of fixation is dependent upon the type of tube.

Care of the insertion/stoma site is a key aspect of nursing care for children with a gastrostomy. The stoma needs to be checked regularly for tenderness, irritation, and leakage and should be cleaned as part of normal washing once the child is two weeks post insertion. The stoma should also be observed for signs of infection such as redness, swelling, or exudate. The tube should be rotated regularly according to the manufacturer's instructions to prevent tube adherence.

The administration of feeds is similar to the procedure for NG feeding. The main differences are:

- There is no need to check the position of the tube.
- The tube must be flushed with water before and after the feed.
- If it is a button device, then the extension set must be fixed on prior to the feed being administered.

Administration of enteral feeds

Enteral feeds can be administered either using gravity or via a pump. They can be given as a bolus (Box 79.1) or continuously (Box 79.2). Prior to administration of a feed, it is important to check that the tube is in the correct position if it is an NG/OG tube (Figure 79.2). The feed should also be checked to ensure it is the correct type for the child and the volume to be administered. More recently there has been evidence to suggest that blended food diets, for example normal family meals, could be beneficial for children who are receiving long-term enteral feeds. Blended food may reduce constipation and other side effects of enteral feeding. Blended food diets also offer families more control over their child's diet. However, there are some limitations to using a blended food diet, such as blockage of the tube if extra care is not taken, so the potential use of blended food should be discussed with the multidisciplinary team and family.

Medication administration

All medication prescribed must indicate the route of administration (Box 79.3). Local policy or guidelines must be followed when administering any medication via an enteral feeding tube. The advice of the pharmacist should be sought at the time of prescribing.

Key points

- Commencing enteral feeding should be a multidisciplinary decision in conjunction with the family.
- Carers need to be involved in the feed whenever possible, from holding the child to learning the full process.
- Safety is paramount. Always check the position of the NG tube before commencing the feed

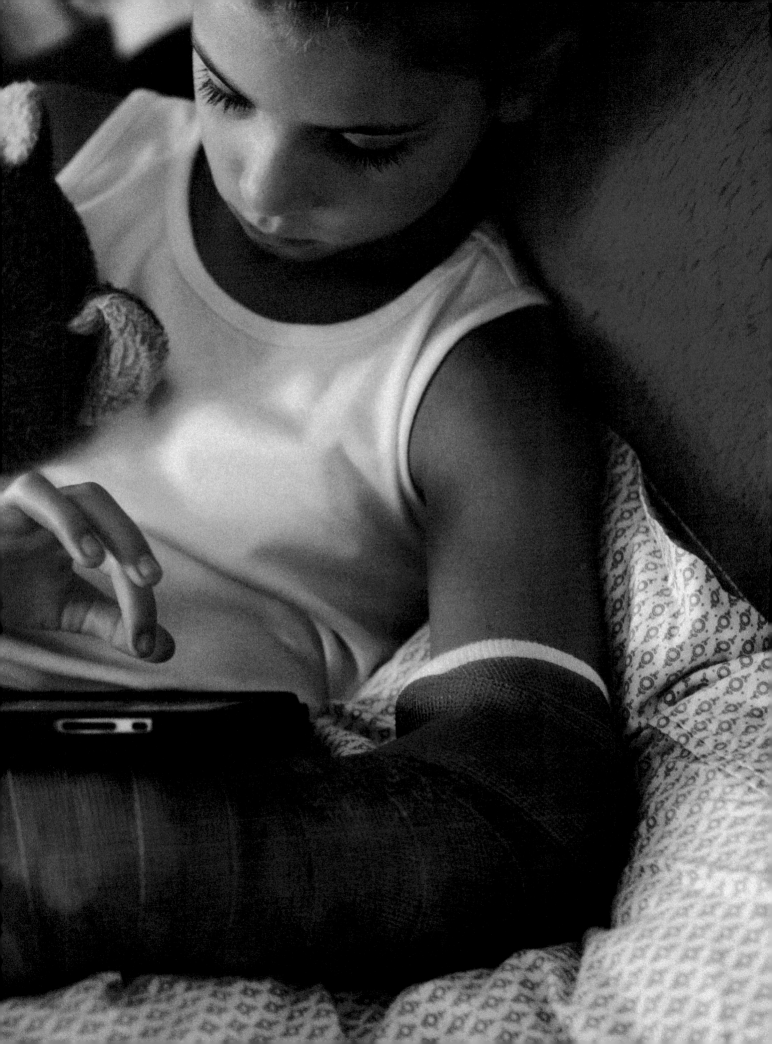

80 The child with a fever

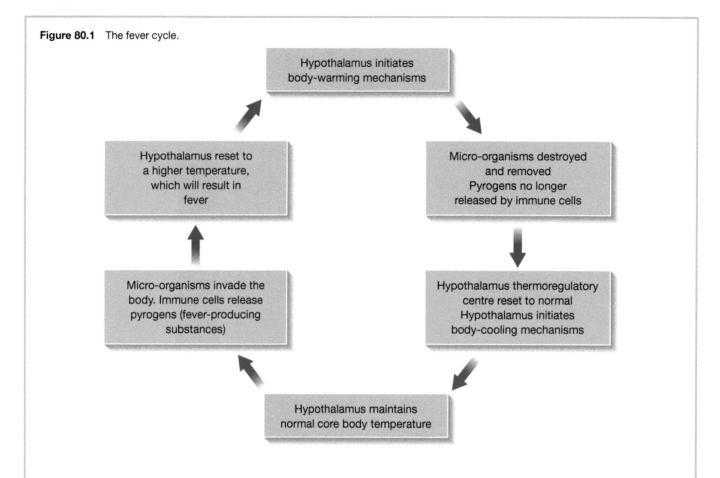

Figure 80.1 The fever cycle.

- Hypothalamus initiates body-warming mechanisms
- Micro-organisms destroyed and removed Pyrogens no longer released by immune cells
- Hypothalamus thermoregulatory centre reset to normal Hypothalamus initiates body-cooling mechanisms
- Hypothalamus maintains normal core body temperature
- Micro-organisms invade the body. Immune cells release pyrogens (fever-producing substances)
- Hypothalamus reset to a higher temperature, which will result in fever

Figure 80.2 The time course of a typical febrile episode.

Shivering and vasoconstriction

Sweating and vasodilatation

Core temperature (°C)

40 — New set point

Patient feels cold as body tries to attain higher set point

39 — Patient feels hot

38 — Normal set point

37

Onset of fever   Fever 'breaks'

Time (hours)

From Pocock G and Richards CD. (2004) Human Physiology: The Basis of Medicine, 2nd edition. With permission of Oxford University Press

Table 80.1 Thermoregulatory responses.

Thermoregulatory responses to cold (body-warming mechanisms)	Thermoregulatory responses to heat (body-cooling mechanisms)
Vasoconstriction	Vasodilatation
Shivering	Sweating
Increase in basal metabolic rate (BMR) mediated by adrenal medullary and thyroid hormones	Decrease in BMR
Warmth-seeking behaviour	Cold-seeking behaviour

Children and Young People's Nursing at a Glance, Second Edition. Edited by Elizabeth Gormley-Fleming and Sheila Roberts.
© 2023 John Wiley & Sons Ltd. Published 2023 by John Wiley & Sons Ltd.

Fever

Fever is defined as a rise in temperature above the normal range 'set point' that is not associated with exercise or a high ambient temperature. It is one of the most common symptoms of illness in children. To facilitate an understanding of fever, it is necessary to review the key points associated with thermoregulation.

Hyperthermia is a significant rise in body temperature and may be non-infectious in origin: drug allergy, status epilepticus, malignancy, heat stroke, and malignant hyperthermia are some of the possible causes.

Thermoregulation

The maintenance of a constant core body temperature is vital for normal cell function, as the rates of all metabolic processes are highly temperature dependent.

A normal core body temperature for a new born infant will be between 36.5 and 37.6 °C. As the child grows, the normal body temperature reflects a decreasing basic metabolic rate, and for an older child a range of 36–37.5 °C may be within normal parameters. This will vary depending on the site measured.

Shell temperature refers to the surface or skin temperature and may vary considerably according to the ambient temperature. The skin can tolerate a wide range of temperature.

Thermoregulation is an example of a negative feedback homeostatic loop. The loop operates to regulate core temperature around a set point. For a normal core temperature to be maintained, it is necessary that heat loss from the body = heat gained by the body. Mechanisms of heat loss include radiation, conduction, and convection. Heat is generated by all the active cellular processes of the body (metabolism).

There are two populations of thermoreceptors: peripheral (located in the skin) and central (located within deeper structures including the central nervous system). Peripheral receptors monitor skin (shell) temperature. Central receptors monitor core temperature. The hypothalamus is the major integration centre for information from the thermoreceptors. It acts as the body's thermostat, set at around 37 °C. When it is informed of a change in temperature, it organizes appropriate effector responses to restore normal temperature. Effector mechanisms are designed to restore normal core temperature and include autonomic, endocrine, and somatic responses closely integrated with behavioural responses (Table 80.1).

Physiology

Fever is usually associated with infectious disease and is caused by chemicals called exogenous pyrogens, which are sometimes derived from bacteria (bacterial endotoxins) or viruses, but more often are secreted by cells of the immune system (monocytes, phagocytes), endogenous pyrogens, in response to infection. In fever, the control centre perceives normal temperature as being too low. Heat conservation and heat production then drive the temperature up to its new set level. The rise in the set point is due to the action of pyrogens that have the ability to readjust the hypothalamus. An example of a pyrogen is interleukin 1 (IL-1). It acts on the hypothalamus to stimulate the production of prostaglandins, which in turn act to reset the set point of the hypothalamus to a higher level. This is a rapid process, the temperature rising within 8–10 minutes of the release of IL-1. Pyrogens appear to induce fever by resetting the hypothalamic thermostat so that heat conservation mechanisms are initiated to raise the core body temperature to the new higher value (Figure 80.1).

Therefore, the child with a rising temperature will shiver, display signs of cutaneous vasoconstriction, and feel cold. Once the cause of infection has been removed from the body, the hypothalamic set point returns to normal and the heat loss mechanism will be initiated. The child sweats, displays signs of vasodilatation, and feels hot until the core temperature returns to normal (Figure 80.2).

Clinical assessment

A mild temperature elevation (less than 38 °C) in an otherwise healthy child should be left to run its course. Temperature measurement in infants and children may be easily measured at several body sites. There are advantages and disadvantages for all sites. A high temperature needs to be investigated and managed:
- Check for any immediately life-threatening features.
- Use the 'traffic light' system to check for symptoms and signs that predict the risk of serious illness.
- Look for a source of fever and check symptoms and signs associated with specific diseases.
- Measure and record temperature, heart rate, respiratory rate, and capillary refill time, and assess for dehydration.

Other points to consider:
- Is child shivering?
- Position of the child: foetal position or splayed out?
- Skin colour: pale or flushed?
- Are they sweating?
- Level of consciousness?
- Urine output?

Note: The traffic light system is a tool for prioritizing children with fever by assessing the presence of certain symptoms. Features associated with fever in children have been categorized by potential seriousness into three groups – 'green' (low risk), 'amber' (intermediate risk), and 'red' (high risk) – to help healthcare professionals identify the risk of serious illness.

Management

Although fever may be regarded as part of the natural response to infection as it reduces the rate at which viruses and bacteria replicate, antipyretic drugs are often used to reduce temperature so that the child feels comfortable. Be aware of the following:
- Do not routinely give antipyretic drugs to a child with fever with the sole aim of reducing body temperature.
- Antipyretics do not prevent febrile convulsions and should not be used specifically for this purpose.
- Do not administer paracetamol and ibuprofen at the same time, but consider using the alternative agent if the child does not respond to the first drug.

Key points
- The ideal technique for measuring temperature should be that it is rapid, painless, and reproduces measurements that accurately reflect core temperature.
- Fever is one of the most common symptoms of illness in children and is often the first symptom that the child is unwell with either a bacterial or viral infection.
- The children and young person's nurse should advise parents to follow evidence-based guidelines in the management of their child's fever.

81 Infectious childhood diseases

Children's nurses will come into contact with a range of infectious diseases as part of their everyday practice. The ability to diagnose these swiftly will result in the quick and safe isolation of the child, providing optimum care for the family while protecting public safety. Infectious diseases of childhood, despite being preventable, are still responsible for significant childhood mortality across the globe, particularly those children under 5 years of age. The common infectious diseases likely to be encountered by a children and young person's nurse will be considered in this chapter (see Table 81.1).

Readers should consider the traffic light system contained within the evidence-based guidelines for the management of the child with fever. This traffic light system provides a framework to assess the severity of the illness encountered by the child.

The notification of certain infectious diseases is a statutory requirement in the UK and it is the responsibility of registered medical practitioners to complete this requirement. Notification is made to local health protection teams or to local councils immediately on diagnosis of a suspected disease.

Table 81.1 Childhood infections.

Rashes and skin infections (incubation period)	Infectious period	Symptoms	What to do
Chickenpox (1–3 wk)	1–2 d before the rash appears, but continues to be infectious until the blister crusts over	Mild flu-like symptoms: • general malaise • aching, painful muscles • moderate to high fever Rash starts as red, itchy spots that blister Fluid in the blister turns cloudy and crusts over The crusting naturally falls off after 1–2 wk	There is no cure for chickenpox as it is a viral infection, but care could include: • Analgesia and antipyretic treatment • Fluids • Strategies to reduce scratching • Cool, light cotton clothing • Those who are newborn, pregnant or immunosuppressed may be administered antiviral treatment
Measles (7–18 d)	Symptoms usually disappear 7–10 d after onset of illness	Symptoms start around 10–12 d with: • High fever • Coryza (runny nose) • Conjunctivitis (non-purulent) • Koplik spots • Rash appears around 4 d after the initial symptoms. Starts with small red spots behind the ears, moving to face and head before clustering and spreading over the body • Photophobia (light sensitivity)	There is no specific treatment for measles as it is a viral infection, but care could include: • Analgesia and antipyretic treatment • Gentle cleaning of the eyes • Regular fluids • Darkened room
Rubella (2–3 wk)	1–5 d after appearance of rash	Cold-like symptoms Distinctive red-pink rash starting behind the ears before spreading around face, neck, trunk, and the rest of the body. Rash last approximately 3–7 d Swollen lymph nodes Moderate to high temperature	There is no specific treatment for rubella as it is a viral illness, but care could include: • Analgesia and antipyretic treatment • Fluids • Strategies to reduce scratching • Cool, light cotton clothing
Impetigo (1–3 d for streptococcal infections and 4–10 d for staphylococcal infections)	If untreated the sores will remain infectious as long as they persist	Can occur anywhere on the body, but generally starts around the nose and mouth Starts as a small, itchy inflamed area that blisters, releasing yellow fluid that forms honey-coloured crusts This fluid is highly contagious	Impetigo is treated with antibiotics that may be administered orally or topically Strict infection control measures should be implemented to reduce the risks of cross-infection within the home, to include the child's own towel and washing equipment

Table 81.1 (Continued)

Diarrhoea and vomiting infections

Rotavirus (1–3 d)	May remain infectious for up to 8 d after the loose stools subside	Starts with a high fever and vomiting, followed by 3–8 d of watery diarrhoea Abdominal cramps Signs of dehydration	Fluid to prevent dehydration such as rehydration drinks Analgesia and antipyretic treatment Good hygiene and possibly barrier nursing
Escherichia coli 0157 (1–10 d)	Several weeks after the symptoms subside	Severe abdominal cramps Diarrhoea (often bloodstained) Moderate fever Most people recover within 5 d, but there is a risk of kidney damage and severe illness	As above
Shigella (12 h–6 d)	During the acute phase and up to 4 wk after symptoms have subsided	Severe abdominal cramps Diarrhoea (often bloodstained) Moderate fever Nausea and vomiting	As above
Cryptosporidiosis (3–12 d after contact)	Should not return to school for 48 h after symptoms have subsided and should not attend public swimming pools for 14 d after symptoms	This is a parasitic infection that may have no symptoms. When ill the child presents with gastroenteritis-like symptoms lasting around 12–14 d	As above
Salmonella (12–72 h after infection)	This can range from several days to several weeks	Severe abdominal cramps Diarrhoea (often severe) Moderate fever Nausea and vomiting	As above

Respiratory infections

Influenza (1–4 d)	One day before and 5 d after symptoms subside	Headache Fever (38–40 °C) Aching muscles and joints Chest pains Lack of appetite Fatigue and weakness Runny nose and sore throat Dry cough Chills and shivering Vomiting or diarrhoea	There is no specific treatment for influenza as it is a viral illness, but care could include: • Analgesia and antipyretic treatment • Fluids • Rest
SAR-CoV Covid 19, see chapter 111			
Tuberculosis (TB) (2–12 wk)	A child is considered at the end of the infectious period when the frequency and intensity of the cough have improved or having received 2 wk of adequate treatment	A productive persistent cough that may contain blood Progressive breathlessness Lack of appetite and weight loss Night sweats Extreme tiredness and fatigue	Pulmonary TB is treated using a 6 mo course of a combination of antibiotics. The usual course of treatment is: • Two antibiotics – isoniazid and rifampicin – every day for 6 mo • Two additional antibiotics – pyrazinamide and ethambutol – every day for the first 2 mo
Pertussis (Average 7–10 d – range 5–21 d)	21 d after onset of symptoms	There are three stages to this illness: • *Catarrhal stage*: usually 7–10 d with coryzal features, low-grade temperature, and a mild occasional cough, progressively deteriorating • *Paroxysmal stage*: usually 1–6 wk, but could last for up to 10 wk. Presenting with frequent, rapid, and productive cough with high-pitched whoop in older children, cyanosis, vomiting, and exhaustion • *Convalescent stage*: usually 7–10 d, presenting with general recovery, less persistent cough that disappears over 2–3 wk period	Treatment is supportive and includes close attention to respiratory effort and exhaustion Small, frequent meals help reduce the paroxysmal cough and fluid management helps with hydration Erythromycin may be prescribed to reduce the period of infectivity, but has little influence on disease progression

(Continued)

Table 81.1 (Continued)

Other infections

Conjunctivitis (1–3 d for bacteria; 1–12 d for viruses)	Usually while symptoms are present, but some viruses could remain infective for 14 d after start of symptoms	The eye appears red and may feel 'gritty', with a watery or yellow discharge One eye is usually involved at first, but both eyes are typically affected within a few hours	Viral infections will resolve without treatment, topical antibiotic drops/ointments may be prescribed for a bacterial infection Eye toilet and strict hygiene help to avoid spread of infection
Meningitis, see chapter 93			
Mumps (Around 17 d)	Just before the swelling of the parotid gland to 9 d after onset of symptoms	Swelling of the parotid glands causing pain and difficulty swallowing Headaches General malaise Moderate to high temperature Loss of appetite and abdominal pain	There is no specific treatment for rubella as it is a viral illness, but care includes: • Analgesia/antipyretic treatment • Fluids • Warm or cool compresses to the swollen glands may reduce discomfort • Soft, light diet

Key points
• Evidence-based guidance should be used to assess the child who presents with fever and a rash.
• Children with infectious diseases may need to be isolated to protect others until they are no longer considered infectious.
• Common childhood infectious diseases are distressing for the child and family and can occasionally be severe, requiring hospitalisation.

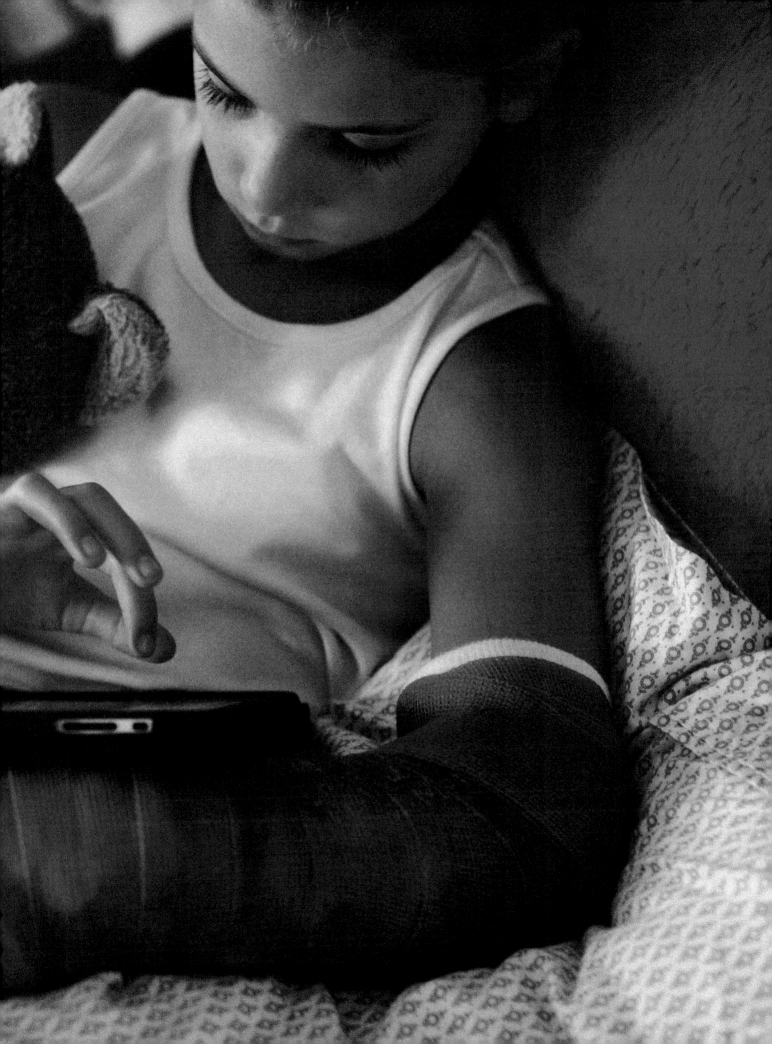

82 Assessing infectious diseases

Figure 82.1 Systematic assessment for infectious disease.

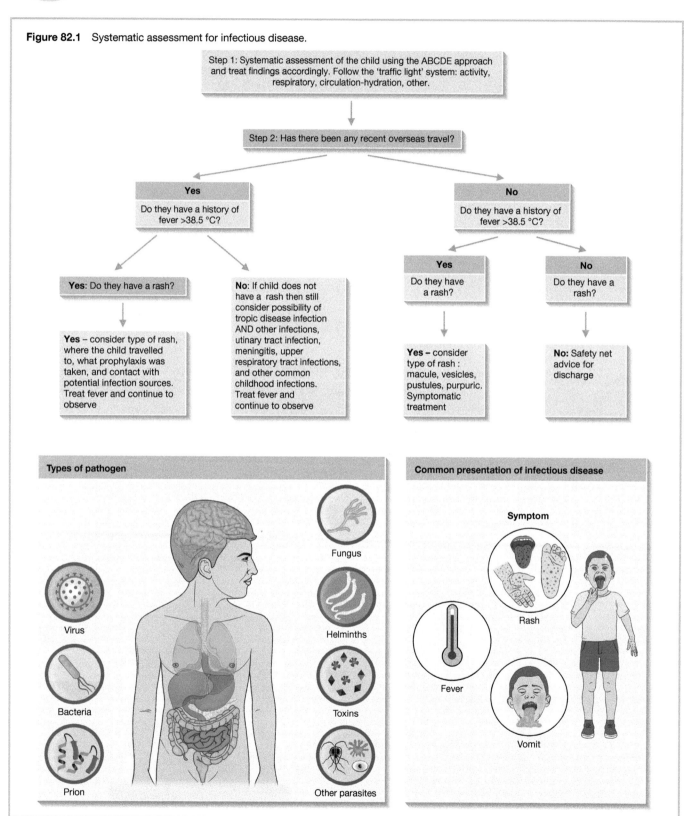

Step 1: Systematic assessment of the child using the ABCDE approach and treat findings accordingly. Follow the 'traffic light' system: activity, respiratory, circulation-hydration, other.

Step 2: Has there been any recent overseas travel?

Yes
Do they have a history of fever >38.5 °C?

No
Do they have a history of fever >38.5 °C?

Yes: Do they have a rash?

No: If child does not have a rash then still consider possibility of tropic disease infection AND other infections, utinary tract infection, meningitis, upper respiratory tract infections, and other common childhood infections. Treat fever and continue to observe

Yes – consider type of rash, where the child travelled to, what prophylaxis was taken, and contact with potential infection sources. Treat fever and continue to observe

Yes
Do they have a rash?

No
Do they have a rash?

Yes – consider type of rash : macule, vesicles, pustules, purpuric. Symptomatic treatment

No: Safety net advice for discharge

Types of pathogen

Virus

Bacteria

Prion

Fungus

Helminths

Toxins

Other parasites

Common presentation of infectious disease

Symptom

Rash

Fever

Vomit

Children and Young People's Nursing at a Glance, Second Edition. Edited by Elizabeth Gormley-Fleming and Sheila Roberts.
© 2023 John Wiley & Sons Ltd. Published 2023 by John Wiley & Sons Ltd.

What is infectious disease?

If the host (the human) sustains injury or pathological changes in response to a parasitic infection, the process is called an infectious disease. The health of the host and the virulence of the microorganism will determine the severity of an infectious disease, which can range from mild to life-threatening. The child who presents with a possible infectious disease should be systematically assessed in order to provide a diagnosis so that a treatment plan can be implemented (Figure 82.1).

Infectious agents

In order to survive, an infectious agent must be able to multiply, emerge from the host, reach a new host, and infect the new host. The agents of infectious disease include viruses, bacteria, rickettsiae, chlamydiae, fungi, parasites, and prions. Some of the key infectious agents are the following:

- *Viruses* can have an immediate effect on the host (e.g. influenza), or they could be latent (or dormant, e.g. herpesvirus and adenovirus, retrovirus [HIV], arthropod-borne virus, enterovirus).
- *Bacteria* are extremely adaptable: streptococcal, staphylococcal, Lyme's disease, Weil's disease, mycoplasmas.
- *Rickettsiae* combine the characteristics of viral and bacterial agents to produce disease in humans and depend on the host cell for essential vitamins and nutrients: arthropods – fleas, ticks, lice.
- *Fungi* are free-living and found in every habitat. They are separated into two groups: yeasts and moulds. Fungi include ringworm and athlete's foot.
- A *parasite* is a member of the animal kingdom that infects and causes disease in other animals and includes protozoa, helminths, and arthropods. Protozoan infections include malaria, amoebic dysentery, and giardiasis. Helminths are a collection of wormlike parasites that include roundworms, tapeworms, and flukes. The parasitic arthropods include ticks, mosquitoes, biting flies, mites, lice, and fleas.
- *Prions* are infective protein agents (e.g. Creutzfeldt–Jakob disease).

Epidemiology

Epidemiology means the study of factors, events, and circumstances that influence the transmission of infectious disease in human populations. It is a science of rates; infectious diseases must be classified according to incidence, portal of entry, source, symptoms, disease course, site of infection, and virulence factors. The purpose of epidemiology is then to predict, avert, and appropriately treat potential outbreaks.

Incidence is the term used to describe the number of new cases of an infectious disease that occurs within a defined population (e.g. 1000 people) over a specified period of time (e.g. monthly).

Portal of entry

The portal of entry refers to the process by which the pathogen enters the body. *Penetration* is a disruption to the integrity of the skin by accident (burn or abrasion), medical procedure (catheterization), skin lesion (impetigo), inoculation, or animal or arthropod bite. *Direct contact* may occur with infected tissue or secretions such as sexually transmitted diseases (gonorrhoea, syphilis) or from mother to child during gestation or birth (rubella, cytomegalovirus, herpes simplex viruses, HIV). *Ingestion* is the entry of the pathogenic micro-organisms or toxins through the oral cavity and gastrointestinal tract. Contaminated water and food are common sources of entry for many bacterial, viral, and parasitic infections (e.g. cholera, typhoid, traveller's diarrhoea, and hepatitis A). *Inhalation* is responsible for the most deaths of children under 5 years because of the vast array of pathogens that invade through the respiratory tract: bacterial pneumonia, meningitis and sepsis, tuberculosis; viruses such as measles, mumps, chickenpox, influenza, respiratory syncytial virus, and the common cold.

The portal of entry does not necessarily dictate the site of infection; ingested pathogens, for example, may cause liver disease.

Symptomatology

The symptoms of an infectious disease may be specific and reflect the site of infection (rash); conversely, there may be non-specific symptoms that are shared by a number of infectious diseases. Symptomatology is the collection of signs and symptoms (the clinical picture) expressed by the host during the course of the disease.

Accurate history taking and documentation are crucial to be able to aid in the diagnosis.

Disease course

There are five distinct stages that the infectious disease takes once entering the host:

1 *Incubation period*: the time taken to produce recognizable symptoms, which could be hours to days.
2 *Prodromal stage*: initial appearance of symptoms.
3 *Acute stage*: the maximum impact of the infectious process.
4 *Convalescent stage*: the containment of the infection and repair of damaged tissue.
5 *Resolution stage*: the total elimination of the pathogen with no residual signs or symptoms.

Site of infection

The site of an infectious disease is determined by the type of pathogen, the portal of entry, and the effectiveness of the host's immunological defence system. Infectious diseases affect one or more of the following systems: respiratory, intestinal, blood, and skin.

Treatment and protection

The diagnosis of an infectious disease requires two criteria: (i) the recovery of the probable pathogen from the infected sites; and (ii) accurate documentation of clinical signs and symptoms.

Most infectious diseases are self-limiting and require little or no intervention. The choice of treatment for an infectious disease may be medicinal by using antimicrobials, immunological with antibody preparations or vaccines, or surgical. The goal of treatment is complete removal of the pathogen from the host and return of normal physiological function to damaged tissues. By far the best treatment of an infectious disease is prevention. Good handwashing techniques, clean water, a healthy diet, and immunizations are fundamental in preventing the spread of infectious diseases.

Key points

- Maintaining the chain of infection control is the most important factor in preventing the spread of disease.
- Risk assessment frameworks exist for the assessment and management of certain infectious diseases.
- The children's nurse needs to be aware of common infectious diseases and the management of children who are required to be nursed in an isolation facility.

83 Prevention of infection

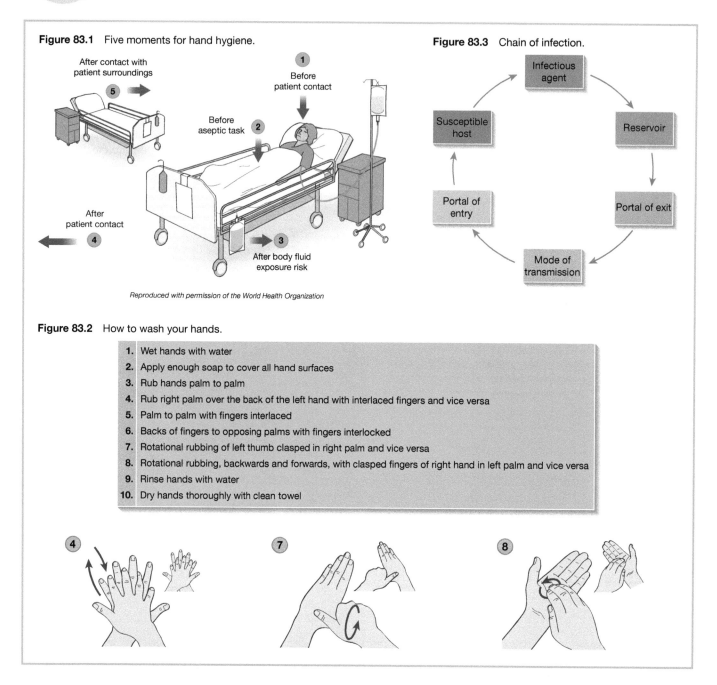

Figure 83.1 Five moments for hand hygiene.

After contact with patient surroundings 5

1 Before patient contact

2 Before aseptic task

4 After patient contact

3 After body fluid exposure risk

Reproduced with permission of the World Health Organization

Figure 83.3 Chain of infection.

Infectious agent → Reservoir → Portal of exit → Mode of transmission → Portal of entry → Susceptible host → Infectious agent

Figure 83.2 How to wash your hands.

1. Wet hands with water
2. Apply enough soap to cover all hand surfaces
3. Rub hands palm to palm
4. Rub right palm over the back of the left hand with interlaced fingers and vice versa
5. Palm to palm with fingers interlaced
6. Backs of fingers to opposing palms with fingers interlocked
7. Rotational rubbing of left thumb clasped in right palm and vice versa
8. Rotational rubbing, backwards and forwards, with clasped fingers of right hand in left palm and vice versa
9. Rinse hands with water
10. Dry hands thoroughly with clean towel

A key clinical priority is to protect patients, visitors, and staff against the risk of healthcare-acquired infections (HAIs). This requirement is in accordance with the Code of Practice on the control and prevention of infection in the Health and Social Care Act 2008 (revised 2014). This code sets out 10 criteria against which all healthcare providers will be judged and includes information and environment management, policy development, and staff education and training.

HAIs are infections that are acquired as a result of a healthcare intervention. These can occur in healthy individuals as well as those with known ill health. The impacts of HAIs are that they:
- Exacerbate underlying conditions, which may delay recovery.
- Require additional pharmacological treatments.
- Have longer-term negative effects on the health of the individual.
- Adversely affect the quality of life.

Children and Young People's Nursing at a Glance, Second Edition. Edited by Elizabeth Gormley-Fleming and Sheila Roberts.
© 2023 John Wiley & Sons Ltd. Published 2023 by John Wiley & Sons Ltd.

- Increase length of stay and therefore cost to the NHS.
- Increase risk of mortality.

Approximately 7% of patients will acquire an infection during an episode of healthcare.

The most common type of HAIs are central line–associated blood-stream infections (CLABSIs), pneumonia (ventilatory-acquired pneumonia), catheter-associated urinary tract infections, surgical site infections (SSIs), and *Clostridium difficile* infection. *Escherichia coli* is the most commonly isolated micro-organism found in HAIs, with *Staphylococcus aureus* the second most common organism identified.

Good infection control is the best way to prevent the spread of infection and this begins with good hand hygiene practices.

Prevention and control of infection

Children are particularly vulnerable to healthcare-associated infection. The younger the child, the more vulnerable they are, as the immune system matures and becomes more efficient across childhood. Some groups of children are particularly at risk of acquiring infections:

- Children with intrinsic immunodeficiency (e.g. severe combined immunodeficiency [SCID]).
- Children with acquired immunodeficiency (e.g. following chemotherapy, radiotherapy, or corticosteroid use).
- Chronically unwell children.
- The unimmunized.

Standard infection control precautions

Standard infection control precautions (SICPs) are the basic infection prevention and control measures required in all care settings by all staff for every patient, irrespective of whether they are known to have an infection or not. This is to promote their safety and that of their families and carers. These measures are necessary to reduce the risk of transmitting infectious agents from recognized and unrecognized sources of infection at the point of care. SICPs have 10 elements:

1 Hand hygiene.
2 Patient placement and assessment of risk.
3 Personal protective equipment.
4 Respiratory and cough hygiene.
5 Safe disposal of waste.
6 Safe management of blood and body fluids.
7 Safe management of care equipment.
8 Safe management of linen.
9 Safe management of sharps and inoculation injuries.
10 Safe management of the care environment.

The application of SICPs during the delivery of care should be determined by assessing the level of risk of all individuals concerned. Identifying the task, amount of interaction, and amount of exposure to potential sources of infection (bodily fluids/equipment) will form part of the risk assessment. It is important that children and young person's nurses adopt a consistent approach to SICPs. The overall aim of SICPs is to break the chain of infection.

Hand hygiene

Hands are one of the most common means of transmitting micro-organisms and causing infection to spread (Figure 83.1). The most effective means of preventing infection is good hand hygiene (Figure 83.2):

- Bare below the elbow, short sleeves, no wristwatch or jewellery (except wedding ring, which should be moved during cleansing to ensure that the area under it is cleansed).
- Care of skin and nails – nails kept short to allow proper cleansing and no nail varnish, which could become a reservoir for contaminants.
- A cleansing technique that covers the whole surface of the hands and wrists.
- Use of sanitizing gel to decontaminate socially clean hands.
- Use soap and water to decontaminate visibly soiled hands.
- Not using hands to operate taps and bins.
- Proper hand drying.
- Appropriate skin care.

Proper use of sterile or non-sterile gloves does not remove the need for hand decontamination.

When is hand decontamination necessary?

- Before touching a patient.
- Before a clean or aseptic procedure.
- After body fluid exposure risk.
- After touching a patient.
- After touching a patient's surroundings.

Hand decontamination technique – gel

1 Palmful of decontaminant into cupped hand.
2 Cover entire surface of hands and wrists.
3 Rub hands palm to palm.
4 Rub right palm over the back of the left hand and vice versa.
5 Rub palm to palm with fingers interlaced.
6 Rub backs of fingers to opposing palms with fingers interlocked.
7 Rotational rubbing of left thumb clasped in palm of right hand and vice versa.
8 Rotational rubbing backwards and forwards of clasped fingers of right hand in left palm and vice versa.
9 Once dry, hands are safe.

Hand decontamination technique – soap and water

See Figure 83.2.

Chain of infection

In order for infection to occur, there are six requirements that are often referred to as the chain of infection (Figure 83.3) The six links in the chain are:

1 The infectious agent has the ability to cause the disease.
2 The reservoir is where the micro-organism lives and thrives. This can be a human, an animal, or an environmental object (food, water, soil).
3 The portal of exit is how the micro-organism leaves the reservoir. For example, a child with rota virus would transmit this in their faeces.
4 The mode of transmission describes how the micro-organisms are transmitted from one person or a place to another.
5 The portal of entry is how the micro-organism enters another individual.
6 The susceptible host is the person who is vulnerable to infection.

Breaking the chain of infection at any time will enable the spread of infection.

Key points

- Hand hygiene is the single most important action for children's and young people's nurses to take to prevent HAIs.
- HAIs are avoidable, but present are a significant risk to the child and family and a cost to the NHS.
- Any break in the chain of infection will enable infectious organisms to be transmitted.

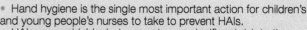

84 Hyponatraemia and its prevention

Figure 84.1 The effects of hyponatraemia and hypernatraemia on the cell.

Normal	Hypernatraemia	Hyponatraemia

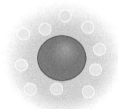 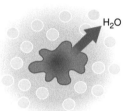 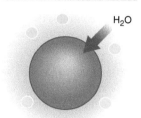

Normal cell size; normal serum Na concentration	Cell shrinks as H_2O is pulled **out** of cell	Cell swells as H_2O is pulled **into** cell

Causes of hyponatraemia include:

- Loss of sodium
- Excess water intake or retention
- Syndrome of inappropriate antidiuretic hormone (SIADH)
- Inappropriate fluid management (e.g. miscalculation, over-infusion of intravenous fluids or oral fluid overload)
- Inappropriate choice of intravenous fluid
- Incorrect reconstitution of formula milk

Signs and symptoms of hyponatraemia

May be asymptomatic but may include:

- Nausea and vomiting
- Headache
- Irritability
- Altered consciousness and lethargy
- Seizures
- Apnoea
- Respiratory arrest

Assessing the child

Ongoing assessment is key and relies on the input of parents/caregivers. Children's nurses should:

- Observe fluid balance status (see Chapter 76) and record/report as appropriate.
- Be able to recognize the signs and symptoms of hyponatraemia.
- Complete clinical observations, using a locally approved Early Warning System chart.
- Weigh the child daily and record/report any changes as required.
- Review regular blood monitoring and results in line with local policy, for example urea and electrolytes.

Children and Young People's Nursing at a Glance, Second Edition. Edited by Elizabeth Gormley-Fleming and Sheila Roberts.
© 2023 John Wiley & Sons Ltd. Published 2023 by John Wiley & Sons Ltd.

Movement of body fluid and electrolytes

Body fluids and associated electrolytes are in constant motion around the body by diffusion, osmosis, and active transport in order to achieve a state of homeostasis. Thus, the body works continuously to achieve optimal fluid and electrolyte balance. Electrolytes, such as sodium and potassium, are substances that develop an electrical charge when dissolved in water. They play an important part in controlling the osmosis of water between body fluid compartments and its movement in and out of the cells.

Sodium

Most sodium is kept outside the cells and potassium inside by the sodium–potassium pump mechanism. The movements of sodium and water are closely related; generally where one goes, the other follows. Thus, under normal circumstances, the sodium–potassium pump prevents too much water entering the cells by closely regulating the concentration of intracellular sodium. In hyponatraemia, a low serum sodium level occurs when more sodium is lost than water through mechanisms such as vomiting, diarrhoea, or stoma loss (sodium depletion) or when the blood becomes over-diluted. Over-dilution may be caused by excessive water intake, inappropriate fluid management, or inappropriate choice of intravenous (IV) fluid (dilutional hyponatraemia). Both mechanisms result in extracellular fluid that is very dilute and therefore water is drawn into the cells by osmosis (Figure 84.1). This can be particularly problematic for the cells in the brain, as there is limited space for expansion, potentially resulting in cerebral oedema and brain-stem herniation. A high serum sodium or hypernatraemia has the opposite effect, but can also have serious neurological consequences (Figure 84.1), although further discussion of this is beyond the remit of this chapter.

What is hyponatraemia?

Hyponatraemia may be acute (duration of less than 48 hours) or chronic (duration of 48 hours or more). This chapter will focus on the nursing management of a child with acute hyponatraemia in the hospital setting.

Normal serum sodium levels are 135–145 mmol/L. Hyponatraemia occurs when levels fall below these limits and may be classified as mild (130–135 mmol/L), moderate (125–129 mmol/L), or severe (<125 mmol/L). Children are more at risk of detrimental effects of hyponatraemia than adults because they have a higher brain : skull size ratio (meaning that there is less space for expansion as the brain cells fill with water) and hormonal changes render female adolescents, in particular, more prone to its development. Other children particularly at risk include those with central nervous system conditions, sepsis, or gastroenteritis, or those in the perioperative period. Stress, pain, nausea, and certain anaesthetics or types of ventilation can cause what is known as the syndrome of inappropriate antidiuretic hormone (SIADH). This hormone normally conserves water in the body in times of dehydration; however, in SIADH it is produced unnecessarily and this can cause the body to retain water and potentially result in hyponatraemia.

Management of the child with hyponatraemia

As with any aspect of children's nursing, a child- and family-centred approach is essential. Careful and appropriate information giving, negotiation, involving the child and family, and open communication will help to reduce anxiety. Good communication within the multidisciplinary team and adherence to local policies are key to ensuring safe and effective care for the hyponatraemic child. Ongoing assessment and monitoring of the child for signs and symptoms of hyponatraemia, clinical deterioration, and fluid imbalance are crucial, and accurate documentation in the nursing notes is essential. In particular, the type, amount, and rate of IV fluids should be recorded accurately, together with any losses (e.g. gastric losses) that may need to be replaced. The child receiving IV fluids should be closely observed and their blood, urea, and electrolytes (including blood glucose) obtained on a regular basis, with results evaluated by the multidisciplinary team. Weight and urinary output require careful monitoring; this may include the collection of urine for osmolality and electrolytes. IV requirements should be adjusted accordingly if the child is also taking oral fluids. Hourly observation of the IV site, for the presence of inflammation and/or phlebitis (using an appropriate tool), is important. The children's nurse has a key role in supporting the family and ensuring that all tests are carried out and results reported back to appropriate medical staff in a timely manner.

Treatment of hyponatraemia may involve the administration of IV sodium chloride (according to local policy) to raise serum sodium levels, and fluid restriction may be required during the initial stages. It must be noted that severe, acute hyponatraemia is a medical emergency and requires management by senior medical staff.

Preventing hyponatraemia

Children's nurses may help prevent hyponatraemia by having a thorough working knowledge of suitable types and amounts of fluids, along with normal serum electrolyte levels. They have a responsibility to listen to and escalate concerns raised by the children and/or families in their care. Children's nurses also need to be aware of the causes of hyponatraemia and the factors that put some children particularly at risk, and to have an understanding of SIADH. Specific clinical guidelines have been developed throughout the UK for local use and it is imperative that children's nurses adhere to such guidance along with other members of the multidisciplinary team. Regular training, supervision, and adequate reporting of incidents or near misses will help to ensure the safety of children at risk of hyponatraemia.

Key points

- The children's nurse should have a thorough working knowledge of local fluid management policies and maintain competence in this area.
- Multidisciplinary working and communication are key, including escalation of child and family concerns as appropriate.
- Accurate assessment, reporting, good record keeping, and ongoing monitoring of the child will help to reduce and manage the risk of hyponatraemia.

Acknowledgements. The authors would like to thank Dr Damien Armstrong for his assistance in the preparation of this chapter.

85 Thermal injuries

Figure 85.1 Classification, assessment, management, and complications.

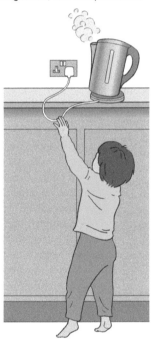

Classification

- Scalds
- Friction or contact burns
- Flame burns
- Flash burns
- Chemical burns
- Electrical burns
- Radiation burns
- Sunburn
- Extreme exposure to cold
- Child abuse

Assessment

Thermal injuries necessitate a structured approach as per Advanced Paediatric Life Support Guidelines (ABCDEFG), and a systematic response. Assessment and overall management of thermal injuries can be subdivided into the following phases of care:
- Rescue
- Resuscitate
- Review
- Resurface
- Rehabilitate
- Reconstruct
- Review

Complications

- Burn shock and hypovolaemic shock
- Fluid and electrolyte imbalance
- Hypermetabolism
- Hypothermia
- Infection
- Contractures
- Compartment syndrome
- Scarring, disfigurement, and disability
- Multisystem organ failure

Management

- Pain assessment and management
- Fluid resuscitation
- Photographs
- Wound assessment using validated assessment tools
- Burns assessment tools
- Blister debridement
- Cleanse wounds according to evidence-based guideline and local policy

Figure 85.2 Zones of injury.

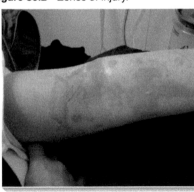

Thermal damage to tissue may be described in three zones:

1. **Zone of hyperaemia:** superficial damage when the damaged skin appears warm and red
2. **Zone of stasis:** the microcirculation is damaged resulting in changes to capillary permeability, which allows fluids to leak from the vascular system into the interstitial space, resulting in local oedema and resultant shock if extensive wounds are present
3. **Zone of coagulation:** the deepest area where damaged cells occlude blood vessels. The obstructed microcirculation prevents the humoral compartments of the immune response targeting the burned tissue

Severity of thermal injury

1. **Local:** oedema, fluid loss, significant circulatory alterations, and development of thrombi
2. **Systematic:** may involve multiple system response including cardiovascular, gastrointestinal, renal, and increased metabolism and body temperature

Box 85.1 The SAFE approach.

Shout for help
Assess the scene for danger
Free the area around the child for danger
Evaluate the casualty

Table 85.1 Lund and Bowden assessment tool.

	At birth	0–1 year	2–4 years	5–9 years	10–15 years
A. Half a head	9.5%	8.5%	6.5%	5.5%	4.5%
B. Half of thigh	2.75%	3.25%	4.0%	4.25%	4.5%
C. Half of leg	2.5%	2.5%	2.75%	3.0%	3.25%

Children and Young People's Nursing at a Glance, Second Edition. Edited by Elizabeth Gormley-Fleming and Sheila Roberts.
© 2023 John Wiley & Sons Ltd. Published 2023 by John Wiley & Sons Ltd.

Thermal injuries have been described as some of the worst injuries for infants, children, and young people. The physical and psychological trauma caused may leave permanent disfigurement and disability. Approximately 50 000 children under the age of 5 years incur thermal injuries annually, the impact of which upon the child and the family cannot be quantified.

The highest incidence occurs in children under 5 years, with the 1–2-year age group more at risk. The most common thermal injury is scalds from hot water (66%). There may be seasonal and regional differences that affect the pattern of burn injuries. Cultural and socioeconomic factors may increase the risk patterns of thermal injuries in any community. Prompt assessment and management are essential (Figure 85.1 and Box 85.1).

Total body surface area

The total body surface area (TBSA) affected can be estimated using a range of methods to assess whether a minor or major thermal injury is involved.

- *TBSA >10% is classified as major burns.* Children whose burns make up 10% or more of TBSA are considered critical and require urgent hospitalization. Fluid resuscitation is calculated using the Parkland Formula, which estimates the amount of fluid required over the 24-hour period following injury. Half the fluid is administered in the first eight hours and the remainder is given over the subsequent 16 hours.
- *TBSA <10% is classified as minor burns* unless there is associated smoke inhalation.

Assessment tools

It is important to remember that the burn itself is being assessed and surrounding areas of redness (erythema) should be excluded.
- *Wallace rule of nines*: An acknowledged formula, but based upon adults (estimates an adult head being 9% of total body area). It has the potential to be adapted for children, but it does not take account of surface area variations for children at different ages.
- *1% rule or rule of palms*: The surface area of a child's palm, including fingers, is considered to be 1% of TBSA. It has been suggested that a more accurate figure for a child's palm is 0.5%, however.
- *Lund and Bowden assessment*: Considered the most accurate tool for assessing percentage burns for children as it takes account of body surface changes with age (Table 85.1).

Burns

Fatal burns in children are often associated with house fires and are the second most common cause of accidents and deaths in childhood, with 50% of fatalities associated with smoke inhalation and the remaining 50% of deaths attributed to burn injuries. Death is attributed to massive fluid loss, hypovolaemic and neurogenic shock, and overwhelming infection.

Classification of burns

Burns are classified according to:
- Depth (Figure 85.2)
- Body surface area affected
- Cause

Depth of burns

First-degree burns (superficial thermal injury)
- Only the epidermis is involved.
- Potential for the formation of serous-filled blisters.
- Pain.
- Blanching of skin when pressure is applied.
- Dry appearance.
- Healing occurs within 5–7 days, generally without scarring.

Treatment
Initiate first aid.

Second-degree burns (partial-thickness thermal injuries)
- Loss of epidermis and partial loss of dermis.
- Potential for blistering.
- May blanch when pressure is applied.
- Red in colour.
- Potential for decrease in sensation.
- Scarring may occur.
- May require skin graft.

Treatment
- Remove burned clothing, clean area with tepid water, and leave blisters intact.
- Pain relief.
- Check immunization status.

Third-degree burns (full thickness)
- Epidermis and dermis are destroyed.
- Absence of serous-filled blisters.
- White appearance of the skin.
- No blanching on pressure.
- Sensation is absent, but may be painful on deep pressure.
- Grafting will facilitate healing.
- Always scars and scarring likely to be severe.

Treatment
- Establish and maintain a patent airway. Initiate advanced life support if necessary.
- Remove burned clothing but keep the child warm.
- Cover burn to prevent contamination.
- Pain management.
- Nil by mouth until transported to specialist burns centre.
- Intravenous fluids and 100% oxygen.

Fourth-degree burns
- Fourth-degree burns are rare.
- Damage extends through deeply charred subcutaneous tissue to muscle and bone.
- No blanching with pressure.
- Will not heal without surgery, severe scarring.
- Fourth-degree burns may be caused by prolonged exposure to flames or high-voltage electrical shock.

Treatment
As per full-thickness burns.

Compartment syndrome

This is a surgical emergency. It occurs when severe oedema causes a tourniquet-like effect that compromises the circulation and entraps nerves.

Scalds

A child becomes scalded far more quickly than an adult, as it takes only one second for a child to sustain a scald when exposed to liquid at 60 °C (the average setting point of thermostats is 55 °C in British homes). The features of any scald are defined by their causal factors such as agent, mechanism, and intent (accidental or intentional), coupled with the physical characteristics of the injury.

• *Accidental scalds in children*: Accidental scalds in children are often described as spill injuries, where the child reaches out and accidentally pulls hot liquid over themselves. This typically leads to a scalded area over the upper trunk, face, and/or arms. The scald usually has an irregular edge and is variable in depth, being deepest at the initial point of contact.

• *Intentional scald/thermal injuries*: Severe burns are reported in an estimated 10–12% of children who have suffered physical abuse. Intentional injuries from hot or boiling water usually affect the back or lower limbs, with or without including the buttocks or perineum. They may also affect the arms and/or both legs in a glove or stocking manner. Forced immersion scald or burn injuries are consistently described as the most common mechanism of intentional thermal injuries. Local safeguarding policies and procedures should be initiated.

Key points

• The children's nurse must always be alert to 'abusive' burns and consider this when history is incompatible with injury and the development of the child.

• Good first aid is important in the management and long-term outcome for the child who sustains a thermal injury.

• Specialist advice should be sought from designated Burns Centres at all times for complex thermal injuries, but it needs to be remembered that all burns have the potential to progress into complex wounds over time.

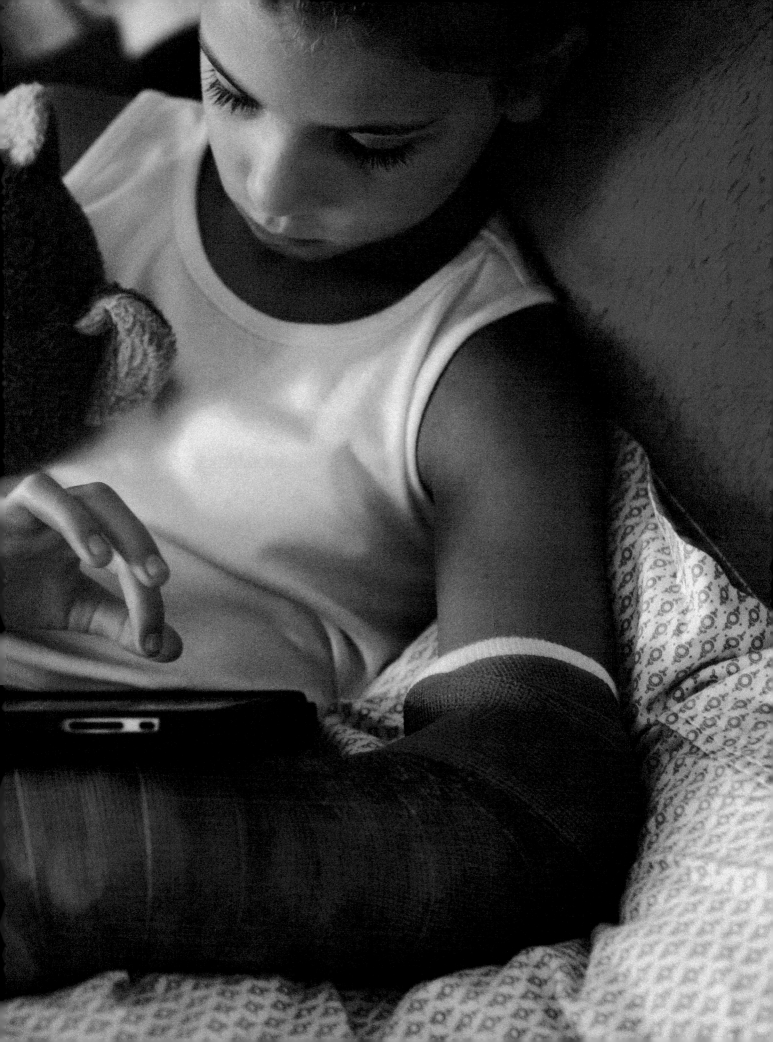

86 Childhood fractures

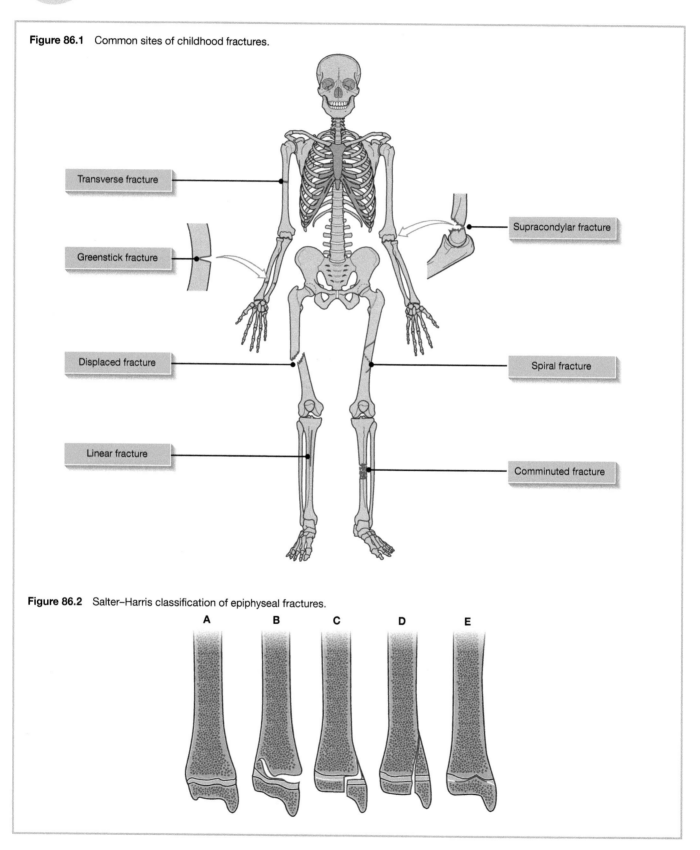

Figure 86.1 Common sites of childhood fractures.

Transverse fracture

Greenstick fracture

Displaced fracture

Linear fracture

Supracondylar fracture

Spiral fracture

Comminuted fracture

Figure 86.2 Salter–Harris classification of epiphyseal fractures.

A B C D E

Children and Young People's Nursing at a Glance, Second Edition. Edited by Elizabeth Gormley-Fleming and Sheila Roberts.
© 2023 John Wiley & Sons Ltd. Published 2023 by John Wiley & Sons Ltd.

A fracture is defined as a break in the continuity of a bone. During play children undertake activities that can increase the risk of injury resulting in a fracture. The child with a fracture may present with pain, swelling, deformity, and loss of function and movement; the diagnosis can be confirmed by X-ray.

There are two main classifications of fractures: closed and open. For a closed fracture the skin remains intact, whereas for an open fracture there is damage to the skin that communicates with the fracture site. This is also known as a compound fracture. Fractures can be displaced, where the bone fragments are not in alignment, or undisplaced.

There are many types of fractures, which are classified according to the nature of the injury and force that caused the fracture (Figure 86.1).

Types of closed fractures

- *Stable*: the bone is broken but the ends are aligned and there is minimal if any displacement.
- *Transverse*: the fracture is horizontal across the bone.
- *Linear*: the fracture is vertical.
- *Oblique*: the fracture is at an angle of <90°.
- *Spiral*: the fracture runs in a spiral around the bone and is a result of a rotational force. Non-accidental injury should be suspected if this type of fracture is seen in an immobile infant.
- *Comminuted*: a fracture that consists of more than two fragments.
- *Compression*: where a bone has been crushed.
- *Avulsion*: a fragment of bone has been pulled away from the site of ligament insertion.
- *Greenstick*: an incomplete fracture where the bone remains intact on one side but breaks on the other. This is like trying to snap a new branch on a tree, hence its name.
- *Buckle or torus fracture*: Compression of a long bone leading to a buckle.

The healing process

The fractured bone initially bleeds, then forms a haematoma. The inflammatory process begins when necrotic bone and the haematoma are removed by macrophages and osteoclasts. Osteoid (bone) tissue develops, forming a callus at the fracture site. There are two types of bone cell: osteoblasts develop new bone and osteoclasts remove necrotic bone and are involved in bone resorption. After a few weeks the callus hardens and the bone develops mechanical strength. This area then consolidates with mature bone. After approximately one year, remodelling has occurred and the normal bone shape is restored. This can occur in children where there has been a significant malalignment of the fracture. This healing process is quicker in children than in adults.

Management

Fracture of a bone is painful, so any child who sustains a fracture should be assessed for pain and given analgesia accordingly. If the fracture is displaced, the bone ends need to be realigned to regain the position and length of the bone fragments and correct deformity. This is known as reduction. Methods of reduction are closed manipulation performed under general anaesthetic, traction, and by open operation. Not all fractures need reducing and some can be treated with simple splintage such as neighbour strapping, the use of a removable splint, or use of a sling/collar and cuff. Following reduction, the fracture needs to be immobilized to maintain the

position. This can be done by the application of a ridged non-removable cast such as a plaster of Paris cast, continued traction, or by internal or external fixation. Internal fixation involves a surgical operation whereby the bone fragments are secured using a metal plate and screws, screws/wires, or an intramedullary nail. External fixation involves the insertion of pins into the fragments of bone, which are then attached to a rigid bar or frame (the fixator). Rehabilitation commences immediately after the initial treatment to promote healing and prevent joint stiffness in order to restore function.

There are concerns if a fracture extends through the epiphyseal growth plate. This can result in interference or complete cessation of growth, and possibly a limb length discrepancy. These fractures are known as epiphyseal or growth plate fractures and are classified according to the Slater–Harris classification system (Figure 86.2). The involvement of the structures surrounding the fracture, such as the epiphysis and the joint, is graded into five types of epiphyseal fractures.

Pin site care

The pins from skeletal traction or an external fixator are a vehicle for hospital-acquired infection due to the nature of the pins penetrating the skin. There has been much debate as to the most effective methods of cleaning pin sites, which led to the Royal College of Nursing developing guidelines based upon consensus:
- Clean pin sites weekly using alcoholic chlorhexidine and non-shedding gauze.
- Cover with a wound dressing that keeps moisture and exudate away from the wound and secure with a bung that gives light compression.
- Increase frequency of dressing changes if an infection is present or the dressing is excessively wet.

Complications

- *Injury to other structures/organs*: injury to the brachial artery following supracondylar fracture of the humerus.
- *Compartment syndrome*: increased pressure within the muscle compartments causing compression of the nerves, blood vessels, and soft tissue by bleeding or tight dressings/cast.
- *Delayed union*: normal healing does not occur as expected. This is less likely in children, especially young children and infants.
- *Malunion*: where the bone heals in an abnormal position.
- *Non-union*: the bone fragments do not heal.
- *Fat embolism*: release of fat from the fracture site of long bones into the circulation and lungs.
- *Osteomyelitis*: an infection of the bone from a contaminated wound of a compound fracture or pin site. This is difficult to eradicate.
- *Avascular necrosis*: death of bone due to loss of blood supply.
- *Growth restriction*: caused by damage to the growth (epiphyseal) plate in children who have not reached growth maturity.

Key points
- Childhood fractures need specialist management if limb integrity and function are to be restored.
- Bones heal by two methods following initial trauma: direct intramembranous or indirect fracture healing.
- There are two main types of fracture: open and closed.

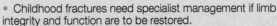

87 Plaster care

Figure 87.1 Equipment required to apply plaster of Paris.

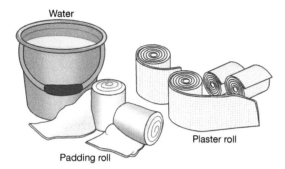

Water

Padding roll

Plaster roll

Figure 87.2 Application of cast.

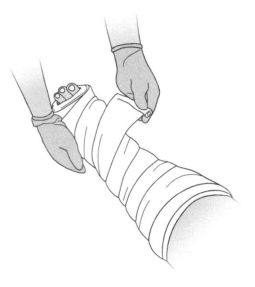

Figure 87.3 Completed cast.

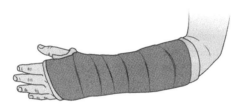

Figure 87.4 Common sites for pressure ulcers to develop.

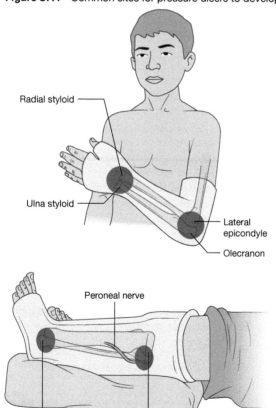

Radial styloid

Ulna styloid

Lateral epicondyle

Olecranon

Peroneal nerve

Lateral malleolus

Tibial tuberosity

Figure 87.5 Splint, cast, fiberglass.

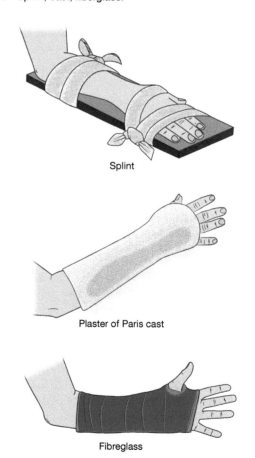

Splint

Plaster of Paris cast

Fibreglass

Children and Young People's Nursing at a Glance, Second Edition. Edited by Elizabeth Gormley-Fleming and Sheila Roberts.
© 2023 John Wiley & Sons Ltd. Published 2023 by John Wiley & Sons Ltd.

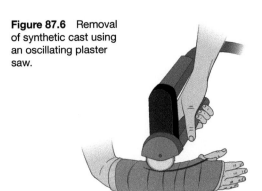

Figure 87.6 Removal of synthetic cast using an oscillating plaster saw.

Plaster casts are applied for a variety of reasons. They can consist of plaster of Paris or synthetic materials such as fibreglass, depending on the reason. It is important for the children's nurse to know the reason why the cast is being applied, what type of material is required, and how long it is to remain in place. Thermoplastic splints are also used in place of plaster of Paris for certain fracture types. The child and family need to understand the function of the cast and the expected duration it will be in situ for. It is also essential when applying lower-limb casts to know whether the child is allowed to bear weight on them.

Reasons for application

- Treatment of fractures.
- Following orthopaedic surgical procedures.
- To improve function by stabilization of a joint.
- To correct and prevent deformities.
- To provide pain relief.
- To permit early ambulation and weight bearing.
- To make a mould of a limb for splints to be made.

Preparation of the child

Prior to cast application, the child and the parent or carer should be provided with an explanation of the process of applying the cast and the reason. Consent should be obtained. Demonstrating the procedure on a doll is a useful method in younger children and can also be used as a means of distraction. It is important to make the child as comfortable as possible; small children may need to be seated on their parent's knee. Clinical holding may need to be considered as safety is paramount.

Applying the cast

The aim is to apply a good cast that fits well, is not too tight, and is smooth on the inside, using only enough materials to provide an effective cast without making it too heavy. The layers also need to be smoothed to ensure bonding (Figure 87.1). It is important to ensure the child has received adequate analgesia before attempting to apply the cast. If the cast is applied following surgery, the child may still be anaesthetized during the procedure. It is important to position the limb correctly and ensure the child has their privacy and dignity maintained throughout, as clothing may need to have been removed to expose the area requiring the cast. The procedure should be documented in the care records.

Indentation should be avoided when handling a wet cast, as this can lead to pressure on the skin under the cast (Figure 87.2). The newly completed cast (Figure 87.3) should be allowed to dry naturally to avoid separation of the layers. This can take 24–48 hours for plaster of Paris; synthetic materials take between 30 minutes and 1 hour. The newly plastered limb should be supported on a pillow to prevent pressure. It may be necessary to elevate the limb to assist in reducing swelling, especially following a fracture. Upper limbs can be placed in a sling, whereas lower limbs should be elevated on a pillow (Figure 87.4). This elevation should be no more than 10 cm above the heart. It is important to check for swelling, which can occur due to the fracture or surgical procedure or if the cast is too tight, and for the neurovascular status of the limb (Box 87.1).

Potential problems

As well as the neurovascular complications, it is important to observe for the following problems:

- Cracking/softening/breakdown of the cast. If areas of the cast are likely to come into contact with bodily fluids, such as for a hip spica, waterproof or absorbent tape should be applied to the edges to keep the cast clean. Parents should be advised to use a smaller nappy that tucks under the edge of the cast and a larger one that goes over the spica. The older child should be advised not to get their cast wet or put weight on it until dry.
- Indicators of pressure. Pressure or cast sores can occur if the underlying padding is uneven or insufficient over bony areas or a poor application technique is used. The cast being too loose or too tight can also be a contributory factor. Damage to the skin can be caused by objects being pushed down the plaster by younger children or to relieve itching by older children. Signs of a cast sore are an offensive smell, staining of the cast from an oozing wound, burning pain, and pyrexia. Younger children may be irritable.
- Allergic reactions to the casting material.
- If it is following a surgical procedure, the cast should be observed for signs of bleeding.
- Children in spica casts may develop bloating of the abdomen.

Caring for a child in a cast or splint (Figure 87.5) can be difficult transition for the child and parents, with many lifestyle adjustments required. Aspects that need consideration:

- *Positioning*: it is important with a child in a hip spica to change position regularly to avoid skin damage due to pressure. The child may not be able to sit up, so needs to be propped up with pillows or on a perch.
- *Hygiene and dressing*: These can be difficult, as the child is not able to be bathed and clothing may not fit so needs to be adapted (e.g. using Velcro fastenings).
- *Feeding*: the previously independent child may need assistance.
- *Sleeping*: this may be disturbed as the child's usual sleeping position will be difficult to achieve.
- *Moving and handling*: parents will need to be given instruction on the best way to carry the child.
- *Mobility*: the child in a spica will not fit into a normal pushchair. Older children will need to adapt to the use of crutches if in lower-limb casts.
- *Travelling*: the child may not fit into a car seat.

On discharge, the child and parents should be given advice both verbally and in writing on what to look for and how to care for the cast. Removal of a synthetic cast is illustrated in Figure 87.6.

Key points

- The child and parents will need to be informed about how to care for their cast. They will need to know what the signs of neurovascular impairment are and have safety-net advice.
- The child and family need to understand the reasons why the cast is required.
- The children's nurse must be vigilant and recognize any alteration to the neurovascular status of the limb in the cast, and take immediate action.

88 Traction care

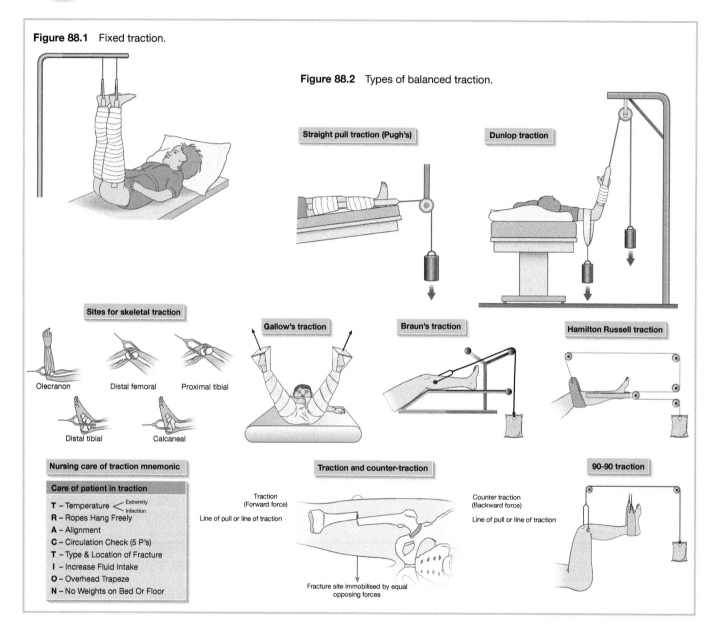

Figure 88.1 Fixed traction.

Figure 88.2 Types of balanced traction.

Straight pull traction (Pugh's)

Dunlop traction

Sites for skeletal traction

Olecranon   Distal femoral   Proximal tibial

Distal tibial   Calcaneal

Gallow's traction

Braun's traction

Hamilton Russell traction

Nursing care of traction mnemonic

Care of patient in traction

T – Temperature < Extremity / Infection
R – Ropes Hang Freely
A – Alignment
C – Circulation Check (5 P's)
T – Type & Location of Fracture
I – Increase Fluid Intake
O – Overhead Trapeze
N – No Weights on Bed Or Floor

Traction and counter-traction

Traction (Forward force)
Line of pull or line of traction

Counter traction (Backward force)
Line of pull or line of traction

Fracture site immobilised by equal opposing forces

90-90 traction

What is traction?

Traction is the application of a pulling force that requires counter-traction in order to be effective. The core principle of traction is the application of an external force to correct a deformity or to reduce a fracture. This follows the principles of gravity. Counter-traction can be achieved by the child's body weight or by elevating the end of the bed. This pulling force is applied to the child's limb with a resultant pull on the bone and soft tissues. The pulling force of traction induces muscle fatigue, which reduces muscle spasm. This minimizes pain and can slow down bleeding at the fracture site and the inflammatory process at the fractured end of the bones commences.

While the traction may not achieve definitive realignment of the fracture, it will reduce displacement, which will improve the pain level and ultimately make the child more comfortable.

Why is traction used?

- To reduce a displaced fracture.
- To maintain alignment of a fracture.
- To reduce muscle spasm.
- To relieve pain.
- To prevent or correct deformity caused by contracture of the soft tissues.

Children and Young People's Nursing at a Glance, Second Edition. Edited by Elizabeth Gormley-Fleming and Sheila Roberts.
© 2023 John Wiley & Sons Ltd. Published 2023 by John Wiley & Sons Ltd.

- To immobilize inflamed or injured joints.
- To aid reduction of a dislocated joint (e.g. developmental dysplasia of the hip).

Types of traction

The type of traction selected is determined by the age of the child, the type and position of the fracture, the amount of displacement, the condition of the skin and soft tissues, and the desired outcomes. The traction should be used to maintain the fracture position until there has been sufficient healing to enable the limb to be immobilized in a plaster cast until complete healing has occurred.

Traction may be used in the management of spinal deformities in the form of halo traction, halter traction, or halo vests.

Fixed

This is achieved by the pulling force being exerted between two fixed points (Figure 88.1). Examples of this type of traction are the application of a Thomas splint and gallows traction.

Gallows traction (also known as Bryant's traction) is used for the conservative treatment of fracture of the shaft of femur in children under the age of 2 years or not weighing more than 16 kg. It is also used for preoperative positioning prior to hip surgery. It is a type of fixed traction. The child's legs are suspended from a Balkan beam attached to the cot by skin extensions. The child's body weight is used to provide counter-traction, achieved by the child's buttocks being raised off the bed. It is therefore important to check that this is maintained. The traction is applied to both legs. Neurovascular observations need to be undertaken, as vascular impairment is a complication of this traction. The child usually adapts quickly to the traction, but involvement of the family and the play therapist to provide distraction is essential.

Balanced (sliding)

This is where the pulling forces are balanced to provide traction and counter-traction between two mobile points – the use of suspended weights and the child's own body weight (Figure 88.2). This is achieved by elevating the end of the bed so that the child moves in the opposite direction to the applied traction.

Methods of applying traction

- *Skin*: adhesive or non-adhesive skin extensions are applied to the limb and bandaged into place.
- *Skeletal*: this involves the insertion of a metal pin through the bone, which is then attached to a stirrup. The traction cord is attached to this. This type of traction may also include the use of a Thomas splint and a Pearson knee flexion piece.

Weights

The amount of weight applied is determined by the following:
- Aim of treatment.
- Degree of displacement.
- Indication for traction.
- Weight of child.
- Tolerance to traction.
- Type of traction.

Generally, approximately 10% of the total body weight of the child is used for skin traction in fractured femurs. The larger the child, the greater the weight required. This will also apply a greater shear force, so underlying skin and soft tissues can be easily damaged. A thorough assessment of the skin should be completed prior to the application of traction.

With spinal traction the weight may need to be applied incrementally so that tolerance can be achieved.

Care of the traction

- Check the traction a minimum of once per shift and after repositioning of the child. This includes ensuring that the frame and attachments are tight, any pulleys are running freely, and the cords are securely knotted and not frayed.
- Check that the weights are securely fastened and are free of the bed or floor and that the correct weight (as documented in the medical notes) is applied.
- Ensure correct alignment of the child and the cords to ensure the pulling forces are maintained.
- Ensure that counter-traction is maintained.
- Ensure that skin extensions are in the correct position and bandages have not become loose or slipped.
- The bandages should be removed at least once daily to enable the skin to be checked.
- If a Thomas splint is used, then this needs to be checked for correct fitting. The area around the ring should be checked for pressure and swelling.
- For skeletal traction the pin sites should be checked for signs of infection and that the pin has not slipped. The ends of the pins should be covered to prevent injury to the other limb.

General care considerations

Traction restricts the child's independence and movement. Young children may regress in their development and adolescents need to adjust to loss of control over their environment. The abnormal positioning required can cause difficulty with the child's activities of living; however, they adapt quickly. Involving the child as much as possible in their care can help with their adjustment as well as encouraging parental participation.
- *Analgesia*: ensure the child receives adequate pain relief.
- *Skin care*: as well as checking the skin for irritation from the traction, areas prone to pressure due to immobilization should be assessed. Changing the child's position is important. Once settled, the child will move position themselves.
- *Eating and drinking*: these can be difficult because of the position of the child, so they may need assistance. Adequate nutrition and fluids are required to aid healing and prevent bladder and bowel problems.
- *Elimination*: the child will not be able to go to the toilet, so will need to use a bedpan. Urinary stasis may lead to urinary tract infections and the reduced level of activity can lead to constipation. Previously toilet-trained children may regress to bed wetting.
- Care of pin sites.
- Neurovascular observations.

Key points

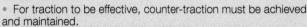

- For traction to be effective, counter-traction must be achieved and maintained.
- Knots must be secure and surgical tape should be used to tape the knot ends to the main traction line to prevent slippage.
- Traction may not fully correct the displaced fracture, but will assist in reducing muscle spasm.

89 Neurovascular assessment

Figure 89.1 Compartment syndrome of the lower limb.

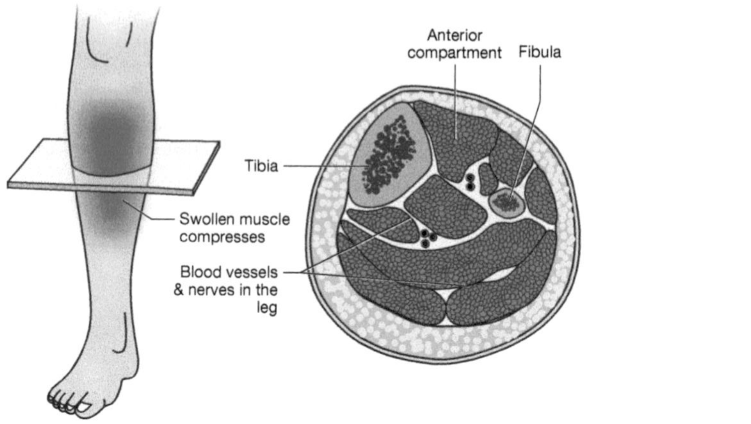

Compartment syndrome

Anterior compartment
Fibula
Tibia
Swollen muscle compresses
Blood vessels & nerves in the leg

Figure 89.2 Neurovascular assessment: sensation and motor function.

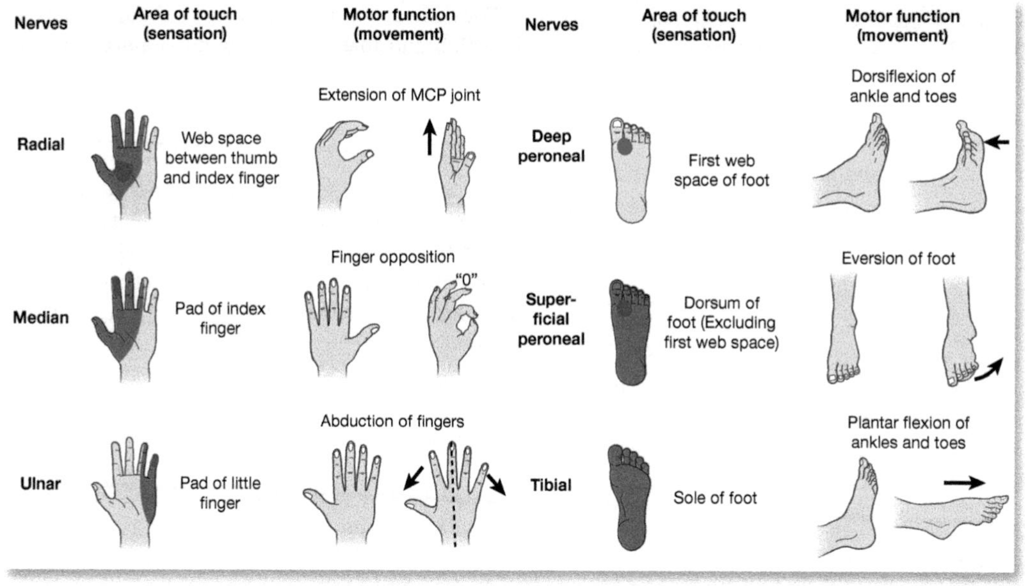

Nerves	Area of touch (sensation)	Motor function (movement)	Nerves	Area of touch (sensation)	Motor function (movement)
Radial	Web space between thumb and index finger	Extension of MCP joint	Deep peroneal	First web space of foot	Dorsiflexion of ankle and toes
Median	Pad of index finger	Finger opposition "O"	Superficial peroneal	Dorsum of foot (Excluding first web space)	Eversion of foot
Ulnar	Pad of little finger	Abduction of fingers	Tibial	Sole of foot	Plantar flexion of ankles and toes

Neurovascular assessment of the extremities is the evaluation of sensory and motor function and the peripheral circulation. Assessment of neurovascular status is important for early recognition of any neurovascular deterioration or compromise. Children's and young people's nurses must be competent in this skill. Neurovascular assessment requires a thorough assessment of the fingers or toes of the affected limb. Neurovascular deterioration may occur following trauma, surgery, or after the application of a cast. The implication of a delay in recognizing neurovascular compromise may be life changing.

Compartment syndrome, neurovascular deficit, and vascular impairment are rare complications of injury and surgery that, if not detected early or if left untreated, may result in disability or death of the child or young person.

Clinical indication for neurovascular assessment

Children and young people who require neurovascular assessment may include those with the following:

- Musculoskeletal injury to the limbs from fractures or crush injuries.
- Orthopaedic and spinal surgery or plastic surgery on the feet or hands.
- Cardiac catheterization.
- Prolonged tourniquet application.
- Application of a plaster cast or a restrictive dressing.
- Infection of a limb.
- Circumferential burns.

Children and Young People's Nursing at a Glance, Second Edition. Edited by Elizabeth Gormley-Fleming and Sheila Roberts.
© 2023 John Wiley & Sons Ltd. Published 2023 by John Wiley & Sons Ltd.

Neurovascular assessment

The components of neurovascular assessment include:
- Perfusion (skin colour, temperature, capillary refill time, swelling, pulses).
- Sensation.
- Motor function.
- Pain.

Perfusion

Capillary refill time is assessed by pressing down on the nail bed of the fingers or toes. The nail bed should blanch and the colour should return within two to three seconds. If it is more than three seconds, this indicates inadequate limb perfusion.

An effective tool to considered in neurovascular assessment is the five Ps:
- Pain
- Pallor
- Paraesthesia
- Pulselessness
- Paralysis

Warmth of extremities should be checked and comparison made between affected and non-affected limbs as well as movement of toes, fingers, and, if appropriate, the affected limb.

Pain

Pain is a very important sign. If the level of pain is inconsistent with the nature of the injury, it is an early indicator of damage or risk. Pain associated with compartment syndrome is constant, not relieved with opioids, and increases on extension and with passive movements. Children and young people should have their pain assessed regularly using an age- and ability-appropriate tool and be managed accordingly. Non-verbal children and young people may indicate their pain through facial expression, guarding, tachycardia, hypotension, increased sweating, tachypnoea, or restlessness.

Pallor

Colour and warmth of the skin of the affected limit are indicators of good perfusion and circulation. It is essential for the nurse to compare the affected limb with the unaffected limb where applicable. Good colour and warmth are provided by a healthy blood supply to the area, but it is important to consider the limb that is overly warm compared with the opposing limb – this could be an indicator of poor venous return caused by obstruction. A cool, pale limb could be indicative of arterial insufficiency. This will be evident below the level of injury.

Paraesthesia

Sensation of the limb and digits is best performed when the child has their eyes closed or is not watching. A light touch by the nurse's finger on the affected limb or digits and the sensation as described by the child or young person should be compared with the non-affected limb. Any numbness or pins and needles could be indicative of nerve damage as well as reduced perfusion.

Pulselessness

Pulses distal to the injury should be assessed to ascertain circulation compromise. Pulselessness is a late sign of potentially irreversible damage to the limb, but it is also important for the nurse to be aware of a strong bounding pulse, which could indicate peripheral obstruction to blood flow. An absent pulse is a late sign and generally indicates tissue necrosis.

Paralysis

Where limbs, feet, or hands are not restricted by casts or traction, flexion and extension of these should be assessed. Even if the child or young person is sleeping, movement should be assessed passively and documented as such. If cast or traction is restricting full movement of foot or hand, then digits should be monitored in the same way to assess nerve function. This is a late sign and results from prolonged nerve compression or damage to the muscle.

Motor function and sensation

Loss of sensation, dysesthesia, numbness, or pins and needles may be reported by the child or young person if there is neurovascular compromise. It is important to note that the young child may not be able to freely express this, as they may not have the language skills to do so. If the child has had surgery, it is important to note if they have had a nerve block or an epidural, as this can cause an altered sensation. A thorough assessment of sensation by palpation is required (Figure 89.1) and of motor function by asking the child to extend, flex, abduct, and adduct the affected limb.

Compartment syndrome

Compartment syndrome (Figure 89.2) usually becomes apparent in the first 72 hours after injury or surgery, but may be as soon as 48 hours or as late as 6 days. There is evidence to suggest that in children it may occur 8 hours after injury.

Muscle, bones, and nerve fibres are surrounded by strong, non-elastic fibrous tissue – fascia – creating individual compartments that join together to form one. When pressure rises within these compartments, the fibrous tissue is unable to accommodate this by stretching, which could result in decreased blood flow to the area, causing the cells to be starved of oxygen and subsequent ischaemia and death to the tissue. A rise in pressure within the compartments may also be caused by direct injury, which would induce an inflammatory response resulting in decreased supply of blood to the tissues and swelling of the limb. This is further impacted by the presence of a cast or traction, which prevents the skin from swelling, putting further pressure on the structures inside. If compartment syndrome is not noticed quickly, it soon leads to necrosis of tissue, which can result in a need for amputation of the limb.

Compartment syndrome is a surgical emergency. The pressure must be relieved or the volume reduced within the compartment in order to preserve the blood supply, enabling tissues to be perfused and function. Failure to recognize compartment syndrome may lead to necrosis of tissue and loss of a limb. A fasciotomy will be required. This requires a surgical incision through the fascia into the compartment. That will release pressure and there should be an improvement to the peripheral neurovascular status, preventing long-term damage.

Further considerations in neurovascular assessment

- *Oozing*: it is essential to monitor any blood or fluid loss from the wound, marking the cast where appropriate, during wound care.
- *Swelling*: new or inappropriate swelling could be an indicator of compartment syndrome.
- *Consent*: as with all nursing procedures, it is imperative to explain to the child or young person and parent the purpose of the observations and how these will be carried out. Time must be taken to assist the child with their descriptions of sensation so that vital cues are not missed.

Documentation

There is no universal tool that is used to document neurovascular observations, but it is the duty of the nurse to ensure that documentation is clear, accurate, and informed.

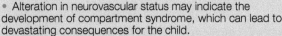

Key point
- Alteration in neurovascular status may indicate the development of compartment syndrome, which can lead to devastating consequences for the child.
- Frequency of neurovascular assessment will be determined by local policy.

90 Neurological problems

Figure 90.1 The International Classification of Functioning, Disability and Health (ICF) framework.

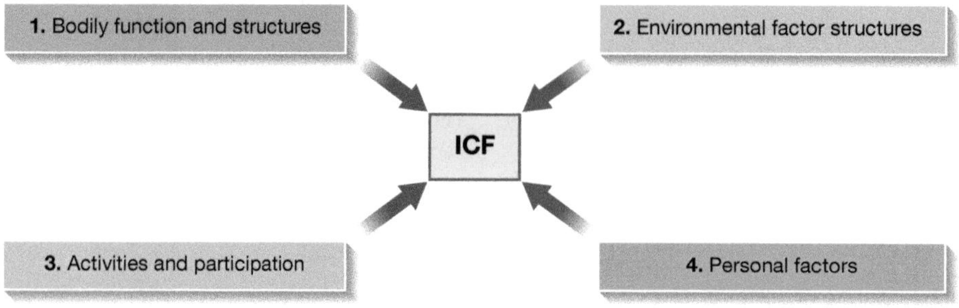

1. Bodily function and structures

2. Environmental factor structures

ICF

3. Activities and participation

4. Personal factors

Table 90.1 Neurological disorders and their origins.

Congenital	Conditions/syndromes
Gene abnormality	Leukodystrophy
Chromosome abnormality	
Change in chromosome number	Turner syndrome (deletion of chromosome) Down's syndrome (extra chromosome)
Change in chromosome structure	Cri-du-chat syndrome Prader–Willi syndrome Angelman syndrome
Metabolic disorder	Phenylalanine (PKU) Homocystinuria
Congenital malformation	Tuberous sclerosis
Perinatal causes	
Toxins and environmental factors: neurotoxins, e.g. alcohol	Foetal alcohol syndrome
Nutritional deficiencies, e.g. folic acid deficiency	Neural tube defects – spina bifida
Infection: TORCH, sexually transmitted infections, hepatitis B, varicella zoster virus, HIV, parvovirus B19, cytomegalovirus, herpes simplex, group B streptococcus	Variable levels of developmental delay, sight loss, deafness, epilepsy, transmission of infections (HIV), encephalitis, meningitis
Hypoxia: perinatal asphyxia from decreased blood flow through the umbilical cord	Hypoxic ischemic encephalopathy
Birth trauma	Physical injury to the brain Hypoxia leading to cerebral palsy
Prematurity/low birth weight	Cognitive impairment: attention deficit hyperactivity disorder, social difficulties
Acquired	
Immune disorders	Autoimmune encephalitis
Post-natal infections	Meningitis/encephalitis
Traumatic brain injury, e.g. closed/open/crushing head injuries	Variable impacts on neurological function
Spinal cord injury	Paralysis
Tumours	Malignant or benign
Toxins, e.g. carbon monoxide poisoning	Variable impacts on neurological function

Chronic neurological disorders in childhood are generally present from birth: congenital in origin or acquired during childhood as a result of trauma or infection. Some may occur for unknown reasons and are termed idiopathic (Table 90.1). They may result in mild deficits or require the child to have significant care needs. The symptoms of neurological disorders vary. They may involve physical, cognitive, behavioural, or emotional alterations, with some disorders having a combination of these. Children with cerebral palsy will have more physical symptoms whereas children with attention deficit hyperactive disorder (ADHD) will have behavioural symptoms.

Neurological disorders present at birth may not always be diagnosed at birth as they are not always apparent. They will emerge during early childhood when the child misses their developmental milestones or has developmental difficulties.

The International Classification of Functioning, Disability and Health (ICF; Figure 90.1) provides a standardized and validated framework on which to base assessment of children with multiple needs, particularly those with neurological or developmental deficits. The ICF is used to measure all aspects of health throughout the child's life and focuses on health and functioning rather than on disability.

Cerebral palsy

Cerebral palsy occurs in 2 per 1000 live infants, with a higher incidence in males, and is one of the most common causes of childhood disability and a major cause of severe disability in children. Cerebral palsy is an umbrella term describing a group of disorders that occur during the development of the foetal or infant brain and result in disorders of movement and posture. Dependent on the cause of cerebral palsy, disturbances of sensation, cognition, communication, perception, or seizure disorder can also occur.

Some 80–90% of children with cerebral palsy will survive into adulthood, causes of death being mainly attributed to seizures and respiratory infections. Management requires interdisciplinary care and therapy and is based on the needs of the individual child, with the focus on enabling functional activity and participation for individuals as well as caring for other clinical conditions. Outcomes are influenced by personal and environmental factors, including the family's socioeconomic status, all of which can serve as barriers or facilitators to functioning.

Headache

Headache is not uncommon in children. The symptoms are dependent on the child's age and the type of headache. The majority of headaches in children are not sinister and are secondary to a viral illness or sinusitis. Chronic headache in childhood is unlikely to be due to serious intercranial pathophysiology. Differential diagnosis can include tension or cluster headaches and migraine. Less commonly, the cause may be raised intracranial pressure, hypertension, trauma, cerebral haemorrhage, or serious infection such as meningitis.

The diagnosis of the aetiology of headache is clinical. However, further investigations including radiology should be considered if the symptoms continue and worsen over days to weeks.

Treatment is based on potential causes and includes identifying and avoiding triggers, the use of appropriate pharmacology, and behavioural and cognitive approaches.

Stroke

Stroke can be defined as a focal neurological deficit with a vascular basis, which lasts over 24 hours and typically presents with hemiparesis and often a visual defect. Transient ischaemic attack (TIA) is similar but lasts under 24 hours.

Headaches, seizures, drowsiness, and neck pain are common symptoms associated with paediatric stroke. Stroke affects hundreds of children each year in the UK and is a common cause of childhood death. Some 50% of children will have a separate medical condition such as sickle cell or cardiac disease, and two-thirds of survivors of childhood stroke will have a residual morbidity. Causes of paediatric stroke are arterial ischaemic stroke (AIS), as a result of blood embolus or dissection of an intracerebral artery, vasculopathic (e.g. moya moya syndrome), thrombotic, post varicella, idiopathic, haemorrhagic stroke, or venous infarction.

Investigations will include a range of radiology imaging. For children with sickle cell disease, exchange transfusion should be undertaken to HbS% <30%.

Treatment for radiologically confirmed AIS is aspirin 5 mg/kg/day, if no haemorrhage or sickle cell disease is present. Treatment for central venous thrombosis is anticoagulation with low weight heparin, although the role of thrombolysis is not clear. Prevention of secondary deterioration (e.g. due to seizures) must be initiated, and early rehabilitation commenced.

Seizures

A seizure is an abnormal electrical discharge and may produce changes in motor, sensory, and cognitive functions. Seizures are of various classifications and require different management protocols. Causes include infection, pyrexia, metabolic, trauma, hypoxia, ischaemia, toxicity, and electrolyte disorder.

Treatment is based around ABCDE to include termination of seizure, maintenance of vital functions, and elimination of any precipitating cause where possible.

Neuromuscular or neuropathic conditions

These can be due to toxins, inflammatory disorders, infection, and genetic causes, and can include hypotonia, abnormal gait, weakness, fatigue, delayed motor milestones, abnormal reflexes, and muscle weakness. Diagnosis can be based on investigations including nerve biopsy, radiology, muscle enzyme analysis, genetic testing, and tests specific to the potential diagnosis.

Muscular dystrophies

Progressive muscle wasting with joint deformity and decreased mobility occurs, but the spectrum varies widely, with Duchenne muscular dystrophy being one of the most severe types. Treatment is aimed at controlling the onset of symptoms to optimize the quality of life and corticosteroids can be beneficial. The genetic mutation in Duchenne is carried by the mother and passed mainly to male children. Diagnosis is made by DNA testing and muscle biopsy. Cardiomyopathy and respiratory failure are common and life expectancy is around 25 years.

With treatment, children with myasthenia gravis have a normal life expectancy.

Metabolic and neurodegenerative disorders

Microcephaly, macrocephaly, developmental delay, hypertonia, hypotonia, abnormal eye signs, and cerebellar signs are among the many symptoms that should alert the paediatrician to the possibility of metabolic or neurodegenerative disorders in children. Radiology, electromyleography, and ophthalmology are among the diagnostic tests undertaken. Treatment is mainly supportive, with a poor life expectancy in these patients.

Key points

- Neurological problems of childhood are congenital, acquired, or idiopathic in origin.
- Neurological disorders present at birth may not be diagnosed until the child has missed the developmental milestones.
- Neurological disorders vary from mild to chronic and life-limiting disorders.

91 Brain injury and coma

Figure 91.1 Traumatic brain injury subtypes.

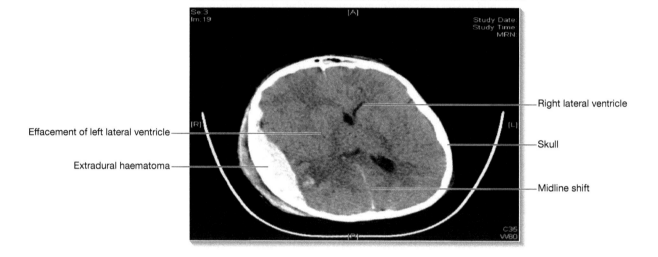

This can constitute a neurosurgical emergency and result in death unless the haematoma is evacuated promptly. Less severe EDHs can be managed conservatively.

Effacement of left lateral ventricle

Extradural haematoma

Right lateral ventricle

Skull

Midline shift

Figure 91.2 Computerized tomographic scan demonstrating extradural haematoma (EDH).

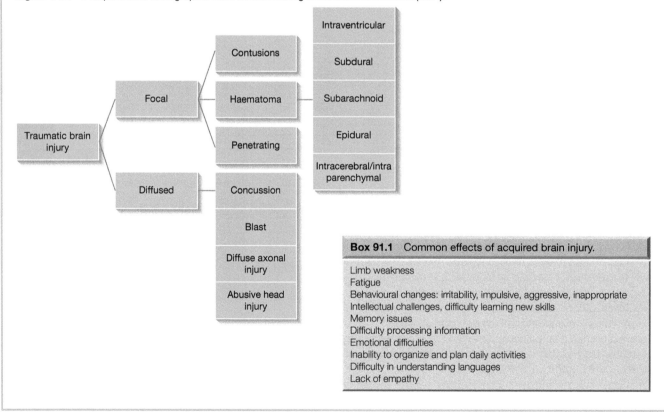

Traumatic brain injury
- Focal
  - Contusions
  - Haematoma
    - Intraventricular
    - Subdural
    - Subarachnoid
    - Epidural
    - Intracerebral/intra parenchymal
  - Penetrating
- Diffused
  - Concussion
  - Blast
  - Diffuse axonal injury
  - Abusive head injury

Box 91.1 Common effects of acquired brain injury.

Limb weakness
Fatigue
Behavioural changes: irritability, impulsive, aggressive, inappropriate
Intellectual challenges, difficulty learning new skills
Memory issues
Difficulty processing information
Emotional difficulties
Inability to organize and plan daily activities
Difficulty in understanding languages
Lack of empathy

Traumatic brain injury (TBI) remains a leading cause of death and disability in children and young people. The survival rate in children with TBI has increased due to improved pre-hospital care, systematic assessment, and early management in specialist centres, with increased use of intracranial pressure monitoring.

The most common cause of head injury is falls, followed by sports-related injury and then motor vehicle accidents. A significant link between head injury and social deprivation has been established.

The age groups most at risk from TBI are newborn infants through to age 4 years, and teens from 15 to 19 years old. Infants carry the greatest risk of abnormality on computerized tomographic scanning. The most common cause is road traffic accidents (motor vehicle, bicycle, pedestrian), followed by falls. The best treatment is prevention and this should be targeted and age specific.

Classification can be mild (based on a Glasgow Coma Score [GCS] of 13–15) with transient symptoms such as dizziness, confusion, headache, and vomiting; moderate (GCS 9–12); or severe (GCS 3–8).

Physiology

The infant skull is relatively large in comparison to the body and the cervical spine is highly mobile, therefore all children with a history of head trauma must have the neck stabilized at the scene of the accident, and this maintained until a cervical injury has been ruled out.

Incomplete myelination and less water content in the infant brain mean that the young brain is more susceptible to acceleration and deceleration injuries, diffuse axonal injury (DAI), and extraparenchymal haemorrhage. Autoregulation is poor in infants and management must be provided accordingly.

Brain injury is acquired and is therefore referred to as acquired brain injury (ABI; Box 91.1). ABI may be as a result of trauma (TBI) or non-traumatic brain injury (Figure 91.1).

TBI results from an impact to the head, for example blunt force trauma, a fall, or a car accident (Figure 91.2).

Non-traumatic brain injury results from infection, tumours, hypoxia, or a cerebrovascular accident.

Primary brain injury

This occurs at the time of injury and includes DAI, brain-stem injury, cortical contusions, and lacerations.

Secondary brain injury

This can occur as a consequence of or independent from the primary injury, minutes to days following the injury as a result of adverse physiology, including cerebral oedema, ischaemia, raised intracranial pressure, hypoxia, hypertension, seizures, pyrexia, hyper- and hypoglycaemia, and seizures.

Immediate management

This must be prompt and systematic, following paediatric life support principles. Cervical spine injury may occur with paediatric head injury and the cervical spine must be immobilized as a priority:

A Check and maintain airway.
B Ensure good oxygenation levels; intubation and ventilation if required.
C Circulation must be maintained and blood pressure and pulse kept within normal ranges.
D Disability: neurological examination, assessment, and treatment; use of paediatric GCS chart and/or AVPU (Alert, Voice, Pain, Unresponsive); management of seizure; electrolytes and glucose.

Evaluation and management of other injuries

The key priorities are to stabilize the child and reduce secondary injury. Published evidence-based guidelines for the management of children with head injury should be followed, including pre-hospital management, inpatient management, and discharge.

Coma

Coma is the most severe impairment of arousal and is defined as an inability to speak, open the eyes to pain, or obey commands. It occurs with head injury, secondary to diffuse changes in the cerebral hemispheres and/or dysfunction of the brain stem, electrolyte imbalance, and/or seizure activity. Treatment is by management of the underlying cause (e.g. raised intracranial pressure, cerebral oedema) and supportive care (e.g. elective mechanical ventilation).

Pharmacologically induced coma may be required for management of children with severe TBI.

Rehabilitation

Rehabilitation may be appropriate in the home setting with community input, but occasionally prolonged inpatient stay is required. Placement at a specialized paediatric rehabilitation centre may be available or appropriate for some children.

Prognosis

The effects of brain injury in the young child may not become obvious until affected skills are called upon, for example during early school years or after the move to senior school. During these early years the immature brain begins to process more complex information, including sensory information.

Long-term deficits may be physical and neurocognitive, the latter including changes in behaviour, mood, speech, memory, learning, attention, and executive functions.

Key points
- Accidental head injury is uncommon in infants under 2 years old, therefore the possibility of non-accidental head injury must be considered in this age group and appropriate measures taken.
- The cervical spine should be immobilized as a priority in children with a severe head injury.
- Targeted age-specific prevention initiatives are required.
- The child with serious head injuries must be transferred to a paediatric intensive care unit where neuroprotection and neurosurgery can be provided if required.
- Rehabilitation can be a long process with an uncertain outcome and should be commenced as soon as possible.

92 Seizures

Figure 92.1 Types of seizure.

Generalized seizures

Rapid onset and spread of abnormal neuronal activity to the brain resulting in a tonic clonic seizure, child becomes unconscious, a vocal noise may be heard, he/she may fall as limbs become stiff (tonic) and convulse in clonic jerking movements.

Focal seizures

Presentation dependent on lobe of location of abnormal neuronal activity:

Frontal lobe: hypermotor movements

Temporal lobe: altered consciousness, oral and hand automatisms, strange smells, tastes and epigastric rising

Occipital lobe: the seeing of flashing lights, vomiting

Parietal lobe: tingling to hand and face

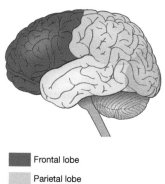

- ■ Frontal lobe
- ▢ Parietal lobe
- ▨ Occipital lobe
- ▢ Temporal lobe

Figure 92.2 First aid care for a child having a convulsion.

1   Stay with the child, stay calm.
Note the time

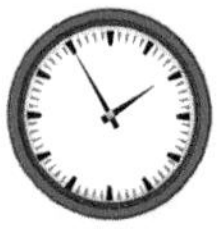

2   Check for medical ID

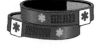

3   Keep the child safe

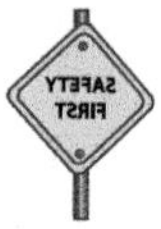

4   Turn child onto their side if they are not alert
Keep airway clear
Loosen tight clothing around their neck
Place something soft and small like a pillow under their head

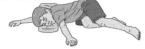

5   Call 999 if seizure lasts longer than 5 minutes, the child does not return to their pre-seizure normal state, has difficulty in breathing, the seizure occurs in water, or there are repeated seizures

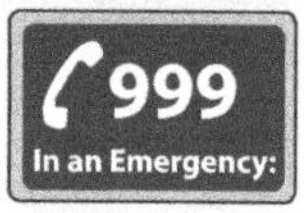

6   Never attempt to restrain or hold the child when they are still seizing
Never attempt to put any object in their mouth

Figure 92.3 Buccal administration of medication.

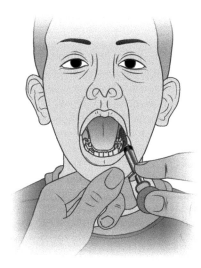

Figure 92.4 Administration of rectal diazepam.

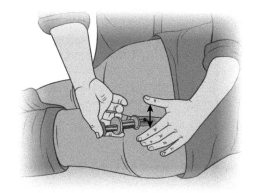

Children and Young People's Nursing at a Glance, Second Edition. Edited by Elizabeth Gormley-Fleming and Sheila Roberts.
© 2023 John Wiley & Sons Ltd. Published 2023 by John Wiley & Sons Ltd.

Causes of seizures

Seizures are quite common and can be attributed to a wide range of causes. Many people think of a seizure as a convulsion-like expression, but some children will have symptoms that are difficult to recognize, such as staring. It is not uncommon for children and young people to have at least one seizure in their lifetime.

Seizures generally present as altered consciousness or change in body motor movements, including tonic (stiffening) and clonic (jerking movements). There is an interruption to the normal electrical activity in the brain resulting in a seizure. Potential causes of convulsions need to be considered when nursing the child presenting with seizures:

- Febrile convulsions, usually observed in the child under 5 years with sudden onset of pyrexia, often associated with viral illness.
- Metabolic imbalance, including hypoglycaemia (low blood sugar).
- Head trauma: a seizure may indicate a rise in intracranial pressure.
- Infection, encephalitis, or meningitis.
- Syncope: a faint caused by a decrease in blood pressure
- Breath holding, hypoxia, or reflex anoxic seizures present with tonic movements in response to a sudden painful stimulus.
- Alcohol or drug toxicity.
- Congenital brain abnormality or tumour may present as focal seizures.
- Epilepsy.

Epilepsy

Epilepsy is the reoccurrence of seizure of primary cerebral origin, and affects 1 in 240 children in the UK (Figure 92.1). The clinical presentation may be as a generalized or focal seizure, with different observed or experienced symptoms dependent on where in the brain the abnormal activity occurs. A very small percentage of children who experience febrile convulsions will go on to gain a diagnosis of epilepsy. Management of the condition will be dependent on cause, type of seizure seen, and epilepsy syndrome.

Nursing care

When caring for a child presenting with seizures, it is essential to ensure safe surroundings, protect them from injury, and use an ABCDE approach. Time the seizure and ensure a patent airway; this can be assisted by placing the child on their side. If the convulsion lasts for five minutes, their own rescue plan or local advanced life support (APLS) guidelines should be followed. It is important to terminate the seizure as soon as possible to reduce the risk of status epilepticus, a continuous seizure of 30 minutes' duration or a cluster of seizures in which the child does not regain consciousness. It should also be acknowledged that many seizures will terminate before admission to the acute setting. In determining the reason for the seizure occurring, a good history from the primary caregiver or a witness is essential; trigger, presentation, and recovery from seizure should be obtained. Birth and family history, educational attainment, and psychosocial and developmental concerns are also relevant.

Further investigations

Further investigations that may be required to ascertain a diagnosis or to reduce the risk of further convulsions include blood and urine tests to rule out infection or metabolic imbalance. A blood sugar (BM) test should be completed to rule out hypoglycaemia.

An electrocardiogram (ECG) should be undertaken to look for cardiac abnormalities, and an electroencephalogram (EEG) may be useful in aiding or excluding diagnosis of epilepsy. However, it is important to be aware that an EEG may be normal in a person with epilepsy and abnormal in a person without epilepsy. The findings should be added to the presentation of seizure history. An EEG would not be indicated in a child with febrile convulsions.

A magnetic resonance imaging or computerized tomographic scan would look for brain abnormalities in a child presenting with focal seizures. National evidence-based guidance informs good practice for diagnosis, treatment, and appropriate referral to tertiary centres.

Treatment

Antiepileptic medication (AED) should only be commenced on consultation with an expert practitioner; this would rarely be indicated following the first convulsion. The prescribing of correct AED will acknowledge the potential reason for seizure and epilepsy syndrome, with the aim of controlling seizures, on a good dose with minimal adverse effects to medication. Other treatment for refractory, difficult-to-treat seizures includes:

- Epilepsy surgery.
- Vagal nerve stimulation (VNS).
- Ketogenic diet.

Follow-up care

On discharge, education for the patient and family is very important. An emergency care plan should be discussed if a potential risk of prolonged seizure is present; that is, a seizure lasting five minutes and over (Figure 92.2). The family should be educated in the use of benzodiazepine buccal midazolam (Figure 92.3) and rectal diazepam (Figure 92.4), and first aid information should be offered for people involved in the care of the child, including their education. Daily management of risk should be acknowledged, including close supervision around water, bike helmets when cycling, and a good sleep pattern. Support should also be offered for the comorbidities of learning difficulties and psychosocial anxiety.

Key points

- Some children may not have very visible signs of seizure activity, so listen to parents if they express concerns about new behaviours/movements that they observe in their child.
- Parents will be extremely frightened when they witness their child having a seizure. They will need education about future management of seizures and reassurance to rebuild their confidence. They will need to know that febrile convulsions are generally harmless and that their child is likely to make a complete recovery.
- Triggers, if known, should be avoided for children with epilepsy and family and school informed about these.

93 Meningitis

Figure 93.1 Recognizing symptoms in babies and young children.

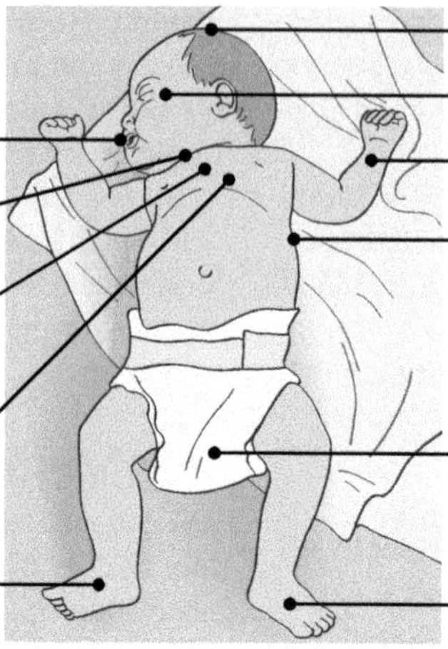
Is the baby's condition deteriorating?
Vomiting? Unable to eat or refusing food?
Airway patent, at risk, or compromised?
Tachypnoea, or with increased work of breathing, such as recession, tracheal tug, nasal flaring?
Tachycardia, with increased central capillary refill time >2 s
Pallor, mottling, cool peripheries, any evidence of non-blanching rash, petechiae, purpura (indicating sepsis)?
Tense or bulging soft spot?
Lethargy/staring expression/too sleepy to wake?
Hyperpyrexia or extreme shivering?
Is the baby or child stiff, with jerky movements or floppiness?
Irritable when handled, with high-pitched or moaning cry? Do carers report the baby or child having reduced interaction or changed behaviour?
Any diarrhoea?
Does the baby or child appear to be in pain? Headache/muscle aches/severe limb/joint pain?

Reproduced with permission of Wiley

Figure 93.2 Recognizing symptoms in young people.

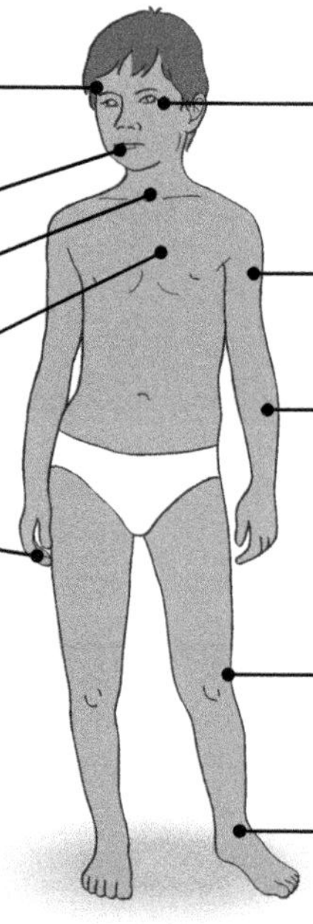
Are they reporting a severe headache, photophobia?
Is their condition abnormal or deteriorating?
Have they been vomiting?
Is their airway patent, at risk, or compromised?
Are they tachypnoeic, do they have increased work of breathing?
Are they tachycardic, do they have a increased central capillary refill time >2 s?
Do they appear confused, delirious, are they exhibiting signs of deteriorating consciousness or altered mental state?
Are they in a toxic moribund state? Teenagers may be combative, confused, or aggressive – you may suspect drug abuse, drunkenness
Do they have focal neurological deficit including cranial nerve involvement and abnormal pupils or pupil reactions?
Do they have a non-blanching rash, petechiae, or purpuric in nature?
Are they exhibiting paresis – muscular weakness caused by nerve damage or disease?
Have they had a seizure?
Are they exhibiting Kerning's sign – extension of the knee on a flexed hip at 90° causes restriction and pain?
Are they exhibiting Brudzinski's sign – such as reflex flexion of a lower extremity on passive flexion of the opposite extremity?

Figure 93.3 Tumbler test for septicaemia.

If a glass tumbler is pressed firmly against a septicaemic rash, the marks will not fade

You will be able to see the rash through the glass. If this happens get medical advice immediately

It is harder to see on dark skin, so check paler areas

Remember someone who is very ill needs medical help even if they have no rash or a rash that fades

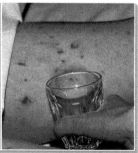

Courtesy of the Meningitis Trust

Box 93.1 Signs of acute raised intracranial pressure.

The Cushing reflex

Symptoms include:

- Increasing blood pressure and decreasing heart rate due to medullary brain ischaemia
- Pupil dilatation
- Coning: the herniation of brain contents: symptoms include worsening bradycardia, hypertension respiratory depression, bilateral papillary dilatation, decerebrate posturing. These will eventually cause death

Children and Young People's Nursing at a Glance, Second Edition. Edited by Elizabeth Gormley-Fleming and Sheila Roberts.

eningitis is a serious infection. Meningitis causes an inflammation of the meninges and cerebrospinal fluid, due to a viral or bacterial infection. While viral meningitis is most common, it is usually self-limiting, therefore the focus will be on the management of bacterial meningitis, which has an overall mortality rate of 5–10% of cases. Once the central nervous system is infected an inflammatory response is stimulated. This may result in vasculitis, thrombosis, infarction, and oedema, which may cause raised intracranial pressure (RICP), brain damage, and death.

Common causes
- Meningococcus – serotypes A, B, C, Y, and W135.
- *Pneumococcus*.
- *Haemophilus influenzae*.

Early recognition, diagnosis, and effective management are vital to improve morbidity and mortality outcomes.

Prevention
Introduction of immunizations has led to a rapid reduction in meningitis cases. Under the UK NHS vaccination programme, all children are eligible to receive vaccines against:
- *H. influenzae* type b (Hib).
- Meningococcus serotype C (Men C).
- Pneumococcus.

The introduction of the Men C vaccine has led to a 99% decrease in the number of people under 20 years diagnosed with serotype C meningitis. Serotype group B meningococcus is now the most common cause of bacterial meningitis, as a vaccine is not yet available.

Assessment
It is essential that children's nurses are able to rapidly assess and recognize any baby, child, or young person who presents with the symptoms of meningitis or meningococcal septicaemia (Figures 93.1 and 93.2 and Box 93.1). The signs may not be easy to detect in the young child. Following a subjective and objective ABCDE systematic assessment will allow effective assessment and evaluation of the child. The Sepsis 6 should be followed if there is a high suspicion of sepsis. This is important, as the child may present at any stage of the illness, from simply being feverish and irritable to being in decompensated distributive shock.

Planning care
Planning care must focus on the effective management of the problems identified during the assessment process and assisting with investigations to confirm the diagnosis.

Primary care
If meningitis is suspected, a tumbler test (Figure 93.3) may be carried out, following which the child should be immediately transferred to an acute hospital environment. If urgent transfer is not possible, the GP may initiate antibiotic treatment in accordance with national recommendations.

Secondary care
Effective communication with both the child and family is vital to allow them to make informed decisions regarding care and treatment.

Diagnosis
- History, subjective and objective ABCDE assessment, consider whether any signs of RICP, or septicaemia such as spreading purpuric rash or "shock."
- Bloods for full blood count, C-reactive protein (CRP), coagulation screen, urea and electrolytes, blood cultures, blood glucose, bone profiling, clotting, blood gas for bicarb, base excess, lactate and blood glucose, and a polymerase chain reaction (PCR) test looking for *Neisseria meningitides* and pneumococcus.
- Urine sample for microscopy, culture, and sensitivity (MC and S).
- Bacterial throat swab.
- Consider lumber puncture; contraindications include a child who is respiratorily, cardiovascularly, or neurologically compromised or unstable, which includes any signs of RICP, seizures, shock, or extensive or spreading purpura. A head computerized tomographic (CT) scan will be required if RICP is suspected. Cerebrospinal fluid will be sent for microscopy and for chemistry.

Management of bacterial meningitis
National guidelines recommend immediate administration of the following:
- Under 28 days – intravenous (IV) cefotaxime plus amoxicillin plus gentamicin.
- 1–3 months – IV cefotaxime plus either amoxicillin or ampicillin.
- Over 3 months – IV ceftriaxone plus corticosteroids as per national guidance.

The bacteria causing meningitis can also result in septicaemia, a life-threatening systemic disease. As with meningitis, the infection triggers an inflammatory response that includes an acute vascular and cellular response, stimulating an immune response. This results in increased vasodilatation and cell permeability as the neutrophils attempt to reach the site of infection. That may result in distributive or septic shock. Close monitoring is vital to allow early recognition and treatment of septic shock. If there is a high suspicion of sepsis or septic shock, then the Sepsis 6 should be commenced within one hour.

Management of fever and pain
Inflammation of the meninges causes pain, headache, irritability, and photophobia. All children with meningitis will also be pyrexial. Treatment with antipyretics and anti-inflammatories is recommended.

Monitoring should be in accordance with the patient's condition; this may be every 30 minutes to 1 hourly initially. It is essential to report any abnormalities immediately. Monitoring must include:
- Patency of airway, respiratory rate, and work of breathing.
- Manual pulse/apex if under 2 years, use of a cardiac monitor.
- Capillary refill time – this should be taken centrally.
- Blood pressure.
- Oxygen saturation if not peripherally compromised.
- Conscious level (AVPU [Alert, Verbal, Pain, Unresponsive]), interaction with carers.
- Paediatric Glasgow Coma Score (PGCS).
- Blood glucose.
- Temperature.
- Completion of Paediatric Early Warning Scores (PEWS).
- Check for new or developing purpuric rash or spreading purpura, as this will indicate the development of septicaemia.

Notification
Meningitis is a notifiable condition. Prophylaxis of close contacts may be required, and the nurse should facilitate this request, as it is important to eliminate asymptomatic carriage of the bacteria and prevent further cases.

Key points
- All elements of the Sepsis 6 should be commenced within an hour if sepsis or septic shock is suspected or confirmed.
- Bacterial meningitis can lead to significant morbidities even if early treatment is commenced.
- Lumbar puncture is contraindicated in the child who is respiratorily, cardiovascularly, or neurologically compromised.

94 Sepsis and septicaemia

Figure 94.1 Signs of septicaemia.

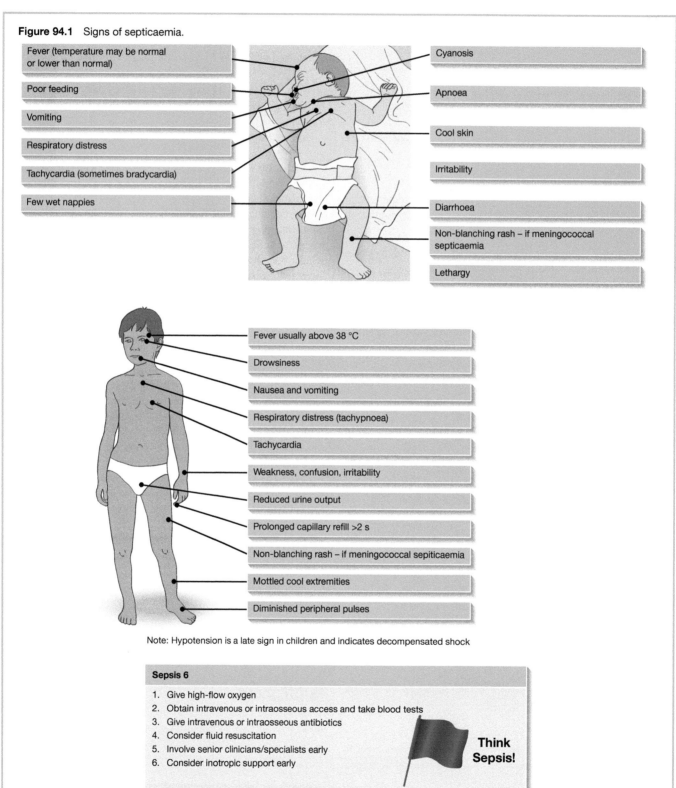

Fever (temperature may be normal or lower than normal)

Poor feeding

Vomiting

Respiratory distress

Tachycardia (sometimes bradycardia)

Few wet nappies

Cyanosis

Apnoea

Cool skin

Irritability

Diarrhoea

Non-blanching rash – if meningococcal septicaemia

Lethargy

Fever usually above 38 °C

Drowsiness

Nausea and vomiting

Respiratory distress (tachypnoea)

Tachycardia

Weakness, confusion, irritability

Reduced urine output

Prolonged capillary refill >2 s

Non-blanching rash – if meningococcal sepiticaemia

Mottled cool extremities

Diminished peripheral pulses

Note: Hypotension is a late sign in children and indicates decompensated shock

Sepsis 6

1. Give high-flow oxygen
2. Obtain intravenous or intraosseous access and take blood tests
3. Give intravenous or intraosseous antibiotics
4. Consider fluid resuscitation
5. Involve senior clinicians/specialists early
6. Consider inotropic support early

Think Sepsis!

Children and Young People's Nursing at a Glance, Second Edition. Edited by Elizabeth Gormley-Fleming and Sheila Roberts.
© 2023 John Wiley & Sons Ltd. Published 2023 by John Wiley & Sons Ltd.

Definitions

Septicaemia (Figure 94.1) is defined as the presence of numerous bacteria in the blood that are actively dividing, and this may lead to sepsis. While bacterial infections are the most common, fungal, viral, and protozoal infections may also lead to septicaemia.

The term sepsis is used to describe a clinical syndrome when a child has an adverse reaction to an infection. The words sepsis and septicaemia may be used interchangeably, but they are two distinct conditions. The immune system will trigger an extreme response to the infection and this may result in a systemic response to the infection, leading to organ dysfunction. It can be complicated by circulatory collapse, myocardial depression, increased metabolic rate, and perfusion abnormalities.

Systemic inflammatory response syndrome

In systemic inflammatory response syndrome (SIRS), two of the following four criteria are present:
- Core temperature >38 °C or <36 °C.
- Severe tachycardia or bradycardia.
- Tachypnoea.
- Raised or reduced leukocyte count.

Septic shock

This is classified as distributive shock and is a combination of issues with the cardiovascular system and fluid. It is characterized by:
- Loss of pre-load.
- Loss of afterload/systemic vascular resistance (SVR).
- Loss of contractility.

At-risk groups

Anyone may develop septicaemia, but it is more common in infants and young children who meet one or more of the following conditions:
- Post surgery.
- Have a central venous access device.
- Previous history of septicaemia.
- Certain long-term conditions – diabetes, cancer.
- Server injury – burns, open wounds.
- Immunosuppressed.

Management principles

The Sepsis 6 pathway should be implemented if the child has any of the red flag sepsis signs:
- Recognition of decreased perfusion and altered neurological status.
- Assessment needs to follow a logical approach.
- Goal of treatment should be resolution of the primary problem, improvement of tissue perfusion, and oxygenation.
- Need to assess and reassess to determine response to therapy, identify need for changes, and detect any deterioration.
  1 Maximize oxygen delivery and administer oxygen:
- Assessment of airway and breathing.
- Is the airway patent?
- Is there respiratory distress?
- Monitor respiratory rate and work of breathing.
- Administer high-flow oxygen to help with oxygen delivery.

- Monitor oxygen saturations, maintain >94%.
- Monitor acid–base balance: acidosis can affect oxygen delivery as well as oxygen utilization.
- Reduce oxygen demand.
- Treat fever.
- Treat pain.
- Eliminate needless stress.
  2 Gain intravenous (IV) or intraosseous (IO) access and take blood cultures:
- Other samples such as urine, cerebrospinal fluid should be considered, as well as blood for lactate level, urea and electrolytes, full blood count, C-reactive protein, blood glucose, and blood gas should be drawn for analysis.
  3 Give IV antibiotics:
- Consider allergies. Adhere to local policy.
  4 Give IV fluids: optimize cardiac output:
- Assess circulation – heart rate, capillary refill, colour.
- Lactate level > 2 mmol/L.
- Correct any acid–base imbalance or electrolyte disturbance as this will affect the ability of the heart to pump.
- Give fluid – 20 mL/kg (usually 0.9% saline) as a rapid bolus, then reassess. Use 20 mL/kg increments. May need up to and over 60 mL/kg in the first hour.
- Neonates: 10 mL/kg as a rapid bolus then reassess. Use increments of 10 mL/kg.
- May need IO access.
- Goal is to restore normal perfusion.
- May have ongoing fluid requirements.
  5 Involve senior clinicians early: may need to seek advice from a tertiary paediatric centre.
  6 Consider use of inotrope support early.

General considerations

- Care of the family.
- Skin care in light of poor perfusion.
- Maintain blood sugar within normal limits.
- Mouth care.
- Prevention of secondary infection.
- Nutrition.

National guidelines should be followed for the specific management of meningococcal septicaemia.

While the Sepsis 6 was an initiative in adult care that was evaluated as being highly effective and showed improved survival rates, it has been adapted for use in the care of the sick infant or child with suspected sepsis. Reduced length of hospital stay has been identified for children with sepsis whose care has followed the Sepsis 6 pathway.

Key points
- Recognition of the sick child and prompt treatment of infection are essential if sepsis is to be avoided.
- The risk of septicaemia can be reduced by good hand hygiene in hospital and in the community.
- Knowing the signs of the Sepsis 6 and the action to take is imperative to reducing mortality and morbidity rates from infants and children.

95 Respiratory problems

Figure 95.1 Assessment of the child with a respiratory problem.

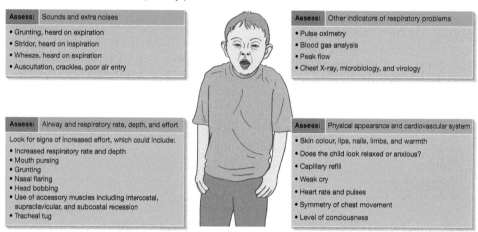

Assess: Sounds and extra noises
• Grunting, heard on expiration
• Stridor, heard on inspiration
• Wheeze, heard on expiration
• Auscultation, crackles, poor air entry

Assess: Other indicators of respiratory problems
• Pulse oximetry
• Blood gas analysis
• Peak flow
• Chest X-ray, microbiology, and virology

Assess: Airway and respiratory rate, depth, and effort
Look for signs of increased effort, which could include:
• Increased respiratory rate and depth
• Mouth pursing
• Grunting
• Nasal flaring
• Head bobbing
• Use of accessory muscles including intercostal, supraclavicular, and subcostal recession
• Tracheal tug

Assess: Physical appearance and cardiovascular system
• Skin colour, lips, nails, limbs, and warmth
• Does the child look relaxed or anxious?
• Capillary refill
• Weak cry
• Heart rate and pulses
• Symmetry of chest movement
• Level of conciousness

History of the presenting complaint	Past history relating to the respiratory problem	Family and social history
• Age of child • Was the onset sudden or was there a preceding illness? • Is there a cough, wheeze, or stridor? • Are there difficulties with feeding? • Are there other symptoms than respiratory? • Is there associated vomiting? • Is there a fever? • Is the child using any medication? Has any medication been administered?	• What is the neonatal history? • Has the child had any similar episodes? • Does the child have a diagnosis of asthma or another recent respiratory illness? • Are the child's immunizations up to date?	• Any history of atopy in the family such as asthma, hay fever, eczema? • Are there any siblings or other family members with similar illnesses? • What are the family's living conditions? • Is the child exposed to tobacco smoke? • Do the family have any pets?

Figure 95.2 Oxygen administration methods.

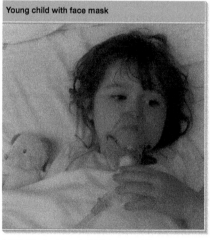

Young child with face mask

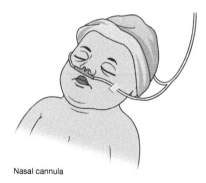

Nasal cannula

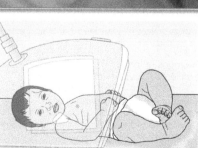

Headbox oxygen administration

Children and Young People's Nursing at a Glance, Second Edition. Edited by Elizabeth Gormley-Fleming and Sheila Roberts.
© 2023 John Wiley & Sons Ltd. Published 2023 by John Wiley & Sons Ltd.

Respiratory assessment

Undertaking a comprehensive respiratory assessment (Figure 95.1) is key in deciding the diagnosis and therefore determining the management of a child who presents with a respiratory problem. The key elements of a comprehensive respiratory assessment are:

- History of the presenting complaint.
- Past history relating to the respiratory problem.
- Family and social history.
- Physical assessment of the child, including respiratory rate, assessment of work of breathing, oxygen saturation, colour, and heart rate.

Once a comprehensive respiratory assessment has been undertaken a diagnosis can be established and treatment and supportive measures instigated.

Bronchiolitis

Bronchiolitis is a seasonal disease that most commonly affects infants aged 3–6 months. The infant presents with breathing difficulties, poor feeding, irritability, wheeze, and, in the very young, apnoea. The symptoms of bronchiolitis are coryzal, a harsh cough, wheezing, and tachypnoea. Only a small number of infants will require hospitalization. The most common cause of bronchiolitis is the respiratory syncytial virus (RSV), which accounts for over 50% of cases. The effects of the virus are to cause inflammation in the small airways, which leads to air trapping and a prolonged expiratory phase. Treatment for bronchiolitis is supportive and includes oxygen therapy and feeding support, either enteral or intravenous. High-flow nasal cannula therapy is effective in treating infants who have severe disease.

Upper airway obstruction

Upper airway obstruction can occur in children of all different ages and there are a variety of causes. It is characterized by stridor, which occurs on inspiration. Symptom progression and severity are assessed in relation to the stridor. Stridor on exertion > stridor at rest > recession on exertion > recession at rest > exhaustion, respiratory failure.

Laryngotracheobronchitis

This is the most common cause of upper airway obstruction in children aged 6 months to 6 years. It most commonly occurs in the 1–3-year age group and is usually viral in origin. The main causative virus is parainfluenza. It is characterized by subglottic inflammation and narrowing. The symptoms are usually worse at night. It is typically benign in course, but some children will need treatment. This can either be oral steroids, usually dexamethasone, or nebulized budesonide. Both of these treatments have been shown to be effective.

Epiglottitis

This is a relatively rare (due to the Hib vaccine) respiratory Haemophilus influenzae (type b) bacterial infection, but it is life threatening. It tends to occur in older children aged 3–6 years and the stridor is accompanied by drooling and a high temperature. The treatment is endotracheal intubation to bypass the obstruction, and intravenous antibiotics. It is important to note that if you suspect epiglottitis you must not extend the neck or place the child in the supine position unless someone is present who can intubate the child, as doing either of these things will often precipitate complete airway obstruction.

Foreign body inhalation

The main diagnostic difference between foreign body inhalation and the other causes of upper airway obstruction is the absence of fever or other systemic symptoms. The child will present with stridor and difficulty in breathing, but there will be no preceding history and the child will normally have been fit and well beforehand. Treatment of foreign body inhalation involves identification and removal of the object, usually by bronchoscope.

Respiratory infections

Most respiratory infections of childhood are viral in origin and on the whole self-limiting. However, it is important to consider bacterial infections in children who have persistent symptoms. Bacterial pneumonia should be considered in children who have a persistent or repetitive fever of 38.5 °C or above and symptoms of respiratory distress. Treatment is with antibiotics, usually oral.

Common respiratory interventions

Much of the treatment and nursing care that children with respiratory problems receive is focused on assessment and support. The most common respiratory interventions are oxygen therapy, suctioning, and positioning.

Oxygen therapy

When choosing the method for administering oxygen, the following factors need to be taken into consideration:

- Age of child.
- Clinical condition of child.
- Percentage or flow rate of oxygen prescribed.
- Compliance of child.

Head boxes, nasal cannulas, and face masks (Figure 95.2) can be used to deliver oxygen to children effectively. Head boxes are most useful in infants and can be used to deliver high concentrations of oxygen and good humidification. High concentrations can also be delivered using a nasal cannula (Optiflow™, Fisher & Paykel Healthcare, Auckland, New Zealand). Nasal cannulas can be used to deliver lower flows of oxygen, as can face masks. Face masks are the most effective method of delivering high concentrations of oxygen to older children who are acutely unwell.

Suctioning

Suctioning is often required for children with respiratory problems. Suctioning can be traumatic for children and it can also cause clinical distress, with decreased oxygen saturations and increased work of breathing. Indications for suctioning include:

- The child's breathing becomes difficult because of vomiting or excessive secretions, in the oropharynx or nasopharynx.
- The child's skin may look pale, blue, or grey, particularly around the mouth or nose.
- The child is coughing excessively and unable to clear secretions.

Positioning

Optimal positioning of children and infants can improve oxygenation and decrease respiratory workload. Positions that can improve work of breathing include:

- Prone positioning.
- Sitting upright.
- Lying over someone's shoulder.

Key points

- Detailed and accurate respiratory assessment is key when assessing a child.
- It is important to identify a suitable oxygen delivery method to match the child's oxygen requirements.
- To ensure the child receives the correct amount of oxygen, oxygen saturation monitoring is vital.

96 Asthma

Figure 96.1 What is asthma?

Symptoms

- Wheeze
- Cough day and night (night-time cough is significant in diagnosis)
- Difficulty in breathing
- Tightness in the chest

Diagnosis

Asthma affects children of all ages and with differing degrees of severity. Diagnosis in the under-3 age group is particularly difficult to give a definitive diagnosis because of the immature smooth muscle in the lungs and therefore its capacity to respond to bronchodilator medication. Diagnosis at any age can be problematic as there is no one definitive gold standard test that can be carried out to confirm this. Diagnosis should be based on:

- Full history, including atopy and other allergies
- Physical examination, bloods for IgE, and rast levels
- Results of spirometry
- Consideration of differential diagnosis
- Response to treatment with a bronchodilator

Physiology

In response to asthma allergens or triggers, the lining of the bronchioles becomes swollen, inflamed, and oedema is present within the bronchial tissue. As the inflammation becomes persistent, a number of changes happen in the airway including epithelial cells sloughing off the airway wall, which mix with mucous resulting in thick plugs being formed. This increase in mucous and narrowing of the airway result in bronchoconstriction, characterized by wheeze, cough, shortness of breath, and difficulty in breathing. Airways can become permanently narrowed as a result of numerous repeated asthma attacks.

What happens to the airways during an asthma attack?

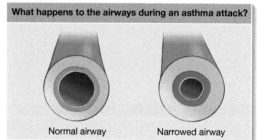

Normal airway   Narrowed airway

Asthma is triggered by a number of environmental factors:

- Grass pollen
- Viral infections, coughs, and colds
- Smoking, passive smoking
- Household dust mite
- Hair and dander from pets and animals
- Stress and anxiety
- Exercise
- Chemicals, perfumes, paint
- Changes in humidity and temperature
- Exhaust fumes, pollution
- Sawdust

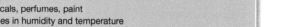

Goals of treatment

- Abolish symptoms during night and day
- Reduce the number of attacks and reduce school absences
- Adequate control with minimal medication, reviewed regularly, stepped up and down regularly
- Prevent hospital admissions, manage condition at home through evidence-based practice, self-management plans, peak flow measurement, education and support. This can be achieved by utilizing the resources within school nursing and specialist nursing roles both within the hospital and in primary care settings

Treatment

The British Thoracic Society and Scottish Intercollegiate Guidelines (2009), updated in 2012, advise on appropriate treatment for children and young people according to age. Treatment usually consists of use of a bronchodilator using a spacer device as and when needed. If this is required on a regular basis, a preventer inhaler (inhaled steroid) will be prescribed, to be taken in the morning and at night using a spacer device. Treatment is stepped up and down as symptoms improve or deteriorate. Regular review of symptoms is essential via primary care and a full table of prescribing is available via the above guidelines

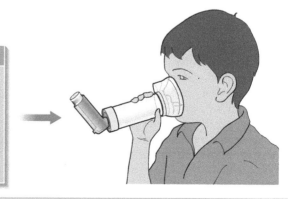

Children and Young People's Nursing at a Glance, Second Edition. Edited by Elizabeth Gormley-Fleming and Sheila Roberts.
© 2023 John Wiley & Sons Ltd. Published 2023 by John Wiley & Sons Ltd.

Asthma

Asthma (Figure 96.1) is the most common long-term condition of childhood, with approximately 10–11% of children in the UK affected. The cause of asthma is still not fully understood, but it is known that the condition has a genetic predisposition combined with environmental factors. There is also a link to related conditions, which include hay fever, eczema, and allergy, and it is common for children to be on several different medications to control each of the related conditions. In the UK more children seek medical admission to the Emergency Department than those in other European countries. Death from acute exacerbation of asthma still occurs in the UK. It is estimated that 80% of all deaths from asthma could be prevented.

Asthma attacks all age groups, but often starts in childhood. It is more common in boys than girls until puberty is reached. It is estimated that 30% of children under the age of 3 years will have sought medical assistance for a wheeze. The condition is characterized by recurrent episodes of breathlessness and wheezing, which vary in frequency and severity from person to person. The condition is due to inflammation of the lining of the bronchioles in the lungs and affects the sensitivity of the nerve endings in the airways so they become easily irritated. During an asthma attack the lining of the small passages becomes inflamed, causing the lumen of the airways to narrow and therefore reducing the flow of air into the lungs.

During an exacerbation of asthma, three factors are involved:
- Bronchospasm
- Inflammation
- Inflammatory cells

Psychosocial impact of asthma

As with any chronic long-term condition, asthma can have a dramatic impact on the quality of life and career choices of many young people. Children with asthma have sometimes been reported to be bullied in school and can have frequent episodes of absence due to poorly controlled asthma. For some children this can lead to academic failure, resulting in low self-esteem. In addition to this, exercise is a known trigger for asthma and poor control of symptoms and incorrect use of inhalers prior to sport and physical exercise can also lead to poor performance, impacting further on a sense of failure. Stress and emotions can trigger asthma, so in some areas of asthma care cognitive behavioural therapy (CBT) is now being used. This has encouraged children and young people to be aware that the concept of CBT combined with good asthma management support from parents, school nurses, primary care health professionals, and teachers can lead to a positive approach that can improve performance, quality, and psychological wellbeing.

Role of asthma UK

Asthma UK is a charitable organization that provides advice, education, information, and support for families and professionals on all aspects of asthma care, from diagnosis and throughout life. Information is evidence based on current research and findings and the organization is seen by all professionals as an excellent and reliable source of information for children, young people, and their families. Its website is updated regularly and information can be requested free of charge in most cases for a variety of reasons. In particular, resources for school staff with regard to education about the condition itself have been particularly useful in promoting good asthma management in schools. Due to several high-profile deaths of school-aged children with asthma over recent years, there has been an increase in the demand for information within schools to promote good asthma care. Asthma UK regularly carries out research with young people who have the condition and acts in an advocacy role in promoting the needs of children with asthma.

Treatment and management

There are many different types of treatment for asthma, but most treatment consists of the use of different types of inhalers. In most instances the child will be prescribed a bronchodilator, usually a beta 2 agonist (also known as a reliever inhaler), which relaxes the smooth muscle in the small airways, making it easier for the child to breathe. This is taken on an as-needed basis and its use should be monitored by a healthcare professional. If the reliever is required on a regular basis, a second inhaler is usually prescribed and this acts as a protector. This inhaler provides protection to the bronchioles and, if taken regularly morning and night, this will help to reduce the inflammation in the lungs and control symptoms such as night-time coughing and recurrent attacks. This type of inhaler is an inhaled corticosteroid (ICS) and the use of this drug should be regularly reviewed by a healthcare professional. There are many other types of inhalers, including combined or long-acting inhalers; oral medication can be used in combination with inhalers. Inhalers are also referred to as pre-measured dose inhalers (PMDI). Evidence-based guidance for prescribers on all aspects of drug therapy, investigation, diagnosis, and symptom management should be adhered to.

Review

Regular review of symptoms and completion of symptom diaries to include use of inhalers can be a useful tool for members of the primary care health team in managing asthma. Self-management plans are advocated for all, with clear instructions and guidance around when to act on an increase in symptoms and how to manage this, avoiding hospital admission and minimizing risk to the patient. Treatment should be stepped up and down according to symptoms, with minimal medication being taken.

Peak flow measurements are seen as a useful tool in assessing lung function within the hospital, home, or school setting and can be used as an additional tool of assessment for some children who are able to manage to use the peak flow monitor appropriately. This should always be considered along with the severity of symptoms in an attack or prior to an attack.

Inhaler technique is poor in children, so PMDIs should be used with a spacer device to maximize inhaled medication. This can enhance the effectiveness of the drug by delivering the full dose and with good technique can ensure that the drug reaches the lungs rather than being swallowed. A face mask can also be used with the spacer for infants and young children.

Inhaler technique should always be checked and reinforced at every opportunity along with continued education about the condition itself, avoidance of exposure to triggers, and a reminder about the different uses of each type of inhaler or medication prescribed.

Emergency management

This should be discussed and reinforced at every opportunity by the healthcare professional. In an emergency, one puff of the child's blue reliever should be given via the spacer, with one puff per minute given for 10 minutes or continued until help arrives. The inhaler should be shaken between each puff.

Key points
- Childhood asthma remains a very common long-term condition that carries a mortality rate that could be reduced by prompt treatment.
- Asthma occurs dur to the hyper-responsiveness of the airways induced by a trigger.
- Inability of a child with asthma to speak is a worrying sign.

97 CPAP and BiPAP

Box 97.1 Causes of respiratory failure.

Category of impairment	Examples
Impaired ventilation	
Upper airway obstruction	• Laryngospasm • Foreign body aspiration • Epiglottitis • Tumour of the upper airways
Weakness or paralysis of the respiratory muscles	• Drug overdose • Injury to the spinal cord • Poliomyelitis • Guillain–Barré syndrome • Muscular dystrophy • Disease of the brain stem
Chest wall injury	• Rib fracture • Burn eschar
Impaired matching of ventilation and perfusion	• Chronic obstructive lung disease • Restrictive lung disease • Severe pneumonia • Atelectasis
Impaired diffusion	
Pulmonary oedema	• Left heart failure • Inhalation of toxic materials
Respiratory distress syndrome	• Respiratory distress syndrome in the neonate

Figure 97.1 Causes of respiratory distress.

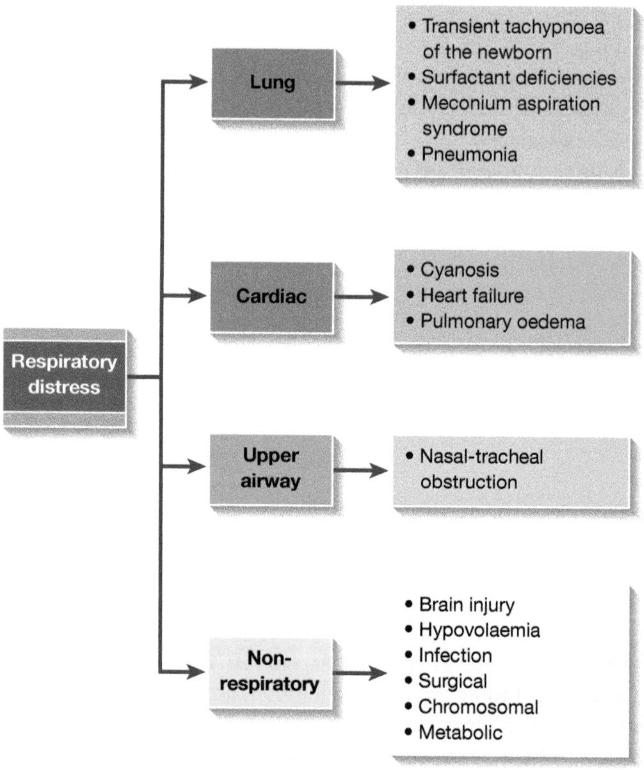

Respiratory distress
- Lung
  - Transient tachypnoea of the newborn
  - Surfactant deficiencies
  - Meconium aspiration syndrome
  - Pneumonia
- Cardiac
  - Cyanosis
  - Heart failure
  - Pulmonary oedema
- Upper airway
  - Nasal-tracheal obstruction
- Non-respiratory
  - Brain injury
  - Hypovolaemia
  - Infection
  - Surgical
  - Chromosomal
  - Metabolic

Figure 97.2 CPAP/BiPAP mask.

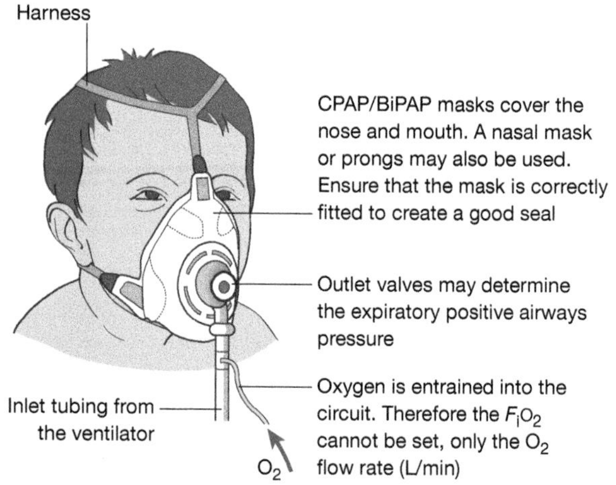

Harness

CPAP/BiPAP masks cover the nose and mouth. A nasal mask or prongs may also be used. Ensure that the mask is correctly fitted to create a good seal

Outlet valves may determine the expiratory positive airways pressure

Inlet tubing from the ventilator

Oxygen is entrained into the circuit. Therefore the F_iO_2 cannot be set, only the O_2 flow rate (L/min)

Figure 97.3 Non-invasive ventilator.

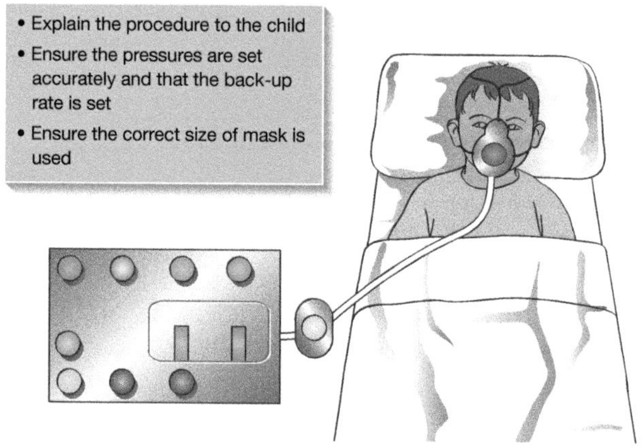

- Explain the procedure to the child
- Ensure the pressures are set accurately and that the back-up rate is set
- Ensure the correct size of mask is used

Respiratory failure

Continuous positive airway pressure (CPAP) and bi-level positive airway pressure (BiPAP) are commonly utilized methods of non-invasive ventilation used to treat both acute (in hospital) and chronic (in the home) respiratory failure in children. Respiratory failure can occur acutely in children who were previously well, or chronically as a result of lung or chest wall disease.

Respiratory failure is not a specific disease and occurs when the lungs are unable to oxygenate the blood adequately or are unable to prevent carbon dioxide retention, even at rest. There are three types of conditions that contribute to the hypoxia in respiratory

Children and Young People's Nursing at a Glance, Second Edition. Edited by Elizabeth Gormley-Fleming and Sheila Roberts.
© 2023 John Wiley & Sons Ltd. Published 2023 by John Wiley & Sons Ltd.

failure: hypoventilation, impaired diffusion across the alveolar–capillary membrane, and mismatching of ventilation and perfusion.

The causes of respiratory failure can be summarized according to each category (Box 97.1).

Obstructive sleep apnoea

CPAP or BiPAP may also be used in the management of obstructive sleep apnoea (OSA), partial or complete upper airway obstruction that is recurrent. There is disruption of normal oxygenation, ventilation, and the child's sleep pattern. OSA is common in children with hypertrophy of the adenoids and tonsils, which is resolved through surgery, so CPAP may be required in the short term. Long-term conditions where the child may require CPAP include Pierre Robin syndrome, craniofacial abnormalities, Prader–Willi syndrome, storage diseases, and some genetic conditions, such Down's syndrome. The age range of children with complex OSA ranges from newborn to young people and on into adulthood. CPAP should be used for the total physiological sleep time, which may be more than 12 hours in young children and for as little as four hours in older children.

Aims and uses of CPAP and BiPAP

The aims of both CPAP and BiPAP are to prevent worsening respiratory failure and respiratory distress, and to alleviate the child's discomfort. Causes of respiratory distress are not always due to a primary respiratory problem or disease (Figure 97.1).

CPAP and BiPAP can be delivered via a face mask, nasal mask, or prongs (Figure 97.2). When considering which mode to use, it is vital to understand the ways in which they work.

CPAP promotes respiratory function by preventing airway collapse and loss of lung volume. The functional residual capacity is increased, thereby increasing the surface area available for gas exchange and so reducing the work of breathing. CPAP is most commonly used for infants with bronchiolitis or apnoea or children with OSA, for weaning from mechanical ventilation, or for upper airway obstruction.

BiPAP combines the benefits of CPAP with keeping the lungs open through the entire respiratory cycle. Both the inspiratory and expiratory pressures can be manipulated on BiPAP machines, along with rate and a back-up breath rate. Using BiPAP can improve minute ventilation and oxygenation, thereby reducing the work of breathing.

CPAP and BiPAP may not be well tolerated by children, causing agitation, cardiovascular instability, and confusion, and further exacerbating the hypoxia. The need for sedation and pain relief should be considered. Further complications include gastric distension or perforation, therefore an orogastric or nasogastric tube should be inserted and kept drainage free; increased airway resistance; and pulmonary air leaks (pneumothorax). The need to commence non-invasive ventilation (Figure 97.3) must be medically ordered and these orders reviewed daily or as indicated by the child's condition.

Monitoring required for CPAP and BiPAP

The following should be monitored once CPAP/BiPAP has been commenced:

- Pulse oximetry, aiming for 94–98% using supplemental oxygen as required.
- Electrocardiogram (ECG).
- Blood pressure.
- Respiratory rate, work of breathing.
- Heart rate.
- Level of consciousness.

- Arterial blood gas.
- Patient comfort.

The monitor device should be reviewed hourly and the positive airway pressure (PAP) and positive end-expiratory pressure (PEEP) observed, humidifier temperature and water level noted, and the circuit rain-out monitored. Tidal volume, minute ventilation, leak, and spontaneous trigger may also be observed along with alarm settings.

It is crucial to monitor the ECG and SaO$_2$ continuously and to document the vital signs hourly. Hourly documentation of the pressure settings and respiratory rate and effort should also be undertaken while the child is receiving CPAP or BiPAP. Blood gas assessment should be conducted regularly, and senior medical help should be close by at all times. The nurse must be vigilant at all times for potential complications. These may be clinical or mechanical complications.

Titration/weaning

Treatment should be continued until the child is improving and the underlying pathology is treated or resolved with clinical improvement. Consisting of short periods of time off CPAP/BiPAP, weaning should be introduced and gradually increased until the child no longer needs the assistance. It is usual that CPAP/BiPAP is discontinued during the day before the night-time requirement is withdrawn.

Contraindications for CPAP/BiPAP

- Vomiting, excess secretions
- Confusion/agitation
- Facial burns/trauma
- Bowel obstruction
- Pneumothorax
- Inability to protect airway
- Impaired consciousness

Further considerations

Ensure accurate sizing of the mask or prongs. The equipment and settings should be checked hourly and documented. Appropriately sized emergency airway equipment and suction should be at the bedside.

Position changes to relieve the pressure of the nasal prongs or mask should be part of the routine care of the child. Trying to cluster care can reduce the oxygen demand and minimize their distress.

The use of CPAP or BiPAP for acute respiratory failure should be carried out in a paediatric high-dependency setting and only those members of staff who are trained and assessed as being competent should be involved in caring for the child receiving CPAP or BiPAP.

If a child requires CPAP or BiPAP, their condition could become worse at any stage and may precipitate the need for invasive ventilation. Therefore, close monitoring, documentation, and communication with the tertiary referral centre (paediatric intensive care) are essential. Treatment of the underlying pathology is crucial.

Key points

- The aims of CPAP and BiPAP are to prevent worsening respiratory failure and respiratory distress due to either acute or long-term conditions.
- The infant or child who needs CPAP or BiPAP requires continuous monitoring of their heart rate and oxygen saturation levels.
- CPAP and BiPAP must only ever be used by trained and competent nursing staff.

98 Cardiovascular assessment and shock

Figure 98.1 Cardiovascular assessment.

Currently, there is no reliable technology to provide exact values for cardiac output or its components. However, assessments can be performed to provide a picture of the child's cardiac output state

Electrocardiogram (ECG)

- Indication of the electrical current moving through the heart muscle to make it function
- Always associate the trace with feeling for a pulse
- *Beware*: pulseless electrical activity (PEA) is when the ECG can appear normal yet the patient no longer has a cardiac output

Pulse

- Feeling for a pulse will provide more sensitive information about cardiac output than a rate alone
- Assessing the quality of the pulse (whether it is bounding or thread or not) will give an indication of:
  - power and regularity of heart beat
  - patient's volume status
  - peripheral perfusion along with patient's colour and warmth of limb
- Good sites to feel for pulses in children are:
  - brachial
  - femoral
  - radial

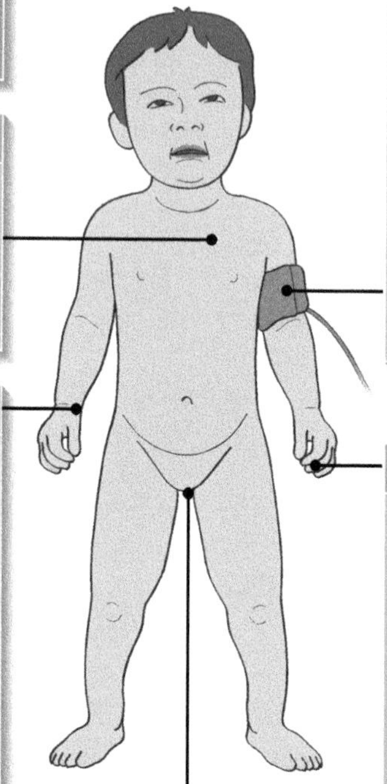

Blood pressure (BP)

- Measures pressure exerted by blood on the walls of the vessel during contraction and relaxation of the heart muscle
- Indicates:
  - circulating volume
  - status of the vessel walls
  - power of the heart muscle
- Helpful to an overall picture of a child's cardio-vascular status
- *Beware*: a low BP is a late sign, suggesting the child is no longer able to maintain their cardiac output

Capillary refill

- Performed by depressing an area of the sternum or a fingertip for 5 seconds and then observing the time it takes for blood to be restored to the area
- Normal is less than 3 seconds
- Note: when assessing a fingertip, it is important that the finger is either in-line or above the heart to ensure it is the power of the heart that is being assessed and not gravity
- *Beware:* capillary refill may be influenced by the environmental temperature

Urine output

A reduction in perfusion to the kidneys causes a chain reaction in the rennin-angiotensin pathway that governs the production of urine. This not only results in increased sympathetic activity and systemic vascular resistance, but also causes the body to retain water to optimize circulating volume. The obvious result of this is a reduction in the child's urine output. Assessment of urine output will also provide further indications of their cardiovascular status

Table 98.1 Stages of shock.

Initial stage	Compensatory stage	Decompensatory stage	Refractory stage
Aerobic respiration becomes anaerobic	Tachycardia	Tachycardia will slow and change to bradycardia	Irreversible cell and organ damage
Lactic acid increases	Tachypnoea BP maintained	Tachypnoea will slow and become bradypnoea	Death
Minor clinical signs	Vasoconstriction seen peripherally and blood diverted to vital organs Urine output reduced Blood glucose levels increased	Hypotension Cold peripheries Agitation Acidosis increases Urine output decreases further or stops	

Children and Young People's Nursing at a Glance, Second Edition. Edited by Elizabeth Gormley-Fleming and Sheila Roberts.
© 2023 John Wiley & Sons Ltd. Published 2023 by John Wiley & Sons Ltd.

Cardiac output

The primary function of the cardiovascular system is to transport gases (oxygen and carbon dioxide), nutrients, and substrates around the body, to ensure that the appropriate amounts of these products are delivered to the cells to meet the cells' metabolic demands.

The prime determinant of the efficacy of the transport system is cardiac output. Cardiac output is the amount of blood that is ejected from the heart every minute and is the product of the equation:

$$\text{heart rate} \times \text{stroke volume}$$

Stroke volume is the amount of blood that is ejected from the heart with each beat. Stroke volume is determined by three factors:

- *Preload:* affected by the volume status of the patient.
- *Afterload:* impacted by the systemic vascular resistance.
- *Contractility:* the power created by the heart muscle to pump the blood around the body.

These factors of heart rate and stroke volume (encompassing preload, afterload, and contractility) adjust to maintain the cardiac output to meet the metabolic demands. Children, in particular, are unable to adjust their contractility in the same way that adults can to maintain their cardiac output. A sudden reduction in preload cannot easily be corrected by the body and alterations to afterload will have a limited affect by themselves. Therefore, the only means younger children have of maintaining cardiac output when compromised is to increase their heart rate.

An increase in heart rate can be very effective in improving cardiac output; however, the heart requires time to fill and eject blood. Therefore, an increased heart rate results in less time for filling and ejection to occur. After the heart rate has reached an optimum point, as it increases further cardiac output will actually begin to reduce. This means that children's nurses should carefully consider the cause of tachycardia, as this is the main compensatory mechanism used to maintain cardiac output. Eventually, an increased heart rate will not effectively maintain cardiac output and the child has no other mechanism to compensate for this.

Cardiovascular assessment

A comprehensive cardiovascular assessment will consist of measurement of heart rate and pulse (in older children), blood pressure, capillary refill time, and observation of the colour and warmth of the peripheries (Figure 98.1).

Shock

Shock is the body's inability to maintain its cardiac output (low cardiac output state), resulting in inadequate delivery of oxygen, nutrients, and substrates to meet the body's metabolic demands. The consequence is anaerobic respiration (cell respiration without oxygen), causing tissue damage and cell death.

Shock is divided into categories that indicate the cause; however, it is more important to recognize that the patient is shocked first and what stage of shock is evident (Table 98.1) rather than focus on the cause.

Hypovolaemic shock

- This the most common form of childhood shock.
- It occurs because of inadequate blood volume in the body.
- Preload is the component of cardiac output that is affected.
- Management is primarily focused on giving fluid to improve the child's volume status.
- Examples of hypovolaemic shock are children with diarrhoea and vomiting or trauma.

Cardiogenic shock

- The heart muscle is not able to generate enough power to pump blood out of the heart effectively.
- Contractility is the component of cardiac output most affected.
- Management focuses on giving drugs to improve the contractility of the heart and where possible reducing the work the heart has to do.
- *Beware:* giving fluid may make the heart work harder so will cause these patients to get worse. As a result, fluid must be given with caution while assessing the impact on the cardiac output.
- Examples are diseases of the heart muscle (cardiomyopathy) or post cardiac surgery.

Distributive shock

- The tone of the vascular system allows for blood volume to be distributed into the wrong areas.
- Causes may be sepsis or anaphylaxis.
- Afterload is the component of cardiac output most affected
- Management focuses on:
  ○ Giving fluids to replace the volume that has moved into the surrounding tissue.
  ○ Encouraging fluid back into the intravascular space.
  ○ Improving blood vessels' tone with drugs or cooling so volume will not leak out.
- Examples are septic shock and anaphylaxis.

Signs and symptoms of hypovolaemic shock

- Tachycardia as the heart attempts to increase blood flow to the body.
- Tachypnoea as the body attempts to increase oxygen levels.
- Agitation may be present if oxygen levels are low.
- During the compensatory stage blood pressure (BP) will be maintained.
- Oliguria, as blood flow is directed away from the kidneys to vital organs.
- Cool peripheries with increased capillary refill time.

  If fluid correction does not occur:
- Compensatory mechanisms will fail, leading to a drop in BP.
- Poor perfusion of organs.
- Low oxygen levels will lead to acidosis and capillary damage.
- Organ failure ensues.

Key points

- An accurate and thorough cardiac assessment is key in assessing a child.
- Diarrhoea and vomiting, especially in young babies, can be a catalyst for hypovolaemic shock.
- Restoring fluid and oxygen levels is vital in the treatment of shock.

99 Inflammatory bowel disease

Figure 99.1 Main inflammatory bowel diseases.

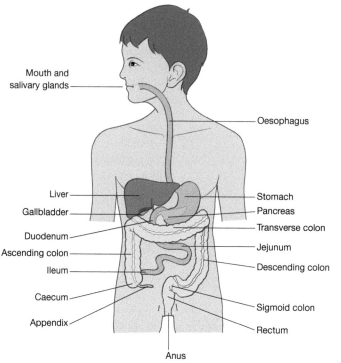

Mouth and salivary glands

Oesophagus

Ulcerative colitis only affects the colon, also known as the large intestine (ascending, transverse, descending, sigmoid colon, rectum, and anus). The inflammatory process involves the lining of the bowel causing superficial ulceration

Crohn's disease can affect any part of the gastrointestinal tract, from the mouth to the anus. The inflammation process is described as patchy transmural inflammation (the bowel lining and the deeper layers may be affected)

Liver
Gallbladder
Duodenum
Ascending colon
Ileum
Caecum
Appendix

Stomach
Pancreas
Transverse colon
Jejunum
Descending colon

Sigmoid colon
Rectum

Anus

Box 99.1 Signs and symptoms of inflammatory bowel disease.

- Abdominal pain
- Diarrhoea
- Urgency to use the toilet
- Passing blood or mucous per rectum
- Blood in stool
- Nausea
- Vomiting
- Loss of appetite
- Weight loss
- Tiredness and lethargy
- Delay in growth and puberty
- Mouth ulcers

Extraintestinal symptoms include skin rashes (erythema nodosum), inflammation of the eye (iritis or uveitis), and joint problems

Box 99.2 Treatments for inflammatory bowel disease.

- Aminosalicylates (mesalazine and sulfasalazine), available in oral and rectal preparations
- Corticosteroids (available as intravenous, oral, and rectal preparations)
- Exclusive liquid diet (first-line treatment for Crohn's disease)
- Immunosuppressants (azathioprine, 6-mercaptopurine, methotrexate, and ciclosporin)
- Biologics (infliximab and adalimumab)
- Surgery (different procedures will be used for ulcerative colitis and Crohn's disease)

Treatment choices will be dependent on the disease activity, extent, and distribution. These treatments may be used on their own or in combination

Inflammatory bowel disease (IBD) comprises two lifelong chronic diseases characterized by episodes of remission and relapse: ulcerative colitis and Crohn's disease (Figure 99.1). It is important to recognize that IBD is not the same as irritable bowel syndrome (IBS) and is not infectious. The cause of IBD remains unknown, but it is thought to be the product of a complex interaction of multiple factors: a genetic predisposition and an abnormal reaction of the immune system to certain bacteria in the intestines, possibly triggered by something in the environment. Triggers such as viruses, bacteria, diet, and stress have been identified, but there is no evidence that any one of these factors is wholly responsible.

Inflammatory bowel disease and children

It is understood that the incidence of IBD has been steadily increasing over recent years. Up to 25% of IBD patients are diagnosed below the age of 18 years. Crohn's disease affects 5.7 cases per 100 000 population, with more females than males affected. IBD is commonly diagnosed during adolescence and puberty, a vulnerable time for growth as well as psychosocial development and education. It is therefore essential that a multidisciplinary team approach is taken when caring for children and families diagnosed with IBD.

Diagnostic tools

Prior to any invasive investigations, it is important that a comprehensive clinical history and examination are completed (Box 99.1). This will enable the clinician to make a differential diagnosis of IBD before proceeding. Although blood tests are not diagnostic, they can give some indication of whether an inflammatory process is occurring. It is essential that stool cultures exclude any infective source that may be contributing to the child's symptoms. All children suspected of having IBD should have an upper and lower gastrointestinal endoscopy with visualization of the terminal ileum, and multiple biopsies from all segments of the intestinal tract should be taken for histological diagnosis. Following this, it is important to establish the extent of the disease process (small bowel and pelvis if clinically indicated) for future care planning; this will be completed with the use of magnetic resonance imaging (MRI). By using a variety of clinical tools, the clinician is able to build a road map of disease extent and activity; this is essential when planning the child's treatment. Specialist care is required once the disease is suspected.

Considerations for children diagnosed with inflammatory bowel disease and their families

Although IBD can be treated with medical and surgical interventions (Box 99.2), there is no cure. Being diagnosed with a long-term chronic condition is hard for both the child and the family to come to terms with, so it is important that appropriate support is offered via a variety of services (specialist nurse, psychological help, and patient support groups). Surgical treatments are extensive and range from partial colectomy to siting of a stoma and refashioning of the anus to form an anal pouch. Support systems encourage the child and family to take ownership of the condition; this has a major impact on compliance and concordance with treatment plans.

Children and young people with Crohn's disease may also have extra-intestinal involvement such as:
- Skin – most common problem is erythema nodosum.
- Eyes – episcleritis.
- Arthritis is a common complication and osteoporosis is also found in people in later life.
- Hepatobiliary system – gallstones.

The aim of treatment for children with a long-term condition is to manage their illness in such a way that they can achieve lifetime goals and make a positive contribution through appropriate education. Maintaining and optimizing growth are also key aims in the treatment and ongoing management of the child or young person with IBD. Enteral feeding may be required initially on diagnosis at periods of acute exacerbation. Treatment with corticosteroids may be required to induce a remission when there is active luminal disease. Other medication may include aminosalicylates, immunosuppressant therapy, and biological drugs, such as anti-tumour necrosis factor-alpha (TNF-α) antibody treatment.

It is therefore vital that effective communication occurs between health and education services. Teachers need to be aware of the special needs that a child with IBD may have and a school care plan should be constructed to include points such as easy and discreet access to the toilet. Teachers need to be aware of the issues that could prime bullying, for example prolonged absences from school, delayed growth and puberty, and rapidly changing body image depending upon disease activity and treatments (steroid treatment can often cause excessive weight gain, spots, and mood swings).

During the childhood years it is commonly the parent's responsibility to ensure compliance and concordance with medication and treatment plans. Adolescence is a tricky time of life for everyone and increasingly so for those with long-term medical conditions. Transitional care programmes are essential for the effective transfer of information, aiming for lifelong support and thus compliance and, ultimately, patient safety. A well-planned transitional care programme can lead to improve compliance with medical therapies, effective planning of long-term life goals, independent living skills, and improved health-related quality of life, not just in the short term but lifelong.

Key points
- Inflammatory activity continues throughout life and the child or young person will have a series of remissions and exacerbation of the disease.
- Care should be planned and delivery coordinated by the multidisciplinary team to enable the child or young person to achieve their life goals.
- Family support is essential and the children's and young person's nurse plays an important role in this.

100 Gastro-oesophageal reflux

Figure 100.1 Gastro-oesophageal reflux.

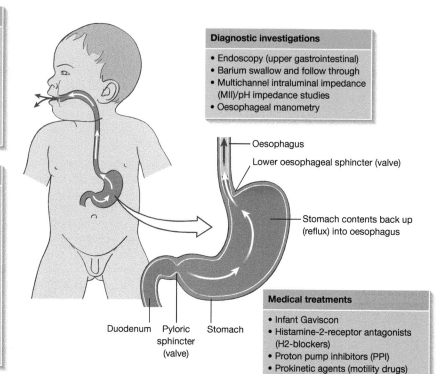

Common symtoms of reflux

- Vomiting (projectile, bile, or blood)
- Excessive crying
- Refusal to feed
- Abdominal distension
- Severe constipation
- Bloody or dark stools
- Weight loss, or poor weight gain
- Lethargy
- Choking or blue spells

Diagnostic investigations

- Endoscopy (upper gastrointestinal)
- Barium swallow and follow through
- Multichannel intraluminal impedance (MII)/pH impedance studies
- Oesophageal manometry

Oesophagus
Lower oesophageal sphincter (valve)
Stomach contents back up (reflux) into oesophagus

Duodenum Pyloric sphincter (valve) Stomach

Non-medical treatments for reflux

- Elimination of cow's milk and cow's milk protein
- Thickening milk
- Avoid over-feeding
- Wind the baby frequently before, during, and after feeding
- Keep the baby upright for at least 30 minutes after feeding
- Where possible try not to lay infant flat – and angle greater than 30° is recommended for sleep time and when changing the baby's nappy
- Avoid using a car seat immediately after feeding

Medical treatments

- Infant Gaviscon
- Histamine-2-receptor antagonists (H2-blockers)
- Proton pump inhibitors (PPI)
- Prokinetic agents (motility drugs)
- Vitamin and mineral

Risk factors for GOR

Prematurity
Parental history of heart burn or acid reflux
Obesity
Hiatus hernia
Known congenital diaphragmatic hernia
Neurodisability (cerebral palsy)

Prognosis in GOR

Length of oesphagus increases
Increase in tone of lower oesophageal sphincter
More upright position become established
Diet becomes more solid

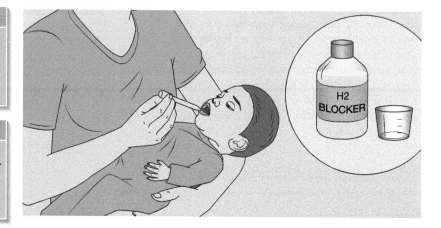

H2 BLOCKER

Children and Young People's Nursing at a Glance, Second Edition. Edited by Elizabeth Gormley-Fleming and Sheila Roberts.
© 2023 John Wiley & Sons Ltd. Published 2023 by John Wiley & Sons Ltd.

What is reflux?

Gastro-oesophageal reflux (GOR) is the passage of gastric contents into the oesophagus. This occurs normally in all infants, children, and adults during and immediately after meals. It is considered physiological when symptoms are absent or not troublesome, and in most cases resolves spontaneously.

Gastro-oesophageal reflux disease (GORD; Figure 100.1) is present when there are symptoms that are troublesome, severe, or chronic, or when there are complications arising from GOR. The most common complication is tissue damage or inflammation to the oesophagus (oesophagitis). In the UK, approximately 0.9% of children younger than 13 years will have GORD.

What causes reflux?

GOR occurs as a result of transient lower oesophageal sphincter relaxation. There are several anatomical and physiological features that make infants (younger than 1 year) more prone to GOR than older children and adults:

- A short, narrow oesophagus.
- Delayed gastric emptying.
- Shorter, lower oesophageal sphincter that is slightly above the diaphragm.
- A liquid diet and high calorie requirement, which can put a strain on gastric capacity.
- A larger ratio of gastric volume to oesophageal volume.

It is also important to consider that GOR and GORD may be caused by an allergy to cow's milk protein.

How is reflux diagnosed?

In the first instance, reflux is usually diagnosed by symptoms alone. Many infants regurgitate part or all of the stomach contents up to the mouth and in young babies, less than 1 year of age, this is considered normal. A feeding history is an important part of the initial assessment. Crying when feeding should be noted and the frequency and estimate volume of any regurgitation as well as vomit and the characteristics of the vomitus should be noted. Effortless spitting up of a few mouthfuls of feed is consistent with GOR. The main symptoms identified are frequent and troublesome vomiting or regurgitation (this may occur up to two hours after feeding), as well as frequent and troublesome crying, irritability, and persistent back-arching during or after feeding. The presence of Sandifer's syndrome (torticollis with neck extension and rotation) is also an important sign of GORD. This may also be accompanied by refusing feed.

Respiratory symptoms or signs such as hoarseness or a chronic cough should be included as part of the overall assessment.

In order to confirm and assess the severity of reflux, and to rule out any abnormalities that could be at the root of the reflux symptoms, specialists may consider conducting diagnostic investigations.

A multichannel intraluminal impedance (MII)/pH impedance test is one of the most commonly used investigations. The test is conducted by passing a tube with multichannel sensors through the child's nostril. The tube has a sensor that sits in the stomach and one that sits just above the lower oesophageal sphincter. The advantage of this test is that it is able to detect both acid and alkaline reflux travels, and investigates the correlation between symptom association, meal times, and patient position (e.g. nocturnal symptoms that may be exacerbated when lying down flat).

Treatments for GOR and GORD

Non-medical therapies for GOR have been proven to be effective in many cases. Reduced-volume feeding with more frequent feeds (while maintaining the total daily amount of milk) should be trialled prior to thickened feeds. Thickened feeds, the elimination of cow's milk and cow's milk protein (from the mother's diet in the case of breastfed infants), as well as other recommended methods should be trialled for two to three weeks. If successful, these should be continued for three months or until weaning. Positioning in an upright position post feeding is thought to help.

Medical treatments include Infant Gaviscon (alginate therapy), which helps thicken the milk; histamine-2-receptor antagonists (H2-blockers), such as ranitidine, which work by blocking or preventing the production of gastric acid; or proton pump inhibitors (PPI), such as omeprazole or lansoprazole, which work by stopping gastric acid production at its source. Prokinetic agents, such as domperidone, work by speeding up the emptying stomach and helping close the lower oesophageal sphincter. A stepped care approach is recommended.

Surgery may be required, a Nissen fundoplication, if pharmacological treatment is unsuccessful or if there are intolerable side effects to the medication. This is usually carried out via laparoscopy.

Do infants grow out of GOR?

Most infants showing signs of GOR will grow out of it between the ages of 12 and 15 months. As young children grow, most cases of reflux will settle when mixed feeding is introduced and when there is an increased effect of gravity on infants as they become more upright and ambulant.

Key points

- GOR is the physiological passage of gastric content into the oesophagus.
- GORD is classified when reflux symptoms become troublesome, causing complications such as oesophagitis.
- Most children will grow out of GOR between the ages of 12 and 15 months.

101 Coeliac disease

Figure 101.1 Normal villi and damaged villi in coeliac disease.

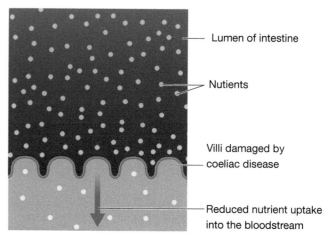

Lumen of intestine

Nutients

Healthy villi

Nutrient uptake into the bloodstream

Lumen of intestine

Nutients

Villi damaged by coeliac disease

Reduced nutrient uptake into the bloodstream

Figure 101.2 Medical treatments for coeliac disease.

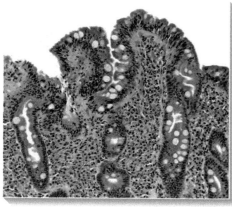

Endoscopy image of person with coeliac disease, showing scalloping of folds and 'cracked-mud' appearance to mucosa

Figure 101.3 The Crossed Grain symbol.

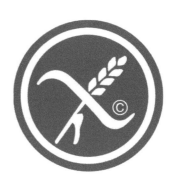

Created by Coeliac UK and promoted by coeliac organizations worldwide – the Crossed Grain is a food labelling symbol that confirms that a labelled food product is gluten free

Box 101.1 What causes coeliac disease?

Coeliac disease is an autoimmune condition that is caused by an abnormal immune reaction to the protein gluten, found in foods such as cereal, bread, pasta, and biscuits

Box 101.2 Common symptoms.

- Diarrhoea, excessive wind, and constipation
- Persistent or inexplained gastrointestinal symptoms (e.g. nausea and vomiting)
- Stomach pain, cramping, or bloating
- Iron, vitamin B12, or folic acid deficiency
- Weight loss
- Lethargy
- Mouth ulcers
- Poor growth

Children and Young People's Nursing at a Glance, Second Edition. Edited by Elizabeth Gormley-Fleming and Sheila Roberts.
© 2023 John Wiley & Sons Ltd. Published 2023 by John Wiley & Sons Ltd.

Coeliac disease is an immune-mediated systemic disorder in which the immune system in a person's gut reacts to a protein, gliadin, that makes up gluten. The antibodies produced against gliadin cause inflammation to the surface of the gut. The damage and inflammation to the gut lining flatten villi (Figure 101.1) that are present in the small bowel.

The villi work by increasing the surface area of the gut and help to digest food more effectively. However, in the case of coeliac disease, the flattened villi are unable to work this way, resulting in an inability to digest nutrients from foods, leading to symptoms such as diarrhoea and weight loss. This is a permanent inability to tolerate gluten. About 1 in 100 people is affected by coeliac disease.

What causes coeliac disease?

It is not fully understood why people develop coeliac disease or why some people's symptoms are more severe than others (Box 101.1). However, there are a number of contributing factors that are known to increase the risk of developing coeliac disease, such as family history, environmental factors, and other pre-existing health conditions.

Who should be tested for coeliac disease?

Children with coeliac disease present with a variety of non-specific signs and the range of symptoms is wide (Box 101.2). Most children present before the age of 2 years. Often these children are failing to thrive and have a history of irritability, poor appetite, mouth ulcers, vomiting, and diarrhoea. The faeces usually have a foul odour and are pale in colour. Abdominal distention and wasting of the buttocks may be noted in physical examination of the child. Symptoms may be very vague in some cases and diagnosis is not made until adulthood. Therefore, it is important to identify and diagnose those children who have a less clear clinical picture in order to reduce and prevent negative health consequences caused by the disease:

• Symptomatic children and adolescents with otherwise unexplained symptoms and signs that suggest coeliac disease such as chronic or intermittent diarrhoea.

• Asymptomatic children and adolescents who have an increased risk of coeliac disease due to pre-existing medical conditions such as type 1 diabetes mellitus, Down's syndrome, autoimmune thyroid disease, and those who have a first-degree relative with coeliac disease.

How is coeliac disease diagnosed?

Screening for coeliac disease involves a two-stage diagnostic process. Blood tests to identify coeliac disease–specific antibodies should be the first diagnostic tool used. The initial tests are immunoglobulin (Ig)A class anti-thyroglobulin (TGN), IgG anti-TGN, and IgG anti-deamidated gliadin peptide (DGP). However, in some cases it is possible to have coeliac disease despite negative blood results. Iron-deficiency anaemia may also be detected in the child with coeliac disease, so this is an important measurement in the diagnostic process. It is therefore important to confirm diagnosis with a histology biopsy. Biopsies are obtained during gastroscopy/endoscopy (Figure 101.2) and should be taken from the duodenal bulb and the second and third parts of the duodenum. NB: Coeliac disease will only be identified from intestinal biopsy if the person being tested is eating gluten regularly.

A detailed history should be taken and family history, risk factors, and associated conditions should be explored. The child should have their weight and height recorded and plotted on an age-appropriate centile chart. Body mass index (BMI) should be calculated for the young person. Nutritional assessment and screening are required. A full abdominal examination is required, as is a full examination of the skin.

How is coeliac disease treated?

Once coeliac disease has been diagnosed, the treatment is a strict gluten-free diet. Children and adolescents should be referred to a dietitian for support and advice in adjusting to the new gluten-free diet and ensuring that a balanced diet containing nutrients is maintained. By sticking to this strict diet, symptoms should improve considerably within weeks. Any relapse in a gluten-free diet will result in symptoms reappearing.

However, a gluten challenge should be given to the child two years after diagnosis, before they are assigned to a gluten-free life. A jejunal biopsy should also be repeated at this stage, as the villi will have had an opportunity to recover through dietary management.

Dermatitis herpetiformis (DH) is a skin manifestation of coeliac disease. This occurs as a rash and is present on the elbows, knees, shoulder, buttocks, and face. The rash is red with raised patches and often with blisters. This is relatively rare and affects 1 in every 3300 people. Referral to a dermatologist is required if DH is present.

Untreated or undiagnosed coeliac disease can cause long-term complications:
• Osteoporosis.
• Malnutrition and developmental delay.
• Lactose intolerance.
• Cancer.
• Ongoing treatment and health prevention are required in the form of annual blood testing for anaemia and nutritional deficiencies. Vaccination for influenza and meningococcal and pneumococcal immunization should be offered to those who are diagnosed with hyposplenism.

Key points
• Coeliac disease is a common digestive condition where a person has an adverse reaction to a protein in gluten.
• The antibodies produced against gluten cause damage and inflammation to the surface of the gut.
• Coeliac disease can be diagnosed with blood tests and histology biopsies.
• Treatment for coeliac disease is a strict gluten-free diet (Figure 101.3).

102 Appendicitis

Figure 102.1 Signs and symptoms of appendicitis.

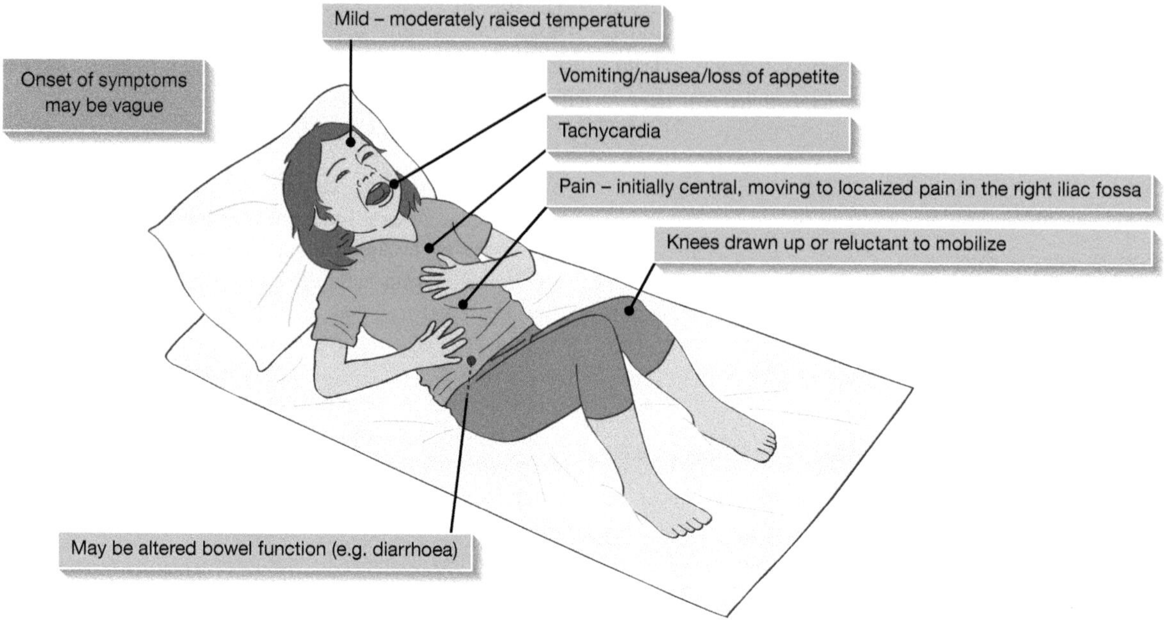

Mild – moderately raised temperature

Onset of symptoms may be vague

Vomiting/nausea/loss of appetite

Tachycardia

Pain – initially central, moving to localized pain in the right iliac fossa

Knees drawn up or reluctant to mobilize

May be altered bowel function (e.g. diarrhoea)

Box 102.1 History and assessment.

- Previous hospital admissions or issues with episodes of abdominal pain?
- How long has the child been unwell?
- Any history of vomiting or diarrhoea or recent gastroenteritis in the family?
- Has the child been pyrexic?
- Any strong smell of the urine?
- Where and when did the pain start?
- Has the child already had analgesia and if so what and when?
- When did the child last eat or drink?
- Any signs of dehydration (e.g. dry mucous membranes, skin, sunken eyes, lethargy)?
- If a female adolescent, has menstruation started and date of last menstrual period?

Box 102.2 Key observations and investigations.

- Temperature, pulse, respirations, blood pressure
- Urinalysis (and culture if positive result to exclude urinary tract infection)
- Pain assessment using an appropriate tool
- Blood tests: for urea and electrolytes, full blood count (usually elevated white cells), C-reactive protein (elevated), group and hold (in the event of needing a transfusion)
- Ultrasound scan of abdomen
- Pregnancy test if female and menstruation has commenced
- Weight

Children and Young People's Nursing at a Glance, Second Edition. Edited by Elizabeth Gormley-Fleming and Sheila Roberts.
© 2023 John Wiley & Sons Ltd. Published 2023 by John Wiley & Sons Ltd.

The appendix is a narrow tube that is attached to the end of the caecum. Appendicitis, or inflammation of the appendix, is a common childhood condition, often caused by an obstruction associated with a kink in the bowel, a faecolith, or a foreign body. Subsequent inflammation causes an accumulation of purulent exudate within the lumen of the bowel. As the appendix swells, the blood supply may become compromised and cause the appendix to become gangrenous. See Figure 102.1 for signs and symptoms of appendicitis. Perforation may occur, resulting in peritonitis and the potential for septicaemia. Sudden relief of pain is usually an indication that perforation has occurred. See Box 102.1 for nursing history and assessment, and Box 102.2 for key observations and investigations required.

Principles of care

Care should be child and family centred. Involving the child and family in decisions and negotiating care in accordance with their wishes will help to build trusting relationships and a sense of control over what is a stressful (and for some a new) situation. Good communication, and a calm, caring, and unhurried approach, will help to alleviate anxiety. Accurate history taking (see Box 'History and assessment') and documentation by all involved and good multidisciplinary working are key to the provision of safe and effective care.

Treatment of appendicitis can vary following the results of medical investigations. Children may be treated conservatively with antibiotics and reviewed at a later date (approximately six weeks' time). If conservative management is not indicated, then surgical intervention is required in the form of appendicectomy (either as open or laparoscopic surgery).

Preoperative care

The aim of preoperative care is to prepare the child and family for appendicectomy safely and effectively. Information should be given to the child in a developmentally appropriate and caring manner and the play specialist has an important role to play in preparing the child for what will happen. Written/informed consent must be obtained by medical staff from the parent (or person with parental responsibility or young person if they have reached the age of consent). Assessment (see Box 'Key observations and investigations') should be ongoing and baseline observations recorded for comparison postoperatively along with a pain score using an appropriate assessment tool (e.g. Wong Baker). Any concerns should be documented and raised with the surgical team. Pain relief should be administered according to local policy and the effect evaluated and recorded.

Prior to the patient attending the theatre department, a preoperative checklist or care pathway should be completed (see Chapter 73). The child should be adequately fasted according to local guidelines. On occasions, intravenous therapy may be requested by the multidisciplinary team. Prior to transfer to theatre, the child should be encouraged to pass urine in order to reduce the risk of bladder perforation.

Postoperative care

Following a comprehensive handover from theatre staff, the nurse should accompany the child and parent(s) back to the ward and set out clearly what will happen. The aim of postoperative care is to provide support, minimize pain, and monitor the child's condition, while being vigilant about potential postoperative complications. Oxygen and suction should be available if needed and the child should be advised not to get out of bed unaccompanied in the early stages of recovery. Bed sides should be used if appropriate and a call bell should be left within easy reach if the parent is not present.

Postoperative observations, such as temperature, pulse, respirations, blood pressure, pulse oximetry, and pain score, should be recorded in line with local policy and any anomalies or concerns escalated to the nurse in charge and subsequently to the medical staff. A rapid, thready pulse, accompanied by falling blood pressure and a restless child, may indicate the presence of shock or haemorrhage. A Paediatric Early Warning System (PEWS) should be in place to detect signs of the deteriorating child. Accurate, ongoing pain and strict fluid assessment and management are key during the postoperative period. The wound (or wounds if laparoscopic) should be observed for signs of infection (redness, swelling, exudate, local tenderness) or dehiscence. Intravenous antibiotics may also be required. The commencement of oral fluids should be based upon direction from the surgical and/or anaesthetic team and is normally detailed in the operation/anaesthetic notes. Once tolerated, a light diet may then be offered. Intravenous therapy is discontinued as directed by medical staff. Discharge advice should include information about the recovery period and a wound check by the community team.

Key points

- Good communication with the child and family and other professionals is key to the provision of safe and effective care.
- Preoperative checks and the use of PEWS are essential to minimize risk in the perioperative and postoperative periods.
- Pain and fluid balance assessment and management should be an ongoing process.

Acknowledgement. The author would like to thank Lynne Leitch, Deputy Sister of Barbour Ward, Royal Belfast Hospital for Sick Children, for her comments on this chapter.

103 Constipation

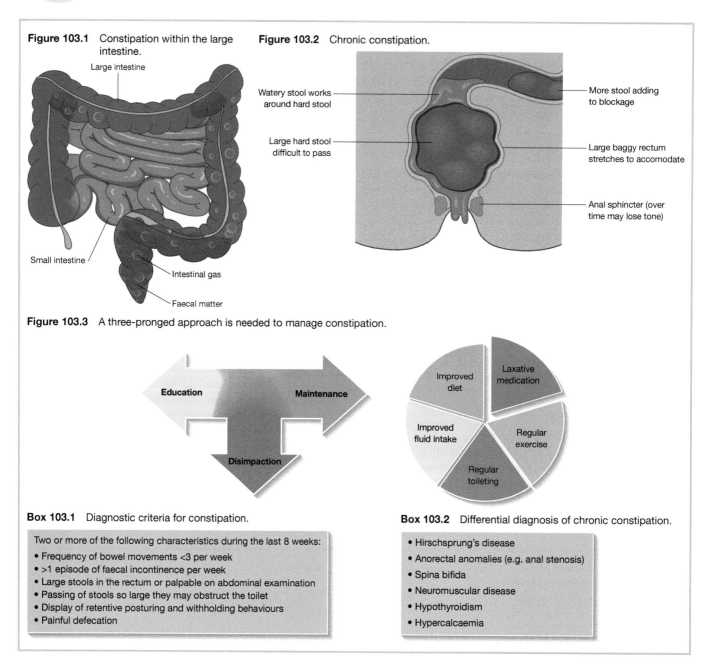

Figure 103.1 Constipation within the large intestine.

- Large intestine
- Small intestine
- Intestinal gas
- Faecal matter

Figure 103.2 Chronic constipation.

- Watery stool works around hard stool
- Large hard stool difficult to pass
- More stool adding to blockage
- Large baggy rectum stretches to accomodate
- Anal sphincter (over time may lose tone)

Figure 103.3 A three-pronged approach is needed to manage constipation.

- Education
- Maintenance
- Disimpaction

- Improved diet
- Laxative medication
- Improved fluid intake
- Regular exercise
- Regular toileting

Box 103.1 Diagnostic criteria for constipation.

Two or more of the following characteristics during the last 8 weeks:

- Frequency of bowel movements <3 per week
- >1 episode of faecal incontinence per week
- Large stools in the rectum or palpable on abdominal examination
- Passing of stools so large they may obstruct the toilet
- Display of retentive posturing and withholding behaviours
- Painful defecation

Box 103.2 Differential diagnosis of chronic constipation.

- Hirschsprung's disease
- Anorectal anomalies (e.g. anal stenosis)
- Spina bifida
- Neuromuscular disease
- Hypothyroidism
- Hypercalcaemia

Constipation is a decrease in the number of bowel movements. It is characterized by the passing of stools that may be hard, and this may be painful for the child. It is a common complaint that presents many therapeutic challenges. It can be associated with faecal soiling, which is the involuntary passing of fluid with some semi-solid material as a result of an overloaded bowel. This is called 'overflow'. Stool retention is also a feature, and this is termed 'faecal impaction'.

Approximately 30% of children aged 4–11 years will have episodes of constipation of less than six months' duration; 5% will continue to have constipation lasting six months or more. The peak time for childhood constipation developing is between the ages of 2 and 3 years, as this is the age at which children are toilet trained. However, not all parents seek help for constipation, so it may be an under-reported condition.

In most cases constipation is functional/idiopathic (has a non-organic aetiology) and can be diagnosed with a careful history and thorough examination. Chronic constipation is when the condition lasts longer than eight weeks.

Children and Young People's Nursing at a Glance, Second Edition. Edited by Elizabeth Gormley-Fleming and Sheila Roberts.
© 2023 John Wiley & Sons Ltd. Published 2023 by John Wiley & Sons Ltd.

Causes

There are a number of contributing factors that may cause the child to become constipated. These include:
- Inadequate fluid intake.
- Pain.
- Reduced dietary fibre.
- Mediation, e.g. antihistamines, iron supplements, opioids.
- Toilet training issues.
- Psychological issues.
- Family history of constipation.
- Physical inactivity.
- Children with impaired mobility or neurodevelopmental disorders are more prone to becoming constipated.

A Paris Consensus on Childhood Constipation Terminology (PACCT) working group published a simplified terminology to standardize and define the diagnostic criteria (Box 103.1).

Pathophysiology

It is important for children's nurse to understand the pathophysiology of constipation (Figure 103.1) so that they can provide explanations to the child and family. Faeces are the end product of digestion. As the chyme passes through the large bowel, water is absorbed. The lumen of the colon is larger than the ileum and it requires the bolus of faeces to be of a reasonable size and consistency if it is to be passed through the colon by peristalsis. If the stools are too watery, they will pass through too quickly, with inadequate time for water to be absorbed, resulting in diarrhoea. When the stools are too hard, they take longer to pass through. This causes more water to be absorbed, resulting in compaction of the faecal material. The end result is a large, hard stool that is difficult to pass. This is constipation (Figure 103.2).

Diagnosing functional constipation

To diagnose constipation (Box 103.1) a detailed history should be taken.

As part of the diagnostic process, it is important to exclude serious or underlying organic causes, for example Hirschsprung's disease, anal stenosis, hypothyroidism, faltering growth, or cow's milk intolerance (Box 103.2).

Management of the child with functional constipation and faecal impaction

The management of functional constipation in children is not just about laxative medication. A three-pronged approach of education, disimpaction, and maintenance is needed (Figure 103.3). All three approaches must be considered and compliance required if constipation is to be resolved.

Drugs used in constipation

Maintenance laxative treatment should be commenced promptly if the child is not faecally impacted. The aim of laxative treatment is for the child to produce soft stools regularly. Laxatives are generally classified according to their mode of action. The British National Formulary for Children (BNFC) divides them into five groups:
- *Bulk-forming laxatives* generally increase faecal mass and thereby stimulate peristalsis.
- *Stimulant laxatives* increase intestinal motility.
- *Faecal softeners* lubricate or soften the stool to try to avoid painful defecation.
- *Osmotic laxatives (macrogols)* increase the volume of water in the large bowel. They act as a softener and have a wash-out effect.
- *Bowel cleansing solutions* are used to prepare the bowel for radiological investigations, surgery, or colonoscopy.

Macrogols are the first line of treatment for children who are constipated. The dose will be dependent on whether the child requires disimpaction or not. If macrogols are not effective, then a stimulant laxative should be added. It may take several weeks to achieve the required effect, hence why concordance is important.

Disimpaction

Clearing a blockage or backlog of hard faeces is a vital component of the management strategy. It must be done prior to establishing a maintenance therapy and the medication used may form part of that maintenance plan in a lower dose.

The oral route is the preferred route of administration, as it is better tolerated and less traumatic for the child and parents. Disimpaction can also be achieved using the rectal route, with enemas and suppositories or manual evacuation in theatre. Although these routes may achieve disimpaction sooner, they are poorly tolerated and may exacerbate stool-withholding behavior and prove too invasive and distressing for the child.

Patient education

Successful management of children with constipation requires parental understanding of the underlying factors and the treatment goals. Parents' understanding of bowel physiology and the mechanism of constipation is a vital component in the management strategy. It will help to demystify the condition and aims to promote cooperation and involvement in resolving the problem. If faecal soiling is a symptom, education will help alleviate blame (i.e. the parents may think their child is 'lazy' or 'dirty' when the child may have no control over the soiling). Reassurance may be needed to help the parents maintain a positive and supportive attitude. It is also about giving ownership of the problem to the child (4 years and older) and encouraging them to take responsibility. The use of picture books, PowerPoint presentations, and appropriate language helps in getting the message across.

Maintenance therapy

Once the child no longer has faecal impaction, the treatment will focus on the prevention of recurrence. Laxative medication may be needed for a prolonged period to facilitate bowel emptying and a return of sensitivity to the muscles and nerves of the rectum.

Medication is only one component of the maintenance therapy and here again education is key. Strategies to improve diet, fluid intake, exercise, and regular toileting are vital ingredients to promote better bowel emptying. It is these life skills that will facilitate a weaning-down of the medication after a sustained period of normal stooling with no soiling.

Key points
- Functional constipation is a common childhood condition.
- Organic causes should always be ruled out as part of the diagnostic process.
- Parental education is essential in achieving the treatment aim.
- A multipronged approach is required to successfully manage and alleviate the condition.

104 Renal problems

Figure 104.1 Renal system.

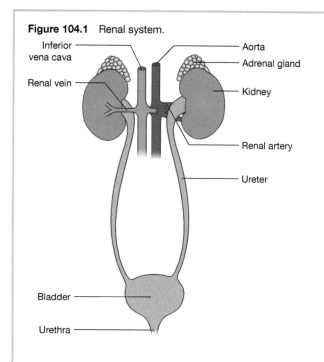

- Inferior vena cava
- Renal vein
- Aorta
- Adrenal gland
- Kidney
- Renal artery
- Ureter
- Bladder
- Urethra

Figure 104.2 Urinalysis.

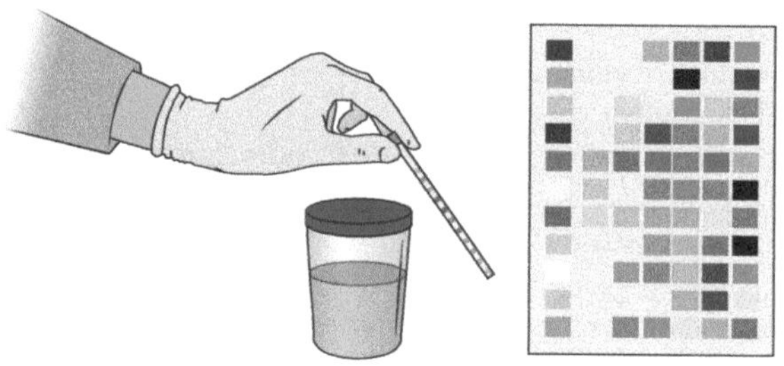

Figure 104.3 Fluid balance chart.

Figure 104.4 Dialysis: haemodialysis and peritoneal dialysis.

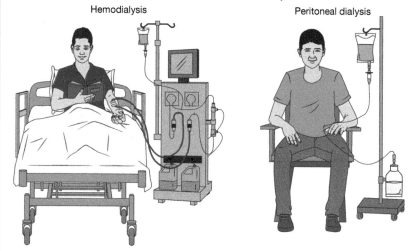

Hemodialysis

Peritoneal dialysis

Box 104.1 Kidney function in children.

- Filters blood to remove waste products
- Maintains fluid and electrolyte levels by selective removal (or reabsorption) and elimination
- Helps to maintain blood pressure (renin)
- Helps to stimulate red blood cell production (erythropoietin)
- Regulates calcium metabolism

Box 104.2 Tests used in renal disorders.

- Prenatal testing (e.g. structural scan with diagnostic ultrasound)
- Diagnostic imaging, X-ray ± contrast media
- Urinalysis – NB blood, protein
- Blood chemistry – electrolytes, blood protein levels, hormones, amino acids

The renal system (Figure 104.1) is very important in determining the overall health status of the individual and it is essential in the maintenance of all the body's systems. The renal system is one of the major excretory systems of the human body and it assists in the maintenance of homeostasis (Box 104.1). Significant changes occur from birth to adulthood in the renal system. The renal system, or urinary system as it is also referred to, consists of:

- Two kidneys that act as filters and produce urine.
- Two ureters that carry the urine to the bladder.
- A urinary bladder that acts a reservoir for urine.
- A urethra that conveys urine out of the body.

Kidney structure

- The kidneys are a pair of organs situated either side of the spine at the back of the abdominal cavity at the level of the T12 to L3 vertebrae.
- They are partially protected by 11th and 12th ribs and the perinephric fat.
- They have a rich blood supply directly from the aorta via the renal arteries, and are very vulnerable to hypoperfusion for any reason.
- The superficial renal cortex and innermost renal medulla form 14–16 renal nodes.
- These contain the filtering and resorbtion functions at the level of the nephron.

Children and Young People's Nursing at a Glance, Second Edition. Edited by Elizabeth Gormley-Fleming and Sheila Roberts.
© 2023 John Wiley & Sons Ltd. Published 2023 by John Wiley & Sons Ltd.

- Urine formed during this process is drained into the renal pelvis and via the ureter into the bladder for excretion.

Structural renal disorders

- Prenatal malformation or non-formation can lead to abnormalities such as horseshoe kidney.
- Strictures in the renal arteries may lead to hypertension.
- Strictures in the renal drainage system can lead to damming back of urine and subsequent pressure damage.
- Ineffective vesicoureteric valves can lead to reflux of urine from the bladder back up the ureters, leaving the child vulnerable to disturbed function and infection.

Acquired renal disorders in childhood

Post-streptococcal glomerulonephritis

This is an immune response to a streptococcal infection (e.g. throat or skin infection) leading to renal damage with reduced function. It generally resolves spontaneously, but sometimes monitoring and supportive therapy are necessary.

Nephrotic syndrome

- Produced by a number of disease processes.
- Leads to damage of the filtering apparatus, resulting in increased permeability allowing protein to be filtered and lost.
- Proteinuria and low blood protein.
- Causes fluid shifts in the body, leading to the characteristic oedema.
- Generally amenable to treatment with corticosteroids.

  Nursing to include the following:
- Make sure that child and family understand what is happening, what to expect, and how they can be involved.
- Monitor constituents of the urine – urinalysis (Figure 104.2).
- Monitor weight.
- Monitor fluid intake and output (Figure 104.3).
- Integrity of skin and oedematous tissue.

Haemolytic uraemic syndrome

- Rare but important cause of severe kidney damage in childhood.
- Often associated with infection with *Escherichia coli*.
- Severely unwell child will need high-dependency/critical care.
- Can lead to acute renal injury and subsequent end-stage renal damage.

Urinary tract infection

- Children are particularly vulnerable; the younger they are, the more vulnerable.
- Symptoms include fever, pain, and vomiting.
- May be recurrent, requiring cause to be investigated; diagnostic imaging may be needed.
- All children with a fever of unknown origin higher than 38 °C should have a urine sample tested,
- Clean catch or urine collection pad should be used,
- Treatment is by appropriate antibiotic therapy. May be long term and may require further investigation once infection subsides.

Acute renal injury (failure)

- Wide range of causative factors (e.g. reduced blood supply [hypovolaemia, hypotension], toxins, physical injury, obstruction).
- As the kidney's vital functions are disturbed or lost the child becomes globally unwell:
  - Lassitude.
  - Loss of appetite and vomiting.
  - Headache
  - Disruptions in vital functions – vital signs.
- Treatment is based on the underlying cause. May be reversible but may lead to chronic disturbed function.

End-stage renal damage (chronic renal failure)

- Devastating end-point of any of the processes that lead to kidney damage beyond repair.
- Severe reduction of glomerular filtration rate for more than three months.
- Treatment based on which systems are primarily affected.
- Long-term supportive nursing is geared to maximal child and family independence in management and minimizing disruption to child and family life and experience.

Renal replacement therapy

Dialysis

See Figure 104.4.

Haemodialysis

- Blood is filtered mechanically to remove waste products and excess water.
- Requires venous access.
- Requires around three sessions per week, each lasting around four hours.

Peritoneal dialysis

- Fluid is instilled into the peritoneal cavity to use the peritoneum as a filtering membrane.
- Adjustment of the composition of the dialysate produces removal of waste products and excess water through osmosis.
- Needs to be performed around four times a day with a dwell time of around 30 minutes. Alternatively, may be carried out overnight.

  Both forms of dialysis are vulnerable to complications such as infection. This therapy can be severely disruptive to the child's and family's lifestyle. Both forms still require some restrictions to fluid intake and nutrition.

Kidney transplantation

Kidney function can be restored with a successful renal transplant. Rejection remains a risk as the body's defensive immune reaction to 'foreign' tissue. This requires long-term suppressant medication.

Tumours

- Some tumours, such as Wilm's, the most common (nephroblastoma), characteristically occur in childhood, some are inherited presentations, but usually of unknown causes.
- Affect around 70 children per year in the UK.
- Most often detected as a painless swollen abdomen.
- Usually unilateral.
- Depending on the stage at detection, the chance of recovery is good: around 90% at five years.
- Treatment involves surgery and possibly radiotherapy and/or chemotherapy.

Renal injury

- Children are particularly vulnerable to renal injury due to:
  - High level of physical activity.
  - Immaturity in judgement.
  - Risk taking and impulsivity.
- May lead to blunt trauma with damage, rupture, and haemorrhage (NB: Kidneys are highly vascular).
- Early identification and surgical intervention are vital.
- May lead to loss of kidney.

Key points

- Urinalysis is a simple but very useful test in diagnosing many renal conditions. However, it is only one of several potential tests (Box 104.2).
- Children's nurses need to have a good knowledge and understanding of the anatomy and physiology of the renal system in order to plan effective care for a child with renal disease.
- Fluid balance is an important aspect of the management of children with renal disease.

105 Haematological problems

Figure 105.1 Bruise formation.

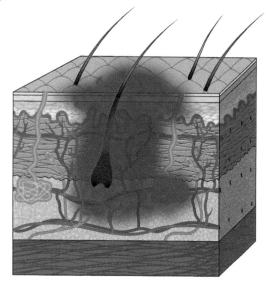

Figure 105.2 Stage in bruise healing and colour scheme.

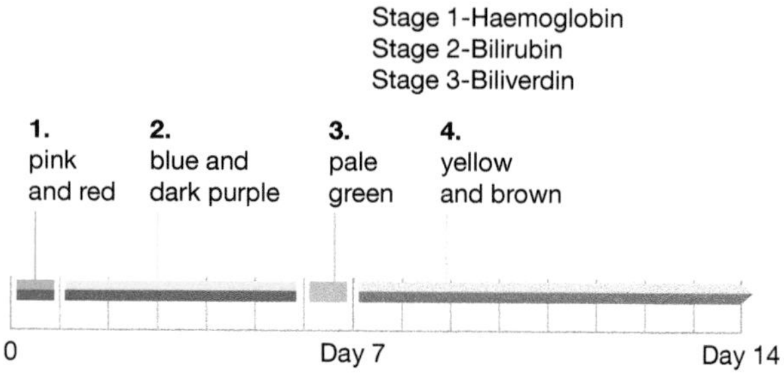

Stage 1-Haemoglobin
Stage 2-Bilirubin
Stage 3-Biliverdin

1.
pink
and red

2.
blue and
dark purple

3.
pale
green

4.
yellow
and brown

0   Day 7   Day 14

Figure 105.4 Complication of β-thalassaemia.

Complication

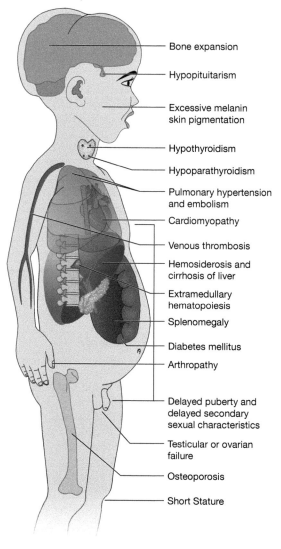

- Bone expansion
- Hypopituitarism
- Excessive melanin skin pigmentation
- Hypothyroidism
- Hypoparathyroidism
- Pulmonary hypertension and embolism
- Cardiomyopathy
- Venous thrombosis
- Hemosiderosis and cirrhosis of liver
- Extramedullary hematopoiesis
- Splenomegaly
- Diabetes mellitus
- Arthropathy
- Delayed puberty and delayed secondary sexual characteristics
- Testicular or ovarian failure
- Osteoporosis
- Short Stature

Figure 105.3 Fanconi's anaemia.

Clinical features

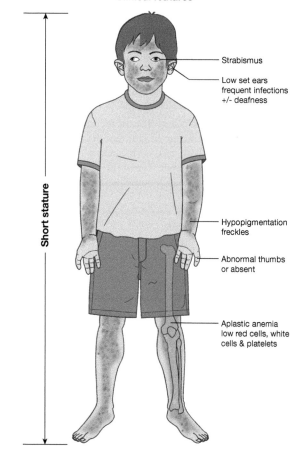

Short stature

- Strabismus
- Low set ears frequent infections +/- deafness
- Hypopigmentation freckles
- Abnormal thumbs or absent
- Aplastic anemia low red cells, white cells & platelets

Children and Young People's Nursing at a Glance, Second Edition. Edited by Elizabeth Gormley-Fleming and Sheila Roberts.
© 2023 John Wiley & Sons Ltd. Published 2023 by John Wiley & Sons Ltd.

Figure 105.5 Sickle cells and normal red blood cells.

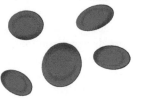

Normal
red blood cell

Sickled
red blood cell

Figure 105.6 Vaso-occlusion in sickle cell crisis.

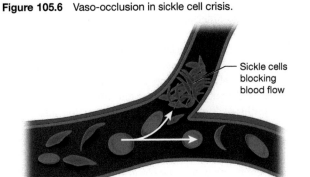

Sickle cells
blocking
blood flow

The most common manifestation of haematological disorder in children is a history of easy bruising and/or bleeding. Bruising is easy to see in Caucasian children, but much harder to see in children of Asian or Afro-Caribbean descent – in these children lumps may be palpable just under the skin.

Bleeding in neonates and young children is abnormal and should always be investigated. A full blood count and clotting screen will identify abnormalities of platelet count and coagulation. Further specialist investigations should then be undertaken following discussion with a paediatric haematologist.

Some rare haematological disorders present with structural abnormalities, such as missing bones/digits and facial abnormalities that are characteristic of the underlying disorder. These may be present without bruising or bleeding. Abnormalities of haemoglobin (sickle cell anaemia and thalassaemia) are now tested for in routine neonatal screening programmes and are thus often diagnosed before symptoms occur.

Treatment of children with diagnosed haematological disorders usually relies on replacement of missing blood components with blood or blood products such as factor VIII (now manufactured using recombinant technology for children in the UK) for haemophilia or red cell transfusions for those with sickle cell anaemia or thalassemia. Some of the haematological conditions described can be cured by bone marrow transplantation; others are long-term conditions where management offers good quality of life.

Easy bruising

This is caused by bleeding into the skin. Bruising is a normal reaction to injury (Figure 105.1). Although painful, bruises are not normally dangerous unless they affect vital organs or are a sign of an underlying bleeding disorder. The majority of bruises will heal within 10–14 days and generally follow a standard patterns of coloration (Figure 105.2). Potential causes include 'normal' childhood trauma, idiopathic thrombocytopenic purpura (ITP), leukaemia, bleeding disorders, and bone marrow failure.

Petechial rash

Petechial rash is small purple or red 'dots' caused by capillary haemorrhage under the skin. Unlike meningitis in bleeding disorders, the rash does not fade with pressure. Potential causes include ITP, leukaemia, rare platelet disorders, and meningitis.

Thrombocytopenia with absent radii

Thrombocytopenia with absent radii (TAR) is a rare congenital disorder characterized by thrombocytopenia in infancy, which improves with age, and shortening or absence of the radial bones.

Babies are born with shortened or absent forearms. This syndrome can also be associated with lower-limb abnormalities.

Fanconi's anaemia

This is an autosomal recessively inherited anaemia associated with growth retardation, and kidney and skeletal abnormalities, which can include TAR, or absent thumbs and bone marrow failure (Figure 105.3). Children experience pancytopenia – reduced levels of red and white blood cells as well as platelets – usually presenting with easy bruising, recurrent infections, and anaemia.

Hermansky–Pudlack syndrome

This is occulo-cutaneous albinism with platelet disorder, an autosomal recessive disorder (both parents carry the gene and are unaffected). Children are fair eyed and skinned and have easy bruising from an early age; they often bleed significantly with surgery.

Haemophilia

Haemophilia affects 1 in 5000–10 000 male infants worldwide. It results in joint bleeding that, without prompt or prophylactic therapy, causes early arthritic damage and reduces mobility, resulting in disability.

Haemophilia A (factor VIII deficiency) affects 80% of those with haemophilia. Haemophilia B (factor IX deficiency) is much rarer. One-third of newly diagnosed children have no previous family history. Treatment involves the use of recombinant factor concentrates. These are genetically engineered so do not contain any plasma or albumin. The advantage of these is that there is no spread of blood-borne viruses. Other treatments involve the use of medication that replaces the function of factor VIII rather than replacing the missing clotting factor directly, such as ACE910 or emicizumab.

Dactylitis

Dactylitis, painful swollen fingers seen in children with sickle cell anaemia, stems from a genetic disorder of the haemoglobin gene that is found in as many as 1 in 4 West Africans. Sickle cell anaemia (or disease) presents in those who inherit an abnormal gene from each parent. It causes painful crises when blood sickles, resulting in occlusion of blood vessels usually related to infection, dehydration, and extremely cold weather. Dactylitis is caused by painful infarction in the small bones, which in turn leads to fingers of differing lengths.

Facial appearance in β-thalassaemia major

This is a genetic disorder of the haemoglobin gene that is found most commonly in people who originate from Mediterranean regions (β-thalassemia) or the far East (α-thalassemia). Carriers of these abnormal genes are not usually affected by anaemia. Inheritance of only abnormal genes in α-thalassemia is incompatible with life. In β-thalassemia, severe anaemia occurs within the first few months of life, when red cell destruction also causes hepatosplenomegaly. Bone marrow overgrowth causes bones to expand and causes the typical features of bossing of the skull and face (Figure 105.4). Children with β-thalassaemia major will require frequent hospital visits for blood transfusion. The majority of children will require a splenectomy during early adolescence or adulthood.

Sickle cell disease

Sickle cell disease (SCD) is the name given to a group of inherited red blood cell disorders. In certain conditions the red blood cells become hard and C-shaped like a sickle (Figure 105.5). Sickle cells have a shorter life span than normal red cells and this leads to a depletion in red blood cells. Due to the changing nature of the shape of the red blood cells, they occlude small blood vessels as they travel through the body (Figure 105.6). This results in pain, infection, and has the potential for acute chest syndrome and strokes. Diagnosis most often occurs during a routine neonatal blood spot screening test. Signs of the disease will start in the first year of life and treatment will depend on the symptoms. Currently the only cure for SCD is bone marrow or stem cell transplant. *Ex vivo* and *in vivo* gene therapy are now revolutionizing treatment and long-term outcomes

Key points

- Children's and young people's nurses should have a knowledge base and understanding of the anatomy and physiology of the blood in order to plan and deliver effective treatments for the child and family.
- Haematological conditions are generally lifelong, so care should be holistic.
- Genetic counselling should be offered to all families and children with a hereditary blood disorder.

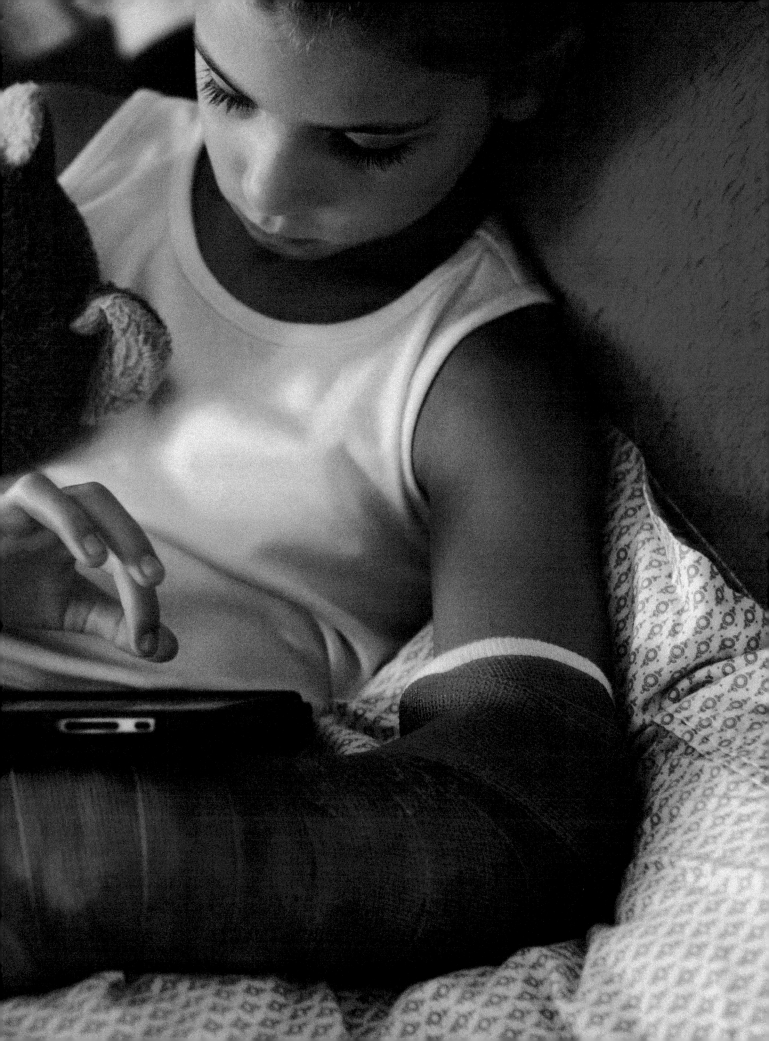

106 Musculoskeletal problems

Figure 106.1 Hip spicas.

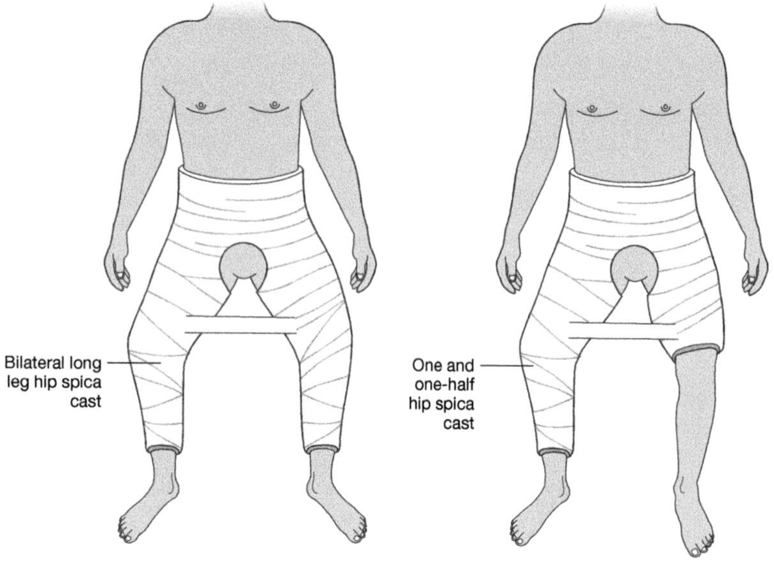

Bilateral long leg hip spica cast

One and one-half hip spica cast

Figure 106.2 Pavlik harness.

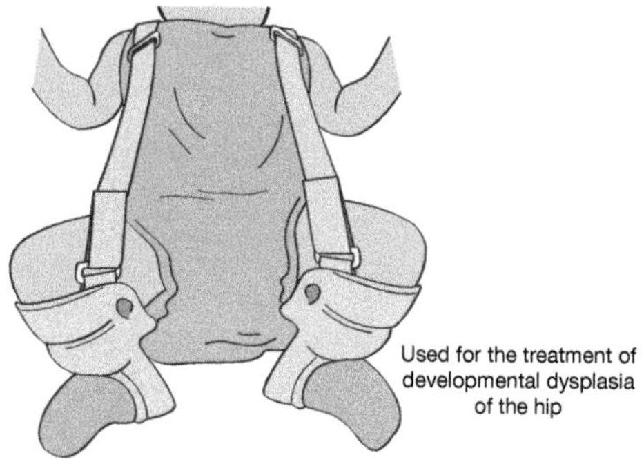

Used for the treatment of developmental dysplasia of the hip

Figure 106.3 Congenital talipes equinovarus, also known as club feet.

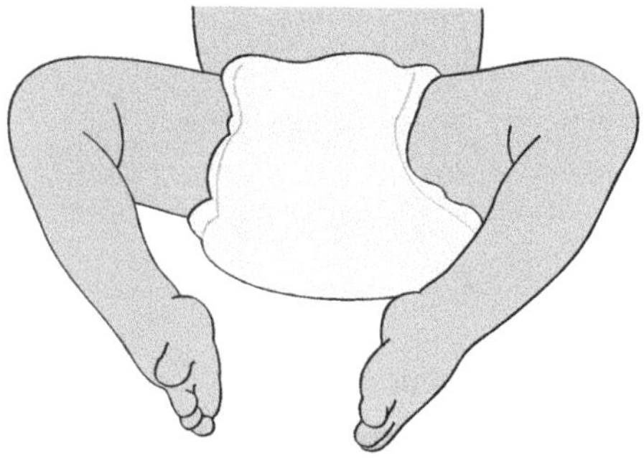

Figure 106.4 Ponseti casting. Note the separate leg plaster used for each leg.

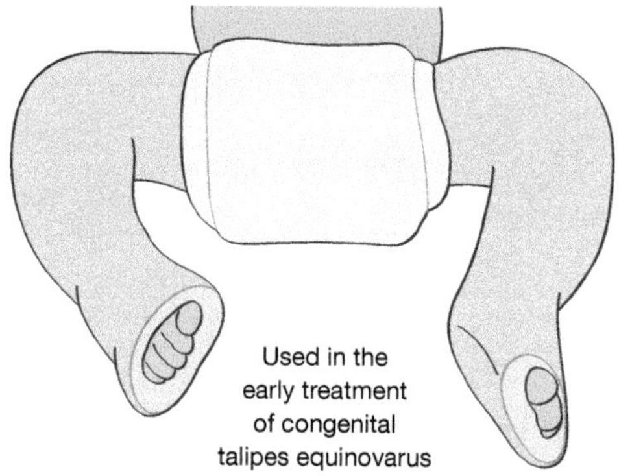

Used in the early treatment of congenital talipes equinovarus

Figure 106.5 Denis Browne boots.

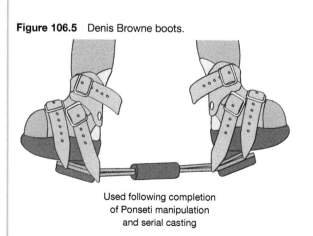

Used following completion of Ponseti manipulation and serial casting

Figure 106.6 Perthes' disease.

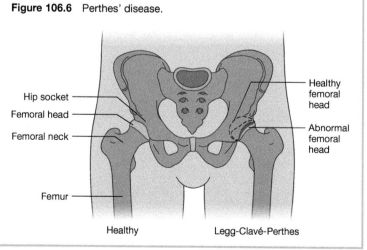

Hip socket

Femoral head

Femoral neck

Femur

Healthy

Healthy femoral head

Abnormal femoral head

Legg-Clavé-Perthes

Children and Young People's Nursing at a Glance, Second Edition. Edited by Elizabeth Gormley-Fleming and Sheila Roberts.
© 2023 John Wiley & Sons Ltd. Published 2023 by John Wiley & Sons Ltd.

Developmental dysplasia of the hip

Developmental dysplasia of the hip (DDH) is a spectrum of disorders related to abnormal development of the hip at any time during foetal life, infancy, or childhood. It ranges from mild acetabular abnormality and joint laxity to irreducible dislocation of the femoral head. The cause is thought to be multifactorial, including heredity with generalized joint laxity and a positive family history; hormonal with increased maternal hormones prior to delivery leading to joint laxity; intrauterine breech position; oligohydramnios (reduced amniotic fluid) during pregnancy; and postnatal positioning – babies who are carried with legs swaddled together are more likely to develop DDH. The condition is more common in firstborn babies and females.

Diagnosis is by postnatal screening, which includes Barlow's test of instability and Ortolani's sign of reduction. The babies should be examined when warm and comfortable, preferably after a feed. Other signs are extra skin creases, shortening of the limb (Galeazzi's sign), limitation of abduction or differences between sides, and limp or waddling gait in an older child.

If suspected, the diagnosis can be confirmed by hip ultrasound or an arthrogram. The aim of treatment is to keep the head of the femur in the acetabulum to enable development of the joint. This can be done by the use of an orthosis (Pavlik harness), a hip spica plaster cast (Figure 106.1), closed or open reduction, or femoral or pelvic osteotomy. The Pavlik harness (Figure 106.2) is a hip flexion-abduction splint that enables the baby to kick while keeping the hips in the correct position. It needs to stay on 24 hours a day initially, but as treatment progresses it can be removed for bathing. Regular checks at a clinic are required for 3–4 months. Parental support is essential as treatment is long term, thus impacting on many facets of normal life.

Congenital talipes equinovarus

This is a congenital deformity in which the foot points downwards and inwards (Figure 106.3); it is often bilateral. It is also known as club foot. The condition affects boys more than girls.

The cause is unknown, but intrauterine moulding, nerve and muscle imbalance, and delayed development have been suggested. It can be associated with other conditions. The condition can be detected on antenatal scans.

Treatment should begin as soon as possible with the aim of correcting the deformity and maintaining the correction. The method used for this is the Ponseti technique of manipulation and serial plaster casting (Figure 106.4). This is done weekly, with correction usually achieved after 5–8 manipulations. The infant may need surgical intervention in the form of Achilles tenotomy. The final cast is worn for three weeks, followed by the application of boots attached to a bar such as Denis Browne boots (Figure 106.5). These have to be worn most of the day for three months and during the night for several years. Relapse is more common when this has not been followed. It is essential for the healthcare team to provide information and support to the parents during this emotional time.

Scoliosis

Scoliosis is a deformity of the spine with marked lateral curvature. It can be classified according to the age of onset: infantile, 0–3 years; juvenile, 3–10 years; adolescent, over 10 years. There is often a family history and girls are affected more than boys.

The risk of progression of the curvature is increased during the rapid growth rate of puberty. The physical signs are one shoulder higher, a protruding scapula, one side of the rib cage higher, one hip higher, and an uneven waist.

An X-ray is undertaken to confirm the degree of spinal deformity. Treatment consists of:
- Observation and regular checks.
- Bracing and/or plaster casts – these prevent progression but do not correct existing deformity.
- Surgery – for curves >40°, fusion of the spine to prevent progression and instrumentation to correct deformity are performed.

Slipped upper femoral epiphysis

This is displacement of the proximal femoral epiphysis on the femoral neck. It is most common in adolescents, with boys affected more than girls. Affected teenagers are usually obese, but they can be tall and thin with delayed maturity. It is thought there may be a possible endocrine dysfunction. The child presents with pain and a limp. There is a possibility that the other hip will also be affected.

Treatment is by insertion of pins or screws to hold the slipped part of the femur in place. Bed rest with traction may be required prior to surgery.

Perthes' disease

This is avascular necrosis of the femoral head where there is disruption of the blood supply, leading to death of the bone, causing it to cease growing. There is swelling of the soft tissues of the hip joint (Figure 106.6). The cause is unknown. It is most commonly seen in those aged 5–9 years, but can occur at any age. Boys are affected more often than girls.

The child presents with a limp and hip or knee pain without a history of injury. This pain follows the pathway of the obturator nerve. It is a self-limiting condition. Following the first stage of interruption of the blood supply, revascularization occurs, where growth of new vessels happens and there is bone resorption. New bone formation takes place that is weak, leading to collapse and flattening of the femoral head.

Reossification is the final stage in the process, where the head of the femur gradually reforms and the necrotic bone is removed.

The aim of treatment is to contain the femoral epiphysis within the acetabulum. This is done by rest and restriction of activity. The child requires analgesia for the pain and is required to be non-weight-bearing. Initially this may be by traction or splintage. Physiotherapy is required to achieve and maintain the range of movement. If the femoral head is not able to be contained in the acetabulum, then surgery in the form of a pelvic or femoral osteotomy may be necessary. All of these conditions may require the use of a plaster cast and traction.

Key points
- DDH is usually diagnosed from screening before the child starts to walk, but should be considered if there is a limp.
- Perthes' disease may follow an episode of transient synovitis.
- Scoliosis is more prevalent in children with neuromuscular disorders such as cerebral palsy and muscular dystrophy.

107 Reproductive and sexual problems

Figure 107.1 Issues of sexual identity.

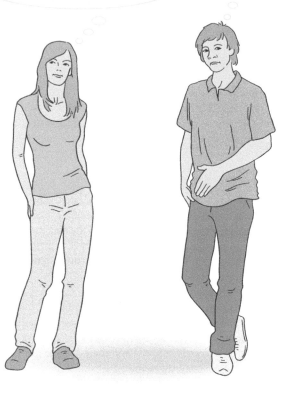

Figure 107.2 Checking the testes.

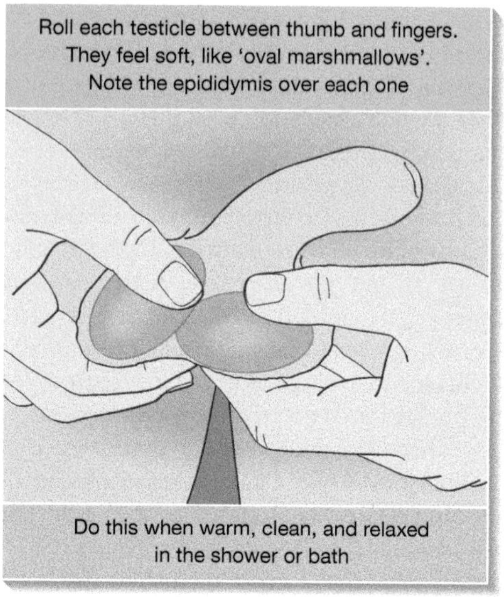

Roll each testicle between thumb and fingers.
They feel soft, like 'oval marshmallows'.
Note the epididymis over each one

Do this when warm, clean, and relaxed
in the shower or bath

Box 107.1 Normal bleeding pattern for established
(~one year) menstruation

- *Frequency:* every 21–35 days
- *Length:* 3–7 days (from spotting to ending with no colour in loss)
- *Amount:* 20–80 mL (up to 4 tampons/day), few small clots

Box 107.2 Causes of delayed puberty.

Males and females

Maturational delay (usually familial)
Lesions of the pituitary gland
Gonadal failure
Chronic and severe disease

Females
Turner's syndrome
Anorexia nervosa
Intense exercising/athletic training

Figure 107.3 Right to healthcare.

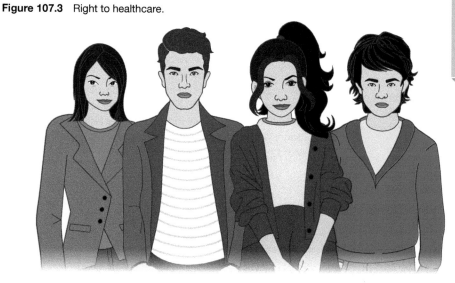

Children and Young People's Nursing at a Glance, Second Edition. Edited by Elizabeth Gormley-Fleming and Sheila Roberts.
© 2023 John Wiley & Sons Ltd. Published 2023 by John Wiley & Sons Ltd.

Structural abnormalities

Congenital anatomical abnormalities within the reproductive, genital or urological organs requiring surgical intervention may include:
- Absence or occlusion of the vagina in females
- Ambivalent or ambiguous genitalia
- Micropenis, hypospadias (urethral opening on underside of penis), epispadias (urethral opeing on upper aspect of penis) or cryptorchidism (undescended testis) in males.

Developmental issues

Reproductive and sexual functioning is a combination of mind and body function. Adolescence is when these processes and functions mature and become a focus of attention. Part of becoming a sexually mature adult may involve difficult decisions about sexual identity (Figure 107.1). Hormone levels are relatively unstable and interlinked with basic drives centrally controlled within the brain: sleeping, eating, drinking, and exercising. The moody, relatively uncooperative and uncommunicative teenager is difficult to establish a rapport with. 'You have an issue – this is a confidential service and we are here to help' facilitates a working relationship.

Signs of puberty may not necessarily be welcomed or understood by the child, despite videos and classroom teaching sessions. Puberty can occur precociously as early as 8 years of age or be delayed beyond 16 years.

Precocious puberty

Precocious puberty in girls is usually idiopathic, whereas in boys it is more likely to be due to an underlying pathological lesion. The child who has precocious puberty has a double challenge as they are undergoing physical, emotional, and social changes at an age when their peers are not, and secondly their adult height potential is jeopardized as their bones will fuse prematurely. Precocious puberty is primarily an endocrine disorder.

Male signs of puberty

Signs of puberty are facial, underarm, and pubic hair, with increases in glandular activity – sweat = odour; sebaceous gland activity – potential acne; voice change and break; growth spurts, which = potential acne; the voice changes or breaks.

Penile and scrotal developmental problems

- *Phimosis*: the foreskin remains too tight for retraction to allow for cleansing underneath glans. Surgical division with conservation of foreskin is now preferred to circumcision. Phimosis may also result from infection, where identification and appropriate treatment are required in addition to surgery.
- *Balanitis*: swelling of the glans (± foreskin). The glans is red and sore as a result of irritation (from for example accumulated smegma; infection – thrush or sexually transmitted; dribbled urine; highly scented shower gels).
- *Paraphimosis*: occurs if a tight foreskin is retracted round the penis, causing the glans to swell and resulting in significant pain. Emergency surgical management and treatment of any infection are required.
- *Varicocele*: swollen veins within pampiniform plexus. Although not a problem in itself, the resultant increases in temperature can cause low sperm counts and male infertility.
- *Hydrocoele*: painless, fluid-filled sacs that enlarge the scrotal contents but feel soft and mobile. These may cause anxiety.
- *Testicular cancer*: the most common cancer in young men, but it is easily treated if detected and diagnosed early. Self-examination of testicles is to be promoted (Figure 107.2).
- *Inguinal hernia*: occurs where a section of intestine has prolapsed into the scrotum through the inguinal canal. This requires surgical repair.

Trauma

- *Frenulum breve* ('short'): this may rupture with masturbation or sexual intercourse and can lead to a haematoma under the glans epidermal tissue, which will resolve. If pain or trauma continues with sexual activity, further surgical division may be necessary, but not circumcision.
- *Testicular torsion* causes acute pain as a result of ischaemia from twisting of the testicle about the spermatic cord.
- *Testicular trauma* causes significant pain.

Female signs of puberty

Signs of puberty are increase in height and weight; female body shape – breast development, widening hips; pubic hair growth; underarms with increased sweat gland activity – odour; sebaceous gland activity – potential acne, particularly linked with menstrual cycle post menarche. A girl's menstrual pattern is one of the major indicators for her general as well as reproductive health (Box 107.1).

Potential problems

- *Primary amenorrhoea*: delayed puberty. Investigations commence if there are no signs of puberty by 14 years.
- *Infrequent or scanty periods (oligomenorrhoea)*: most frequently caused by polycystic ovarian syndrome (PCOS), examine for hirsutism and virilism. PCOS treatment includes weight loss, metformin to counteract insulin resistance, combined oral contraceptive pill (COCP) when the body mass index is under control to protect endometrium.
- *Excess bleeding (menorrhagia)*: dysfunctional bleeding (DUB) is the most frequent diagnosis of exclusion in young women: local (e.g. fibroids, polyps, endometritis, or endometrial carcinoma), a clotting disorder, or endocrine. Treatment for DUB includes COCP and/or non-steroidal anti-inflammatory drugs.
- *Pelvic pain*: a good history helps determine potential causes, including:
  - Early pregnancy problems such as miscarriage or ectopic.
  - Pelvic inflammatory disease (sexually transmitted infection (STI) – chlamydia and/or gonorrhoea)
  - Contraceptive post intrauterine device or termination.
  - Trauma – surgical, adhesions, infection, consider abuse.
  - Menstrual – the first day of the last menstrual period is vital information and relationship of pain to cycle could indicate endometriosis, which often goes undiagnosed and untreated but is a significant cause of distress.
  - If COCP or Depo-Provera injection therapy is unsuccessful, specialist treatment centres are now available.
- *Other pelvic pain causes*: ovarian cysts (rupture, haemorrhage, and torsion), fibroids, and gynaecological malignancy are possible but rare in the adolescent age group. Non-reproductive tract causes need to be considered, such as urinary tract infection, renal calculi, irritable bowel, and diverticulitis.
- *Vaginal discharges*: most are physiological, but associated itch, malodour, colour change, or consistency may indicate abnormality. Causes could be foreign body (e.g. tampon), infection (non-STI, e.g. *Candida* or bacterial vaginosis). Likelihood of these is increased with excess washing (>1/day) and shaving pubic hair, or an STI.

Key points

- Puberty is considered to be delayed if there are no physical signs by the age of 14 years in males and 13 years in females, or if periods have not commenced by the age of 16 years (Box 107.2).
- Chronic and severe illness can delay puberty.
- Sexual activity is occurring at a younger age, so the rate of sexually transmitted infections in young people continues to increase.
- Young people have a right to supportive and relevant healthcare. (Figure 107.3)

108 Skin conditions

Figure 108.1 Classification of skin disorders.

Figure 108.3 Quality of life considerations.

Figure 108.4 Acute skin conditions.

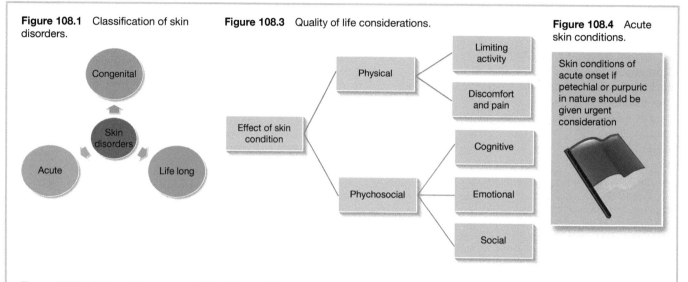

Skin conditions of acute onset if petechial or purpuric in nature should be given urgent consideration

Figure 108.2 Systematic assessment of a skin condition.

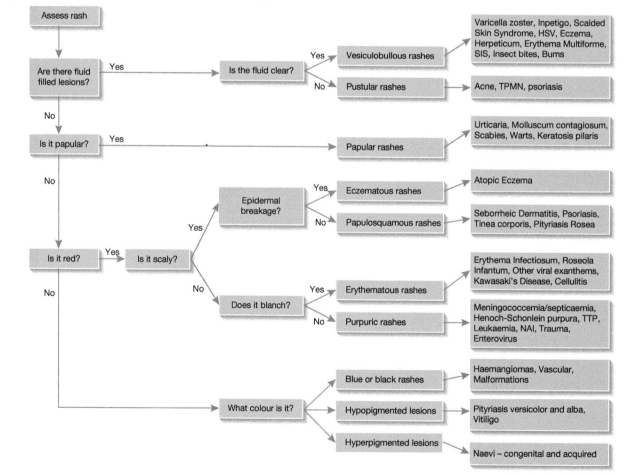

Children and Young People's Nursing at a Glance, Second Edition. Edited by Elizabeth Gormley-Fleming and Sheila Roberts.
© 2023 John Wiley & Sons Ltd. Published 2023 by John Wiley & Sons Ltd.

The skin is a complex organ that is essential for human survival due to its physiological functions. It undergoes significant changes from birth to adulthood, and the children and young person's nurse will need to have a good understanding of the anatomy and physiology of the skin if they are to plan effective nursing care for the child and family. Skin conditions in children (<14 years of age) comprise about 21% of all those consulting with skin disease; this age group represents 19% of the population. Skin conditions may be inherited (epidermitis bullosa), acute (urticaria, petechia in meningococcal disease), or long term (atopic eczema) (Figure 108.1).

Assessing the child with a rash

The skin should be examined in a warm, well-lit room, preferably with natural lighting or artificial lighting that will not change the natural colour of the skin (Figure 108.2). The assessment should be systematic, using a structured approach. A focused history and appropriate investigations are essential in arriving at a correct diagnosis and therefore treatment plan.

Clinical history

- Onset: acute or chronic.
- Systemic symptoms (fever).
- Duration of rash.
- Change in rash over time: flare and remission.
- Symptoms of rash (itching, pain, soreness).
- Family history of skin disease.
- Recent contact with individuals with a rash (scabies, chickenpox).
- Drug history.
- Allergies.
- Other medical history (atopy: asthma, hay fever).
- Does it occur at different times of the year?
- School and hobbies – do they have an impact?
- Pets – contact with animals/birds?
- Medications – applied to the skin, taken by mouth, or purchased by the parents.
- Previous and present treatments and their effectiveness.
- Are there any treatments, actions, or behavioural changes that have influenced the condition?

Coping with the skin condition

The impact of the skin condition on the child and family is an important consideration irrespective of the duration of the condition. They child may be withdrawn, not sleeping, or be very conscious about their appearance and the reactions of others: staring, name calling, or bullying. This will also impact on the parents' wellbeing. There are several psychological and disease-specific scores that can measure the impact of skin disease. Quality of life assessment is an important consideration in the management of both acute and long-term skin conditions (Figure 108.3).

Clinical examination

When examining the child, use a gown or sheet to maintain their dignity as each area of the skin is exposed for examination. Touching is an important aspect of the examination. It provides information about skin texture and temperature and also breaks down the physical barrier and stigma associated with skin disease. The skin should be examined thoroughly from the scalp to toes, including hair, nails, and flexures, looking at the following:

Distribution

Is it acral (hands, feet), extremities of ears and nose, in light-exposed areas, or mainly confined to the trunk?

Character

Is there redness (erythema), scaling, crusting, exudate? Are there excoriations, blisters, erosions, pustules, papules? Are the lesions all the same (monomorphic, e.g. drug rash) or variable (polymorphic, e.g. chickenpox)? Lesions can further be defined as primary or secondary. Primary lesions are present at the initial onset of the disease:

- *Macule*: flat mark; circumscribed area of colour change: brown, red, white, or tan.
- *Papule*: elevated 'spot'; palpable, firm, circumscribed lesion, generally <5 mm in diameter.
- *Nodule*: elevated, firm, circumscribed, palpable; can involve all layers of the skin, >5 mm in diameter.
- *Plaque*: elevated, flat-topped, firm, rough, superficial papule >2 cm in diameter. Papules can coalesce to form plaques.
- *Wheal*: elevated, irregular-shaped area of cutaneous oedema; solid, transient, changing, variable diameter; red, pale pink, or white in colour.
- *Vesicle*: elevated, circumscribed, superficial fluid-filled blister <5 mm in diameter.
- *Bulla*: vesicle >5 mm in diameter.
- *Pustule*: elevated, superficial, similar to vesicle but filled with pus.

Secondary lesions are the result of changes over time caused by disease progression, manipulation (scratching, rubbing, picking), or treatment:

- *Scale*: heaped-up keratinized cells; flaky exfoliation; irregular; thick or thin; dry or oily; variable size; silver, white, or tan in colour.
- *Crust*: dried serum, blood, or purulent exudate; slightly elevated; size variable.
- *Excoriation*: loss of epidermis; linear area usually due to scratching.
- *Lichenification*: rough, thickened epidermis; accentuated skin markings caused by rubbing or scratching.

Shape

Are the lesions small, large, annular (ring-shaped), or linear?

Skin types

With different skin colours and hair types, lesions that appear red or brown in white skin appear black or purple in pigmented skin, and mild degrees of redness (erythema) may be masked completely. Inflammation commonly leads to pigmentary changes – both lighter (post-inflammatory hypopigmentation) and darker (post-inflammatory hyperpigmentation) – which may persist for a long time after the initial skin condition has settled.

Investigations

- Samples of scales, crusts, hair, and nails – yeast, fungus, virus, bacteria.
- Skin biopsy (blistering rashes or when diagnosis uncertain).
- Blood investigations, depending on diagnosis and assessment.

The acute rash

Children who present with fever and irritability and a purpuric rash should have urgent assessment (Figure 108.4) to rule out sepsis or meningococcal disease. Other acute conditions that need rapid treatment include scaled skin syndrome, acute haemorrhagic oedema of infancy, and skin conditions associated with drug eruptions or Stevens–Johnson syndrome.

Key points

- Skin conditions will inevitably impact on the quality of the child's and family's life.
- A holistic systematic assessment is required in order to make an effective treatment plan.
- Some rashes are acute and require immediate treatment.

109 Atopic eczema

Figure 109.1 Managing eczema.

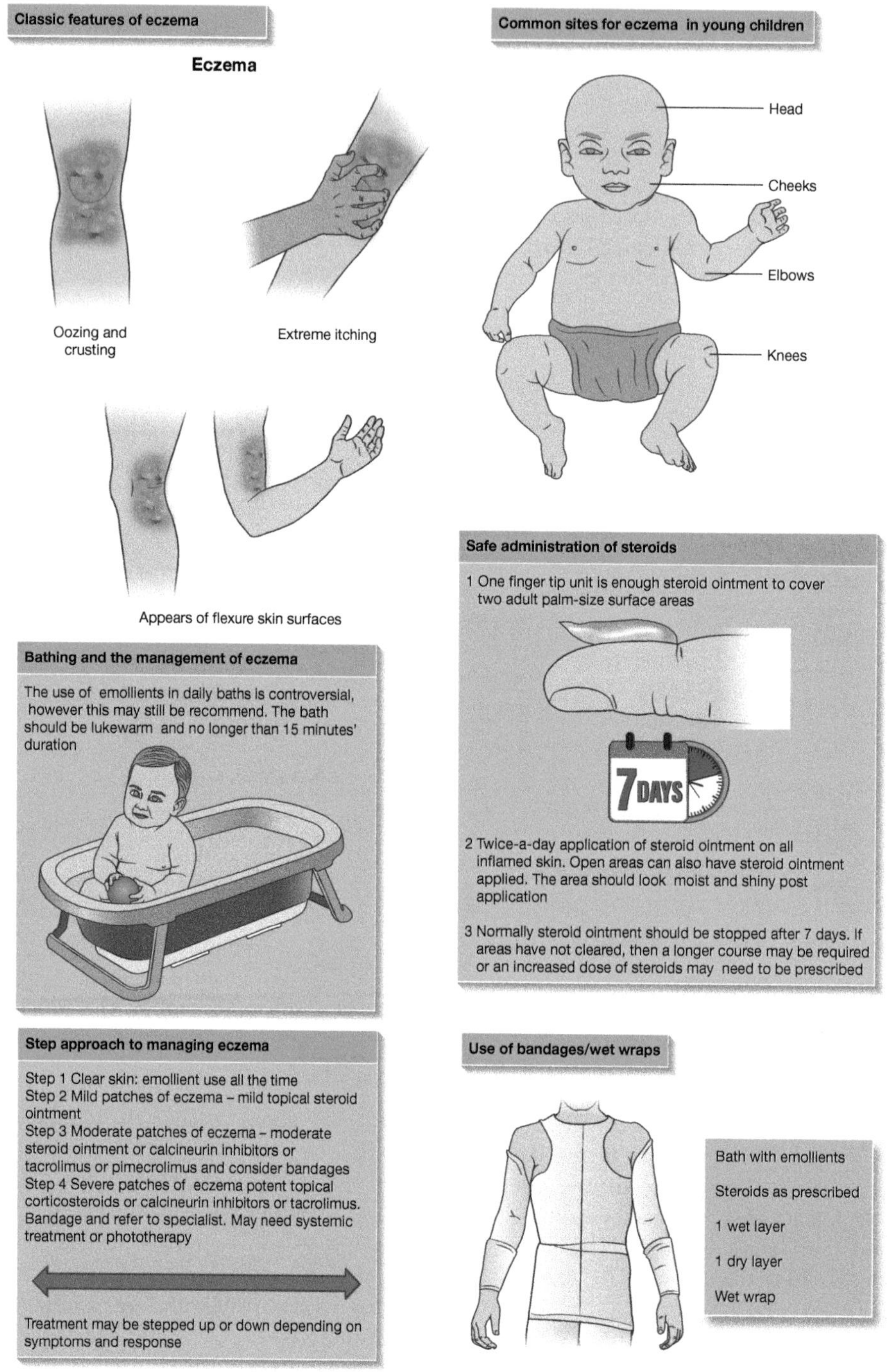

Classic features of eczema

Eczema

Oozing and crusting

Extreme itching

Appears of flexure skin surfaces

Common sites for eczema in young children

Head

Cheeks

Elbows

Knees

Bathing and the management of eczema

The use of emollients in daily baths is controversial, however this may still be recommend. The bath should be lukewarm and no longer than 15 minutes' duration

Safe administration of steroids

1 One finger tip unit is enough steroid ointment to cover two adult palm-size surface areas

7 DAYS

2 Twice-a-day application of steroid ointment on all inflamed skin. Open areas can also have steroid ointment applied. The area should look moist and shiny post application

3 Normally steroid ointment should be stopped after 7 days. If areas have not cleared, then a longer course may be required or an increased dose of steroids may need to be prescribed

Step approach to managing eczema

Step 1 Clear skin: emollient use all the time
Step 2 Mild patches of eczema – mild topical steroid ointment
Step 3 Moderate patches of eczema – moderate steroid ointment or calcineurin inhibitors or tacrolimus or pimecrolimus and consider bandages
Step 4 Severe patches of eczema potent topical corticosteroids or calcineurin inhibitors or tacrolimus. Bandage and refer to specialist. May need systemic treatment or phototherapy

Treatment may be stepped up or down depending on symptoms and response

Use of bandages/wet wraps

Bath with emollients

Steroids as prescribed

1 wet layer

1 dry layer

Wet wrap

Table 109.1 Management of eczema.

Clear	Emollients					
Mild	Emollients	Mild-potency topical corticosteroids				
Moderate	Emollients	Moderate-potency topical corticosteroids	Topical calcineurin inhibitors	Bandages		
Severe	Emollients	Potent topical corticosteroids	Topical calcineurin inhibitors	Bandages	Phototherapy	Systemic therapy

Children and Young People's Nursing at a Glance, Second Edition. Edited by Elizabeth Gormley-Fleming and Sheila Roberts.
© 2023 John Wiley & Sons Ltd. Published 2023 by John Wiley & Sons Ltd.

A topic eczema (atopic dermatitis) is a chronic inflammatory skin condition characterized by itching, which usually develops in early childhood and follows a pattern of remission and relapse. It often has a genetic component that leads to the breakdown of the skin barrier. This makes the skin susceptible to trigger factors, including irritants and allergens, which can make the eczema worse. Although atopic eczema is not often thought of as a serious medical condition, it can have a significant impact on quality of life.

Diagnosis

Diagnose atopic eczema when a child has an itchy skin condition plus three or more of the following:
- Visible flexural dermatitis involving the skin creases (or visible dermatitis on the cheeks and/or extensor areas in children aged 18 months or under).
- Personal history of flexural dermatitis (or dermatitis on the cheeks and/or extensor areas in children aged 18 months or under).
- Personal history of dry skin in the last 12 months.
- Personal history of asthma or allergic rhinitis (or history of atopic disease in a first-degree relative of children aged under 4 years).
- Onset of signs and symptoms under the age of 2 years (do not use this criterion as one of the three in children under 4 years).

In children of Asian, black Caribbean, and black African ethnic groups, atopic eczema can affect the extensor surfaces rather than the flexures, and discoid or follicular patterns may be more common with post-inflammatory hypo- or hyperpigmentation.

Assessment

History:
- Time of onset, pattern, and severity.
- Response to previous and current treatments.
- Possible trigger factors (soap, detergents, weather, seasons, skin infections, animal dander, pollens, house dust mite, foods, and stress).
- Impact of the condition on children and their parents or carers.
- Dietary history.
- Growth and development.
- Personal and family history of atopic disease

Take into account the severity of the atopic eczema and the child's quality of life, including everyday activities and sleep, and psychosocial wellbeing. There is not necessarily a direct relationship between the severity of atopic eczema and its impact on quality of life.

Also consider the impact of atopic eczema on parents or carers as well as the child.

Clinical findings

The appearance of eczema varies and is related to the age of the child, their ethnic background, and the presence of infection. The distribution changes with age; the face is a common site in infants followed by flexural involvement. It can affect the extensor surfaces rather than the flexures and a discoid or follicular pattern may be seen. It can be localized or widespread (Table 109.1). There may be dry skin and fine scale, areas of ill-defined erythema (redness), excoriations, lichenification vesicles, weeping, and crusting, which may be signs of infection. Infections may be bacterial or viral (eczema herpeticum).

Table 109.2 Severity index.

	Absent – 0	Slightly – 1	Moderately – 2	Severe – 3
Redness of skin				
Oedema/ swelling				
Oozing/ crusts				
Scratching traces/injury				
Thickened skin				

Assessing severity

To assess severity a severity index scoring system may be used (Table 109.2). Each section is scored 0–3.

Management

Use a stepped approach for managing atopic eczema, and tailor treatment steps to severity. Use emollients all the time and step treatment up or down as necessary. All aspects should be supported by education and demonstrations.

Referral

Refer immediately (same day) for specialist dermatological advice if you suspect eczema herpeticum.

Refer urgently (within two weeks) for specialist dermatological advice if:
- The atopic eczema is severe and has not responded to topical therapy after one week.
- Treatment of bacterially infected atopic eczema has failed.

Refer for specialist dermatological advice if:
- The diagnosis is uncertain.
- The atopic eczema is not controlled based on a subjective assessment by the child or parent or carer.
- Atopic eczema on the face has not responded to appropriate treatment.
- Contact allergic dermatitis is suspected.
- The atopic eczema is causing significant social or psychological problems.
- The atopic eczema is associated with severe and recurrent infections.
- The child, parent, or carer might benefit from specialist advice on treatment application.

Refer for psychological advice children whose atopic eczema has responded to management but for whom the impact on quality of life and psychosocial wellbeing has not improved.

Refer children with moderate or severe atopic eczema and suspected food allergy for specialist investigation and management.

Refer children with atopic eczema who fail to grow at the expected growth trajectory, as reflected by the UK growth charts, for specialist advice relating to growth.

Key points
- Parents and the child need to be aware that treatments can help ease the symptoms but not cure them.
- Compliance with treatment is important and this needs to be understood.
- Triggers must be avoided if known.

110 Clinical holding

Figure 110.1 Holding a child in a supportive manner.

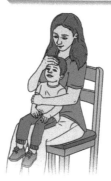
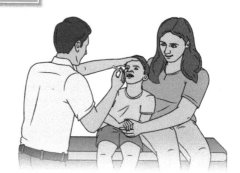

Comfort holding positions

Supportive holding position

Definitions

Holding still means the immobilization of a limb, for example using limited force in order to manage a procedure such as cannulation or venepuncture. This implies consent

Restraining is defined as the positive application of force with the intention to overpower the child. This implies that the child's consent is not required

Swaddling/wrapping technique

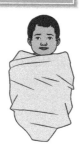

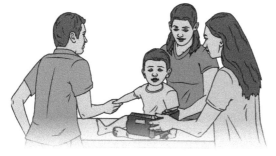

Good practice principles

1. Care and respect for the child's rights are paramount
2. Consent is required
3. Staff are confident and competent in holding techniques
4. Agreement is sought on the method used and for how long the child will be held still
5. Age-appropriate techniques will be used – swaddling, wrapping, splinting
6. The least force for the shortest duration should be practised
7. Infection control principles are adhered to
8. Consider non-pharmacological methods, e.g. sucrose for babies
9. Parental presence and involvement are established pre-procedure
10. Safety of all staff is maintained at all times
11. Hospital play specialists are available to provide pre-, inter- and post-procedural preparation and distraction play
12. Documentation reflects procedure and concerns are recoded on risk reporting systems

Child-centred approach to clinical holding

Their long-term psychological wellbeing is the priority
Their rights are respected and their voice is heard
They are involved in making decisions and have choice

Distraction play is essential as it comforts the child and parents

Physically holding a child for a procedure may also be described as restraining, supportive holding, clinical holding, therapeutic holding, retracing movement, immobilization, and restricting physical intervention. These terms are based on presumptions of force and suggest that nurses have a common understanding of what constitutes the use of force in the clinical setting. Irrespective of the name given, this practice must always be justified. As more children with complex needs, including intellectual disabilities, autism spectrum disorders, and mental health needs, are admitted to children's services, the children and young person's nurse must be conversant in safe practice with regard to clinical holding. Children, parents, and children's nurses find many types of procedures stressful and

Children and Young People's Nursing at a Glance, Second Edition. Edited by Elizabeth Gormley-Fleming and Sheila Roberts.
© 2023 John Wiley & Sons Ltd. Published 2023 by John Wiley & Sons Ltd.

sometimes traumatic, and often have questions around why, when, and how restriction happens.

Restricting a child's movement for routine clinical procedures is distressing for the child and may have an impact on their later psychological development. Parents have also expressed feelings of helplessness and powerlessness when their child was restricted for a clinical procedure. Explanations about safety are essential prior to the procedure for the parent and child. The parents are in a very vulnerable position, often unable to adequately comfort or care for their child, and not questioning practice because they feel disempowered in an unfamiliar environment. In addition, it is often a fine balance between the parent knowing the importance of the procedure being carried out in order to assist with treatment or diagnosis, and parental guilt that the child is unwell or has sustained injury.

There are a number of considerations for the nurse when caring for a child who needs to be held still for a clinical procedure, relating to the care of the child, care of the parents, and self-care for the nurse. All practices must comply with the professional code of practice and local policies. There are three main phases: the lead-in to the procedure, care during the procedure, and the post-holding phase.

Considerations

Caring for a child undergoing a clinical procedure requires the nurse to consider the individual needs of the child and the family. This includes questioning the necessity for restriction, considering alternatives to restriction, establishing the potential for parental involvement, considering the child's physical and emotional needs, and affording the child and parent(s) the opportunity to debrief after the procedure if they wish. It is possible that younger children are more likely to be restricted for a clinical procedure because of the nurse's anticipation that such children are more difficult to keep still.

Children need to have some sense of control when undergoing a clinical procedure, in order to help them cope. Addressing the child's comfort and need for control may encourage greater compliance from the child, thus enhancing the delivery of safe care. This is supported by the work of many theorists on child development, who identified the need for young children to have a sense of control in their environment, to have a sense of participation, and to trust those caring for them.

Pre-holding considerations

In the lead-in to holding the child, the nurse should consider the needs of the child, the parent, and their own professional needs, as follows.

Child-focused considerations

• Is it necessary for this child to be held still for this procedure?
• Is this decision influenced by the procedure to be performed, the child's age, or the child's cognitive ability?
• Is the procedure urgent or necessary?
• Are there any alternatives to holding the child still that are appropriate to the child's stage of development? What are they (e.g. distraction, imagery, sedation)?
• What will it mean for this child to be held still?
• How are they likely to react and how will I manage and support them through that?
• What is the child's understanding of what will happen? What are their information needs?

Considerations for the nurse

• How do I feel about holding a child still?
• Do I have the education, experience, and skill to do this safely?
• Is there any policy that should guide my involvement in this?

Parent-focused considerations

• Are the child's parents present?
• What is their understanding of what will happen?
• Do they have an expectation of being involved? If so, how will this work in practice?
• What guidance do they require?
• Is there a named person to care for their needs if I am involved in holding their child?

Care during clinical holding

If a decision is made to hold the child still for a clinical procedure (Figure 110.1), it is important that the child is very clear on who their lead person is, what they can do if they are distressed, and where their parents are.

Some questions for your consideration:
• Who is giving direction to the child?
• Is the child being held for the shortest time possible?
• Are the child's and parents' physical and emotional needs being met?

It is very likely that a child will object to being held still; when this happens the focus is always on gaining cooperation through de-escalation. This can evoke a wide variety of feelings, so it is worthwhile considering what this might mean for you. Did you agree with the need for clinical holding? Are you in a hurry to complete the procedure due to time pressures? Do you feel you have enough support? Is the child or parent not cooperating to the extent you would wish? Why do you think this is? It is very important to think about these issues, as you may communicate your feelings through your verbal or non-verbal actions to the child and parents.

In the event of non-cooperation, it is essential to try to establish what the child's motivation for their behaviour is. Think back to the earlier prompt questions. Were all information and comfort needs of the child and parent addressed? What has changed? What are their needs now, and who is best placed to address them?

Post-holding considerations

The aftermath of clinical holding is an opportunity for the nurse to consider what went well and what aspects of the care could be improved on. Consideration should be given to the following:
• Was there an appropriate rationale for clinical holding?
• Were the method and length of holding suitable in this situation?
• Are there any potential effects for the child or parents?
• Were they addressed and how can they be addressed in future?

It is very important that notes on all of the above are documented to enhance continuity of care and to communicate the child's particular preferences, and the coping strategies employed that were found to be particularly useful.

Key points

• Pre-procedural expectations of clinical holding must be explained, and the child and parent(s) allow to ask questions.
• The children and young person's nurse must have an understanding of professional accountability in relation to clinical holding.
• There must always be sufficient staff available to undertake the procedure; that is, holding the child, assisting with the procedure, and comforting the child and parent(s).

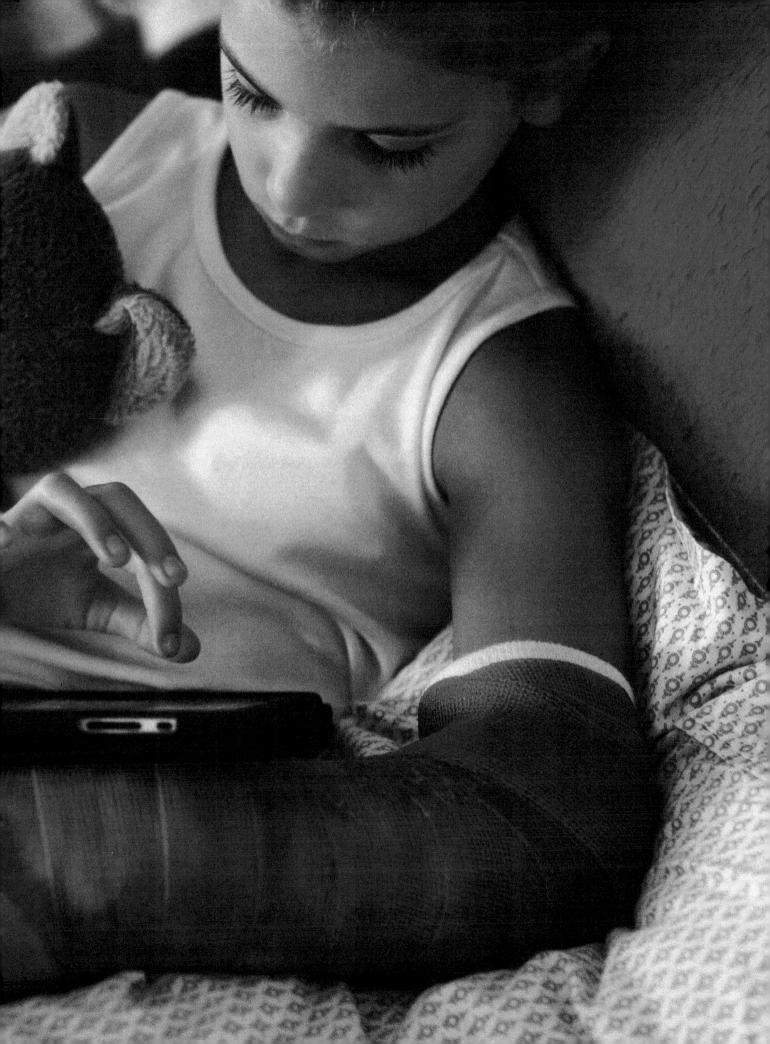

Part 7

111 Coronavirus, Covid-19, and children

Figure 111.1 SARS-CoV-2.

Spike glycoprotein (S)
Membrane protein (M)
Nucleoprotein (N)
Genomic RNA
Envelope small membrane protein (E)

Figure 111.2 Transmission of coronavirus.

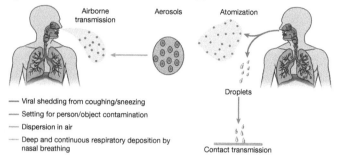

Airborne transmission   Aerosols   Atomization

Droplets

— Viral shedding from coughing/sneezing
— Setting for person/object contamination
— Dispersion in air
— Deep and continuous respiratory deposition by nasal breathing

Contact transmission

Figure 111.3 Clinical signs and symptoms of multisystem inflammatory syndrome in children (MIS-C).

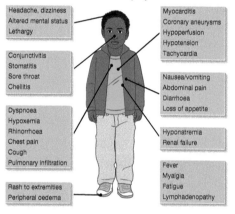

Headache, dizziness
Altered mental status
Lethargy

Conjunctivitis
Stomatitis
Sore throat
Chelitis

Dyspnoea
Hypoxemia
Rhinorrhoea
Chest pain
Cough
Pulmonary infiltration

Rash to extremities
Peripheral oedema

Myocarditis
Coronary aneurysms
Hypoperfusion
Hypotension
Tachycardia

Nausea/vomiting
Abdominal pain
Diarrhoea
Loss of appetite

Hyponatremia
Renal failure

Fever
Myalgia
Fatigue
Lymphadenopathy

Table 111.1 Human and novel coronaviruses.

Human coronavirus	Novel coronavirus
229E	SARS-CoV-1
HKU1	MERS
NL63	SARS-CoV-2
OC43	

Table 111.2 Personal protective equipment (PPE) requirements for level of airborne risk and general patient contact.

PPE requirements	Low risk General patient contact	Low risk Aerosol-generating procedure	Medium risk General patient contact	Medium risk Aerosol-generating procedure	High risk General patient contact	High risk Aerosol-generating procedure
Full face shield/eye protection	√ (If risk of body fluids or blood splash to face)	√	√ (If risk of body fluids or blood splash to face)	√	√ (If risk of body fluids or blood splash to face)	√
FFP3 respirator						√
FFP3 mask				√		
Fluid-resistant surgical mask	√	√	√		√	
Long-sleeve fluid-repellent gown		√		√	√	√
Disposable plastic apron	√	√	√		√	√
Gloves	√	√	√	√	√	√

Aprons and gloves are single-use items and should be disposed of after each patient contact. Good hand hygiene is vitally important.

Other PPE, fluid-resistant surgical masks, respirators, eye protection can be subject to single sessional use

Box 111.1 The R value.

Covid alert level = rate of infection (R value) + number of infections

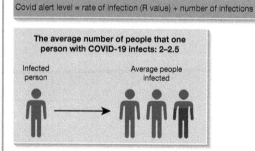

The average number of people that one person with COVID-19 infects: 2–2.5

Infected person   Average people infected

Initially described in December 2019, coronavirus disease progressed quickly into a global pandemic. This new coronavirus originated from Wuhan, China.

By March 2020, Covid-19 had reached pandemic status. A pandemic is defined as the worldwide spread of a new disease. The impact of the control measures taken to prevent the spread of this deadly disease has led to significant global economic and social disruption. The burden on health services has been felt globally. The impact of this pandemic has been far reaching in relation to the health and wellbeing of children and young people, their families, and their communities.

Coronaviruses

Seven coronaviruses are known to infect humans. Four of these human coronaviruses (hCoVs; Figure 111.1) are in global circulation and typically cause mild respiratory disease in children. The three novel coronaviruses of zoonotic origin (Table 111.1) have appeared in the last decade and are responsible for endemics and more recently a pandemic.

Severe Acute Respiratory Syndrome (SARS-CoV-1), Middle Eastern Respiratory Syndrome (MERS), and SARS-CoV-2, known as Covid-19, are known to cause a range of severe illnesses and mortality in the

Children and Young People's Nursing at a Glance, Second Edition. Edited by Elizabeth Gormley-Fleming and Sheila Roberts.
© 2023 John Wiley & Sons Ltd. Published 2023 by John Wiley & Sons Ltd.

elderly with pre-existing comorbidities. Children and young people are generally less severely affected than adults and mortality rates among them are significantly lower. Asymptomatic infection in children is not uncommon. SARS-CoV-2 has been identified in newborn babies.

Transmission

SARS CoV-2 is a highly infectious disease. It is transmitted from person to person via respiratory droplets and direct or indirect contact with infected secretions (Figure 111.2). Respiratory droplets normally do not travel more than 1–2 m. Aerosol generation can occur during certain medical procedures: bronchoscopy, intubation, non-invasive ventilation. Airborne isolation precautions are required during any of these procedures (Table 111.2).

Polymerase chain reaction (PCR) testing is widely used for confirming the presence of SARS-CoV-2 from nasopharyngeal swabs, aspirates, and throat swabs from children and adults. Non-respiratory fluids – blood, conjunctival fluid, stools, and anal swabs – have tested positive for SARs-CoV-2 using PCR testing. Lateral flow testing has become commonplace.

Children and young people are thought to comprise 1–2% of all cases worldwide and up to 5–13% of reported cases where testing is more extensive. It remains challenging to get accurate figures.

A disproportionate burden of disease has been noted in certain ethnic groups. This has been characterized by higher infection rates, prolonged hospitalization, and death in adults. Disparities are complex and thought to be related to social and structural determinants of health, economic and educational disadvantage, discrimination, and disparities in access to healthcare.

The R value

The R (reproduction or regeneration) value represents the number of people that an infected patient can infect (Box 111.1). If the R value is 1, then every person who is infected will infect one other person in the right conditions. SARs-CoV-2 has an R value of between 2 and 2.5. If no action is taken to stop the spread of SAR-CoV-2, then one infected person can potentially infect up to three others. Hence the need is always to try to reduce the R value and thereby reduce the risk of spreading infection.

The infection rate is said to be stable if the R value is less than 1. If the R number is 0.5, then on average for each two people infected only one will have a new infection. The infection rates are then said to be shrinking. If the R is greater than 1, infection rates are increasing.

Signs and symptoms of coronavirus infection

Children appear to play a significant role in the transmission of SARS-CoV-2. The incubation period in children is on average 6.5 days, whereas it is 5.4 days in adults. Nasal and pharyngeal detoxification in children is up to 21 days, with an average of 12 days.

Because children and young people may be less seriously ill or be symptom free, everyday preventative behaviors remain important as they play an important role in disease transmission.

Symptoms in children

The main symptoms of coronavirus in children are:
- High temperature.
- A new continuous cough, coughing a lot, three or more coughing episodes in 24 hours.
- A loss of taste (ageusia) or smell (anosmia) – younger children may not be able to recognize this.
  Other symptoms may include:
- Vomiting.
- Diarrhoea.

- Headache.
- Abdominal pain.
- Rash (vesicular eruptions, urticaria, maculopapular, livedo).
- Myalgia.
- Fatigue.
- Sore throat – pharyngeal erythema.
- Rhinorrhoea.
- Neurological manifestations.
- Covid toe (discoloration and swelling of a toe or toes).
- Conjunctivitis.
This list is not exhaustive.

Multisystem inflammatory syndrome in children

A number of children have required intensive care for the management of multisystem inflammatory syndrome in children (MIS-C). A significant number of cases of Kawasaki disease have also been reported in children since the start of the Covid-19 pandemic. MIS-C is rare but a serious condition (Figure 111.3). It may appear a number of weeks after the child has been infected with SARs-CoV-2.

Diagnosis

In addition to the standard history taking and physical assessment, cardiac testing is more frequently assessed given the association of Covid-19 with MIS-C. The assessment is likely to include electrocardiogram (ECG), echocardiogram, cardiac enzymes (troponin), and B-type natriuretic peptide levels. Other assessments will be determined according to the signs and symptoms the child presents with.

Treatment

Standardize treatment for MIS-C has yet to evolve. Treatment is symptom based. Multispecialty consultation is required. Fluid resuscitation and inotropic support may be required along with respiratory support. Intravenous immunoglobulins and systemic steroids have been used to date. Aspirin has also been used for the anti-platelet effect. Antibiotics are routinely used to treat potential sepsis until bacterial cultures are negatives. Thrombotic prophylaxis may also be required.

Control measures

Unprecedented control measures in terms of scale and duration were put in place during the Covid-19 pandemic. Lockdown required closure of all but essential services. Outdoor activity was either banned or limited to once-a-day exercise. Visiting family or friends was not allowed for many months and then restricted in both number and location. Home schooling was required. All of this was required to keep the R value down and to 'flatten the curve'. Social distancing measures were put in place and face masks became mandatory. Children have been exempted from wearing masks under the age of 11 years in the UK, and certainly mask wearing may be a health and safety issue in the younger child age group. A test and trace programme was implemented.

The Covid-19 vaccine was developed in haste and a mass vaccination programme has enabled a relaxation of the control measures. There is worldwide variance in the vaccination of children. Currently vaccinations are available for all children aged 5 years and above in the UK.

Impact on children and young people

The unintended consequences of the measures taken to control the pandemic on children and young people may not yet be fully realized. However, it is known that there is an increase in eating disorders and in mental health problems in these age groups.

112 Living with long-term and life-limiting conditions

Figure 112.1 Family challenges.

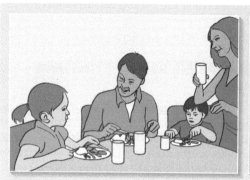

- Learning to integrate the restrictions of disease and treatment with other more routine aspects of their lives
- Developing knowledge and understanding of the child's condition and needs
- Living with uncertainties and knowing how to deal with emergencies
- Continuing to see the child as a child first and foremost
- Practical adaptations: home, location, work, lifestyle, finance
- Avoiding disruption to relationships
- Ensuring that siblings receive the same level of care and attention and feel involved
- Providing the extra time and support needed to help their child cope with the demands of the condition
- Having confidence in receiving support from other carers and professionals
- Finding time for themselves

Figure 112.2 Role of the children's nurse.

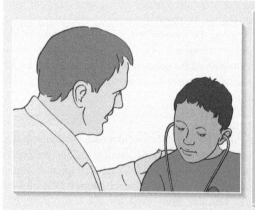

- Sensitive breaking of news to parents; helping parents to see their child as a unique individual who is a child first and the condition or disability as secondary
- Continuing to share evidence-based information at a pace that suits
- Helping the family to understand their emotional responses and coping strategies and coordinate specialist support as appropriate; ensuring sensitive and responsive family-centred care at times of challenge or crisis
- Acting as an advocate for the child; ensuring their rights are upheld and they are involved in decisions; working in partnership to prepare the child and family to deal with 'normal' life transitions as smoothly as possible; enabling the child or young person to self-manage their condition as far as they are able
- Collaborating with other professionals and services to ensure holistic family needs are met (e.g. regarding housing and finance)
- Planning ahead with the young person and family, enabling them to cope with transition from children's to adult services; ensuring well-coordinated and holistic end-of-life care and bereavement support as appropriate

Box 112.1 Emotion- and problem-focused coping strategies.

Emotion-focused coping strategies Dealing with *feelings* about the situation	• Not focusing on the condition; perspective seeking • Unburdening and explaining stress • Maintaining an image of the healthy child; normalizing • Thinking positively and clinging to hope • Taking one day at a time and staying calm • Seeing the child happy • Trusting others
Problem-focused coping strategies Dealing with child's *needs* *(adapted from Lazarus and Folkman 1984)*	• Being assertive; taking charge of situations; learning and understanding • Advocating for child • Maintaining family integrity • Talking to other families and developing social support networks • Cooperating with professionals; adhering to treatment • Sharing responsibilities

Definitions

Long-term conditions in childhood affect a relatively high proportion of the population. In England, it is thought that this group constitutes about 17% of the population. Globally the number is less clear. A long-term condition is a generic term that relates to a wide range of health conditions, including those that have a biological basis and consequent effects on the physical functioning of body systems; sensory or physical disabilities; conditions that impact on long-term mental health and wellbeing; and those that affect cognitive and psychological development, communication, and learning.

Children and Young People's Nursing at a Glance, Second Edition. Edited by Elizabeth Gormley-Fleming and Sheila Roberts.
© 2023 John Wiley & Sons Ltd. Published 2023 by John Wiley & Sons Ltd.

Some children and young people may be affected by more than one condition or disability or have symptoms that affect a number of body systems, leading to complexity in management, self-care, and appropriate support provision and development towards independence. Some conditions may be life-limiting and lead to early death.

Many conditions present at (or before) birth and others develop during childhood or the teenage years. Common features include the ongoing nature of the underlying disease; wide-ranging consequences for the life of the individual child and family; possible limitations in daily living requiring some care in hospital (with continuing care ideally provided at or closer to home); medication; dietary restrictions or special feeding regimes; special assistance, equipment, mobility aids, or adaptations at home. Living with uncertainty may also be a feature, for example for the parents of the toddler who has Down's syndrome who are unsure how the child will respond to heart surgery; for the boy who has haemophilia and is worried he may have a joint bleed during a PE lesson; for the teenage girl who has epilepsy and fears she may have a seizure while out at the cinema with friends; or for the young person who 'hears voices'.

Impact on the child and family

Learning that a child has a long-term or life-limiting condition will have a very significant effect on parents and must be handled with skill and sensitivity. The professionals involved must recognize that parents may be experiencing shock and grief and will need time and repeated opportunities to ask questions in order to be able to come to terms with the news. Implications may be far-reaching, affecting everyday routines, hopes and ambitions, and the relationships between family members (including siblings) and the outside world (Figure 112.1). These vary, for example from the child who has mild asthma that is well managed by the GP with few limitations on lifestyle, to the young person who has to learn to self-manage diabetes through daily injections of insulin, blood glucose monitoring, and a carefully controlled diet. More extensive restrictions will be experienced by children who are dependent on technologically complex equipment to sustain their lives, for example children who require dialysis or those who are dependent on assisted ventilation because of a complex breathing problem. Chronic illnesses also include mental health problems such as anorexia nervosa and potentially progressive or life-limiting conditions such as cystic fibrosis, muscular dystrophy, and leukaemia.

For many children and young people with more severe conditions, there will be numerous challenges: the management of symptoms; being active; maintaining optimal health and wellbeing despite limitations; exercising choice in how care is managed; and participating in as full a life as possible. Professionals will need to consider the support needed by a family learning to integrate the restrictions of disease and treatment with other, more routine aspects of their lives, recognizing the impact of a parent's anxiety about the child's condition and wellbeing and the child's right to as 'normal' a childhood as possible. The reactions and support of brothers and sisters and other family members will also be an important consideration.

Parents need to consider their own emotions, which will not only involve the initial shock and ongoing increased stress, but feelings of guilt. 'Why my child?' and 'What have I done to cause this?' are frequent questions parents ask. Financial implications may add to the stress: one parent may have to give up work to care for the sick child,

and more hospital visits bring additional costs in the form of travel and parking. Stress and guilt, along with a fear for the future, put additional strain on the relationship. Parents need to be able to understand that these feelings are normal (Box 112.1).

The impact on siblings of a child with a chronic illness should also not be overlooked. Siblings may go through a range of emotions such as feeling left out or jealous, when all the attention is focused on the sick child. They may feel guilty for being well or feel as if they are being punished for perhaps being unkind to their sibling. Emotions will vary depending on the child's age and their level of understanding. Their behavior may regress, such as bed-wetting or reverting to thumb sucking. Older siblings may have nightmares or behavioural issues at school. Adolescents may develop mental health issues such as eating disorders as a means to have some control over their lives. Siblings need to be included in all aspects of the sick child's life at home and during periods of hospitalization.

Child and young person first and foremost

According to the Children Act (2004), the child or young person with a chronic illness will be considered to be a child in need of additional support and will require ongoing coordinated services, perhaps involving a number of professionals and agencies working together to ensure that the child is safe, healthy, and achieving their full potential. The role of the children's nurse (Figure 112.2) is central in ensuring that children, young people, and families receive the most supportive, responsive, and empowering care possible and that this leads to optimal health, wellbeing, and development. It is important to remember that the child who has a chronic illness is a child first and foremost. They share the same rights as healthy children and have similar concerns: about their relationships with other children, siblings, and parents; fitting in; their ability to succeed; play and leisure interests; hopes, dreams, ambitions, and fears. Life course transitions such as moving from nursery, through school, to further or higher education and employment may present particular challenges. Friendships and intimate relationships, or establishing social and financial independence, may be more challenging for young people with chronic illness than their peers as they progress to young adulthood. Transition between services (for example paediatric clinic to adult services) will require a coordinated and carefully planned approach starting in the early teenage years, with consideration of all aspects of the young person's development and wellbeing. The current NHS Longer-Term Plan sets out transformational reforms to community-based care for children with long-term conditions. The aim is to improve outcomes for young people and reduce the demand on emergency hospital services.

Key points

- First and foremost, the child with a long-term or chronic illness is a child/young person.
- The impacts for the child of having a long-term condition are individual, but may include concerns for the future, everyday disruption to school and social life, and concerns with body image.
- The impact on the parents is also significant, with added stress and guilt.
- Siblings and other extended family members should not be forgotten.

113 Cystic fibrosis management

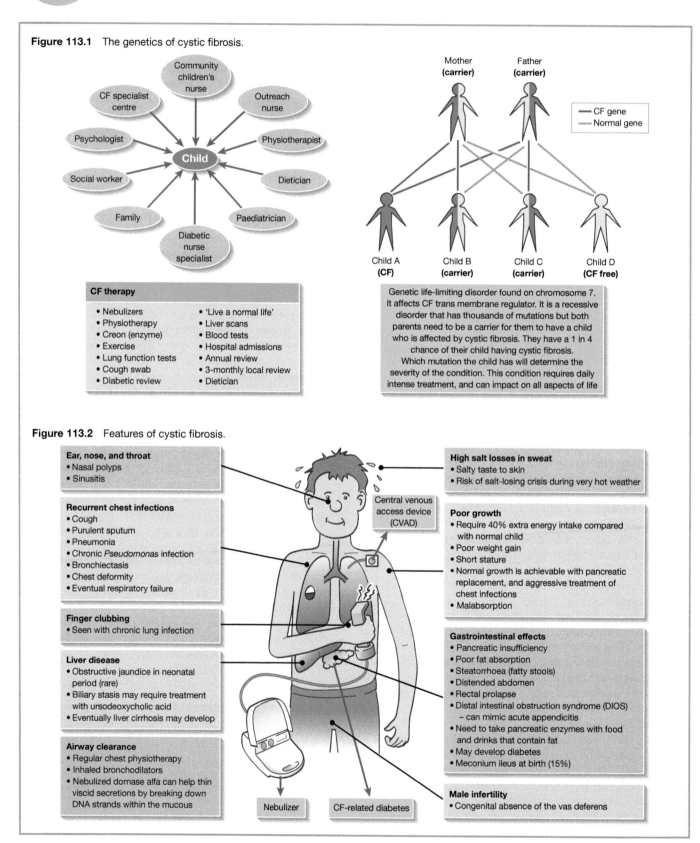

Figure 113.1 The genetics of cystic fibrosis.

CF therapy

- Nebulizers
- Physiotherapy
- Creon (enzyme)
- Exercise
- Lung function tests
- Cough swab
- Diabetic review
- 'Live a normal life'
- Liver scans
- Blood tests
- Hospital admissions
- Annual review
- 3-monthly local review
- Dietician

Genetic life-limiting disorder found on chromosome 7. It affects CF trans membrane regulator. It is a recessive disorder that has thousands of mutations but both parents need to be a carrier for them to have a child who is affected by cystic fibrosis. They have a 1 in 4 chance of their child having cystic fibrosis. Which mutation the child has will determine the severity of the condition. This condition requires daily intense treatment, and can impact on all aspects of life

Figure 113.2 Features of cystic fibrosis.

Ear, nose, and throat
- Nasal polyps
- Sinusitis

Recurrent chest infections
- Cough
- Purulent sputum
- Pneumonia
- Chronic *Pseudomonas* infection
- Bronchiectasis
- Chest deformity
- Eventual respiratory failure

Finger clubbing
- Seen with chronic lung infection

Liver disease
- Obstructive jaundice in neonatal period (rare)
- Biliary stasis may require treatment with ursodeoxycholic acid
- Eventually liver cirrhosis may develop

Airway clearance
- Regular chest physiotherapy
- Inhaled bronchodilators
- Nebulized dornase alfa can help thin viscid secretions by breaking down DNA strands within the mucous

Central venous access device (CVAD)

Nebulizer

CF-related diabetes

High salt losses in sweat
- Salty taste to skin
- Risk of salt-losing crisis during very hot weather

Poor growth
- Require 40% extra energy intake compared with normal child
- Poor weight gain
- Short stature
- Normal growth is achievable with pancreatic replacement, and aggressive treatment of chest infections
- Malabsorption

Gastrointestinal effects
- Pancreatic insufficiency
- Poor fat absorption
- Steatorrhoea (fatty stools)
- Distended abdomen
- Rectal prolapse
- Distal intestinal obstruction syndrome (DIOS) – can mimic acute appendicitis
- Need to take pancreatic enzymes with food and drinks that contain fat
- May develop diabetes
- Meconium ileus at birth (15%)

Male infertility
- Congenital absence of the vas deferens

Children and Young People's Nursing at a Glance, Second Edition. Edited by Elizabeth Gormley-Fleming and Sheila Roberts.
© 2023 John Wiley & Sons Ltd. Published 2023 by John Wiley & Sons Ltd.

Cystic fibrosis (CF) is one of the most common inherited (Figure 113.1) life-limiting conditions that impacts on the quality of life of a child and their family. The condition can affect multiple organs, not only the lungs. CF affects the transfer of salt between the cells, and where salt goes water follows via the process of osmosis. This alters the environment and effective motility within the organ. Earlier diagnosis improves prognosis.

Diagnosis of cystic fibrosis

Cystic fibrosis is diagnosed generally by either a positive test result in asymptomatic children, or other clinical manifestations supported by a positive sweat or genetic test, or by symptoms alone in the presence of a negative sweat or genetic test, although the latter is very rare (Figure 113.2). Screening of newborn babies for CF is now a routine part of neonatal blood spot screening and the majority of cases are diagnosed this way.

Children who present with the following should have an assessment that includes screening for CF:
- Meconium ileus.
- Recurrent chest infections.
- Chronic sinus disease.
- Congenital intestinal atresia.
- Distal bowel obstruction.
- Failure to thrive and malabsorption.

CF diagnosis can be confirmed via a sweat test, gene testing, or a stool sample. Further tests are required to determine the mutation and severity of the condition.

Common problems and management

Chest infections

The lining of the lungs is covered in thick, sticky mucous in CF patients, making it more difficult to clear the lungs of the mucous that contains bacteria and fungus. This leads to recurrent chest infections.

Pseudomonas aeruginosa is the most common fungal infection and causes scarring on the lung. It is hard to eradicate and so, once identified using a cough swab, lifelong treatment begins to suppress its growth and prevent scarring. Children with CF have daily prophylactic oral antibiotics to help prevent infection. Oral antibiotics are changed to a treatment regimen when the child becomes symptomatic. If the child remains unwell, they will require hospital admission for intravenous antibiotics. It is a constant battle to prevent infection and maintain lung function. Failure to do so results in scarring of the lungs and the eventual need for a lung transplant.

A daily intensive physiotherapy regime also helps to clear the lungs of mucous in conjunction with nebulizer therapy.

Pancreatic insufficiency

Some children with CF have a deficiency in breaking down fatty foods, which causes bowel obstructions. In the same way as their lung lining is thick and sticky, the gastric lining is also unable to pass food and break down any waste products. They produce foul-smelling sticky stools and require enzyme capsules (Creon) to aid in the digestion and absorption of vitamins and minerals. They require a high-calorie diet to meet their metabolic demands, as children with CF are constantly fighting infections. If they are unable to maintain a good weight, they may have a gastrostomy device fitted to enable artificial feeding directly into the stomach. They may also need additional salt in their diet to replace salts lost through sweating.

Cystic fibrosis–related diabetes

CF-related diabetes can develop as a result of blockages in the pancreas in the same way as the lungs become sticky and do not work efficiently. Some CF children require glucose monitoring and high blood sugars can be controlled by diet or insulin. Most patients with CF who go on to develop CF-related diabetes find it hard to fit blood glucose monitoring and insulin injections into an already hectic treatment regime. To have both CF and CF-related diabetes can be hard to come to terms with.

Liver

Liver damage can be caused in the same way as the lungs: the bile ducts become sticky and the liver can develop cirrhosis. Patients need annual liver scans to detect any liver damage early.

Infertility

Most men with CF will go on to have problems with infertility and may require interventions to conceive.

Women with CF can have problems with fertility, but most can go on to have children. They need to be monitored closely throughout their pregnancy.

Carriers of the CF gene are offered genetic counselling prior to starting a family when the risks are explained.

Impact on family

Diagnosis of CF is a life-changing event that impacts on all aspects of life. The treatment is not a cure, but compliance with all forms of treatment can extend life expectancy, currently 38 years.

Everything is a constant battle and young adults find it hard to comply with all the treatment, attending school, and taking control of their CF. Families struggle financially and parents become carers.

Segregation is required in CF clinics and on hospital wards to prevent cross-contamination. This helps to prevent infections, but results in CF being a very isolating condition where peer support is hard to obtain. Parents can mix but patients are advised not to.

Transitional preparation begins around the age of 10 years and is based on preparing the young person for independent living. Most hospital wards only cater for under-16-year-olds and so CF patients need to be prepared for taking ownership of the condition, learning their medication routine, and knowing when to seek medical interventions. This can be a hard time for everybody, as parents have to take a back seat and allow their child to take more control, which the child may not be ready for.

The burden and compliance with treatment are not only on the child or young person but on the whole family. Every day is impacted by CF, whether the child is unwell or not. Having a child with CF causes constant uncertainty. The biggest uncertainty for the child or young person and their family is living with a reduced life expectancy.

Box 113.1 Living with cystic fibrosis

The severity of CF is determined by the particular mutation. Therefore, treatment varies from daily oral antibiotics and physiotherapy, to nebulizers three times a day, intense physiotherapy, up to 20 different tablets throughout the day, Creon with every meal, and artificial feeds overnight. This is in conjunction with three-monthly admissions onto the ward for intravenous antibiotics for two weeks at a time, or sometimes three weeks. CF patients also attend regular clinics and undertake an annual assessment, which involves a whole day of tests and lung function monitoring. Patients with severe CF have 24-hour oxygen therapy and a long wait on the transplant list. The disease is a battle for survival and a normal life.

Key points

- Expertise and expert advice are required for the child and family who have a diagnosis of cystic fibrosis (Box 113.1).
- A shared care model of care is desirable, with specialist centre available to the child and family at all times.
- Conversation about transition to adult services needs to start as early as possible, ideally in the pre-teenage years.

114 Juvenile idiopathic arthritis

Figure 114.1 Juvenile idiopathic arthritis.

Criteria for diagnosis of juvenile idiopathic arthritis (JIA)

- Patient under 16 years
- Arthritis (joint swelling or effusion) or two of the following: limitation of range of movement; tenderness or pain on motion; increased heat in joint
- Duration of 6 weeks or longer
- Exclusion of other causes

Diagnosis is on clinical findings. Antinuclear antibodies, rheumatoid factor, human leukocyte antigen typing, or ultrasound aid assessment. X-ray and MRI may be considered

Possible complications

- Joint contractures
- Growth failure
- Leg length discrepancy
- Osteoporosis
- Joint damage requiring replacement
- Blindness from associated uveitis
- Scoliosis (secondary)
- Macrophage activation syndrome and amyloidosis (rare)

Many complications have been shown to be avoided with early recognition and aggressive treatment

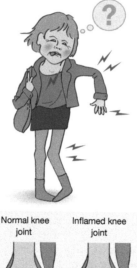

Normal knee joint   Inflamed knee joint

Treatment

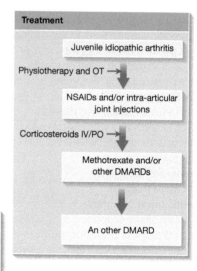

Juvenile idiopathic arthritis

Physiotherapy and OT →

NSAIDs and/or intra-articular joint injections

Corticosteroids IV/PO →

Methotrexate and/or other DMARDs

An other DMARD

Effects of arthritis on joints

- Synovitis
- Pannus formation
- Cartilage and bone erosion

Paediatric rheumatology team

- Consultant
- Specialist nurse
- Physiotherapist
- Occupational therapist (OT)
- Ophthalmologist
- Psychologist
- Orthotist
- Play specialist

Differential diagnosis

- Biomechanical joint pain
- Reactive/post-infectious arthritis
- Septic arthritis/osteomyelitis
- Trauma/haematological disorders
- Malignancy including leukaemia, lymphoma
- Pain problems

Triangle of care

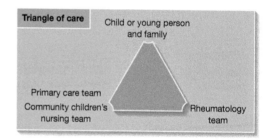

Child or young person and family

Primary care team
Community children's nursing team

Rheumatology team

Disease subtypes	Classification (research purposes)
Oligoarticular JIA (previously known as pauciarticular)	Up to four joints in first 6 months of disease (usually larger joints, e.g. knees, ankles, and wrists). After 6 months if more than four joints become affected, classified as extended oligoarticular, or if arthritis remains in fewer than four joints classified as persistent oligoarticular. More common in females (5 : 1)
Polyarticular JIA	Affects five or more joints during the first 6 months of disease. Often includes involvement of large and small joints; may have symmetrical pattern. Classified as rheumatoid factor negative or positive. More common in females (3 : 1)
Systemic-onset JIA (previously known as Still's disease)	Arthritis in one or more joints (may not be present initially) with 2-week history of fever (usually quotidian), and one or more of the following: evanescent erythematous rash; lymphadenopathy; hepatosplenomegaly or serositis. Equal incidence in males and females (1 : 1)
Psoriatic arthritis	Arthritis and psoriatic rash or if no evidence of rash, arthritis, and at least two of the following symptoms: dactylitis; nail pitting; psoriasis in a first-degree relative. Arthritis is usually asymmetrical
Enthesitis-related arthritis	Arthritis with enthesitis (inflammation where tendons or ligaments attach to bone), or enthesitis with at least two of the following: sacroiliac tenderness and/or lumbosacral pain; presence of HLA B27 antigen; onset of arthritis in a male over 6 years of age; acute anterior uveitis; family history of HLA B27-associated disease. Most common site is calcaneal insertion of Achilles, tendon, plantar fascia, and tarsal area
Undifferentiated arthritis	Arthritis does not fulfil any of the above subtypes. Can occur with arthritis-associated conditions (e.g. inflammatory bowel disease)

DMARD, disease-modifying anti-rheumatic drugs; IV, intravenous; MRI, magnetic resonance imaging; NSAID, non-steroidal anti-inflammatory drug; PO, per os (orally).

Children and Young People's Nursing at a Glance, Second Edition. Edited by Elizabeth Gormley-Fleming and Sheila Roberts.
© 2023 John Wiley & Sons Ltd. Published 2023 by John Wiley & Sons Ltd.

Juvenile idiopathic arthritis (JIA) is a term used to describe a group of autoimmune diseases characterized by arthritis. The UK prevalence is 1 in 1000. Subtypes devised by the Paediatric Standing Committee of the International League for Rheumatology (ILAR) are described in Figure 114.1.

Patient history characteristically includes reports of morning stiffness with gradual improvement during the day. Increasing pain with activity in the absence of morning stiffness is usually indicative of a biomechanical problem. Active joints are typically painful on active or passive movement and can be swollen and warm. Other symptoms include fatigue, increased sleep requirements, increased irritability, loss of appetite, and weight loss. These are more common in polyarticular or systemic disease.

Although the ultimate aim of treatment is to obtain disease remission, many children will continue to have flares of arthritis, so with persistent disease the aim may be to decrease the frequency of flares.

Joints commonly affected are:
* Jaw 30%
* Neck 10–40%
* Shoulder 50–60%
* Elbow 50%
* Wrist 80%

Management

Aims of management are to prevent joint damage and to maintain joint function in order to promote independence and improve quality of life.

Exercise and physiotherapy are important aspects of treatment, aiming to prevent complications by maintaining full joint range of movement, improve muscle strength, and prevent reduction in cardiovascular fitness. Educating families and professionals involved in the child's care about exercise is vital to minimize exclusion from activities and isolation from peers. Children with JIA may have trouble with balance and will often have weaker motor skills. This means they have less control over large muscle groups, so strengthening muscle through exercise and activities is important.

In younger children, it is important to ensure that normal developmental milestones are met. Education should also prepare them for the possibility of disease flares and consider pain relief, support, and advice for management during these periods.

Occupational therapy support and advice may be required for children with multiple joint involvement, including joints of wrists and hands. Therapists can provide handwriting assessment and advice for exams. They can also liaise with schools and provide information and guidance for teachers about how children can be supported in school to reach their full potential.

Pharmacological management varies depending on the severity of disease (see the treatment flow chart in Figure 114.1). Medication is divided into two categories: drugs that relieve symptoms and drugs that are referred to as disease-modifying anti-rheumatic drugs (DMARDs). Non-steroidal anti-inflammatory drugs (NSAIDs) and intra-articular steroid injections may adequately control oligoarticular disease, but when multiple joints are involved or if the arthritis reoccurs after joint injection, long-term therapy may be required. Methotrexate is the first-choice drug, but if ineffective or not tolerated then other DMARDs including biologic drugs are required. Steroids (intra-articular, intravenous, or orally) can provide short-term relief or bridging until longer-term therapy becomes effective. All drugs used require appropriate monitoring. Support and advice are usually provided by the specialist centre; shared care protocols may facilitate local support for prescribing, administering, and monitoring, to minimize disruption to school and family life.

Many children will not require surgery, but a small percentage will. Surgery is usually required to enable improved joint functions, for instance arthroscopies. However, some children will require full joint replacements.

Specialist nurses have a pivotal role in coordinating care, holistic assessment and education, psychosocial support, drug advice, and monitoring and liaising with primary and secondary care teams.

Key points

* Juvenile arthritis is the most common rheumatic disease of childhood and a major cause of disability.
* Each form of arthritis – systemic, poly-, and pauci- – has its own distinctive features.
* The main aim of management is twofold: to preserve joint function and to help the child achieve optimal psychosocial acceptance of their disease.

115 Epilepsy

Figure 115.1 Features of epilepsy.

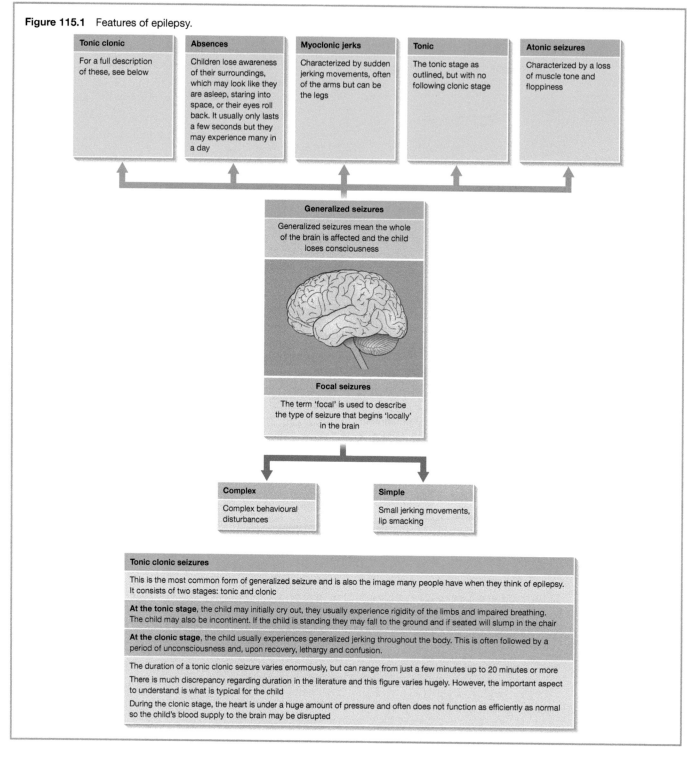

Tonic clonic

For a full description of these, see below

Absences

Children lose awareness of their surroundings, which may look like they are asleep, staring into space, or their eyes roll back. It usually only lasts a few seconds but they may experience many in a day

Myoclonic jerks

Characterized by sudden jerking movements, often of the arms but can be the legs

Tonic

The tonic stage as outlined, but with no following clonic stage

Atonic seizures

Characterized by a loss of muscle tone and floppiness

Generalized seizures

Generalized seizures mean the whole of the brain is affected and the child loses consciousness

Focal seizures

The term 'focal' is used to describe the type of seizure that begins 'locally' in the brain

Complex

Complex behavioural disturbances

Simple

Small jerking movements, lip smacking

Tonic clonic seizures

This is the most common form of generalized seizure and is also the image many people have when they think of epilepsy. It consists of two stages: tonic and clonic

At the tonic stage, the child may initially cry out, they usually experience rigidity of the limbs and impaired breathing. The child may also be incontinent. If the child is standing they may fall to the ground and if seated will slump in the chair

At the clonic stage, the child usually experiences generalized jerking throughout the body. This is often followed by a period of unconsciousness and, upon recovery, lethargy and confusion.

The duration of a tonic clonic seizure varies enormously, but can range from just a few minutes up to 20 minutes or more

There is much discrepancy regarding duration in the literature and this figure varies hugely. However, the important aspect to understand is what is typical for the child

During the clonic stage, the heart is under a huge amount of pressure and often does not function as efficiently as normal so the child's blood supply to the brain may be disrupted

Epilepsy is the most common chronic disabling neurological condition and is where a child has repeated seizures. Seizures occur in the brain and occur when the function of the brain is interrupted or becomes 'disordered'.

It is reported that approximately 1 in 131 people in the general population experiences epilepsy, but it is more common in the learning disabled population, where the prevalence is approximately 1 in 3 and this figure increases as the severity of the learning disability increases.

Everyone has the potential to have a seizure at different times in their lives and many people do due to illnesses or accidents. One seizure would not result in a diagnosis of epilepsy; a person would experience two or more seizures prior to receiving a diagnosis of epilepsy. Of those who experience epilepsy, approximately 5% will have photosensitive epilepsy. This is where seizures can be triggered by flashing lights.

Symptomatic epilepsy can be caused by any damage to the brain. This can be a result of central nervous system (CNS) infections such as meningitis or encephalitis, tumours, neurosurgery, or head injury. Many people have idiopathic epilepsy, which means it arises spontaneously and the specific cause is unknown.

Seizures

During a seizure a person may experience changes in awareness, involuntary movement, or confused behaviours. The clinical presentation (what the seizure looks like) depends on a number of factors:
- Part or parts of the brain affected.
- Pattern of spread of the disordered activity through the brain.
- Cause of the epilepsy.
- Age of the individual.

There are approximately 40 different seizure types, so just knowing that a child has epilepsy does not really tell you much about what they experience or what a seizure will look like. To understand that, we need to know more about what type of seizure the child has. Although there are 40 different seizure types, they are usually divided in two main groups: generalized and focal seizures (Figure 115.1).

Generalized seizures

Generalized seizures mean that the whole of the brain is affected and the child loses consciousness. It is really important to remember this, that the child is unconscious during the seizure – although in some cases what we see may seem small and insignificant, this is not what the child is experiencing.

Focal seizures

The term focal is used within the literature to describe a type of seizure that begins 'locally' in the brain, in other words in one part of the brain. Focal seizures are often categorized as simple or complex. This type of seizure occurs without loss of consciousness; however, consciousness may be impaired and the child will not be in control of what is happening. Although focal seizures can originate anywhere, the most common sites are the frontal and temporal lobes.

Focal seizures can result in the person experiencing abnormalities of taste, smell, auditory and visual hallucinations, changes in pallor, or small jerking movements of the limb. Simple focal seizures generally last less than one minute. The child's muscles are more commonly affected, so the seizure is often limited to an isolated muscle group. The child may also present with strange mutterings and lip smacking. If the occipital lobe is involved, for example, the child may have altered vision temporarily. Additionally, in some cases focal seizures can manifest as complex behavioural disturbances.

Complex focal seizures

Some children experience complex focal seizures. The temporal lobe of the brain is more commonly affected. This section of the brain controls emotion and memory function. A variety of behaviours may occur, including screaming, running, strange mutterings, crying, laughing, and lip smacking. These generally last between one and two minutes and consciousness may be lost. The child is typically sleepy post seizure, and this is referred to as being post ictal.

Treatment

Antiepileptic drugs taken on a daily basis are always the first-line treatment option for children with epilepsy, but becoming seizure free can be a long process with a range of medication combinations being trialled. This can be a frustrating time for the child and their family and can take many years. Even after several years of medication combinations, some people are unable to control their epilepsy and this is referred to as chronic or refractory epilepsy. To enable effective medication regimens, accurate recording of seizure activity is vital.

Status epilepticus

Normally, when a child has a seizure they will recover naturally and the seizure will end of its own accord. However, sometimes this is not the case – this is called status epilepticus. Status epilepticus is when the seizure is longer than normal for that child or the child has several seizures straight after each other. Status epilepticus is an emergency situation, as the child is unconscious and the blood supply to the brain can be affected and lead to brain damage.

The medication used in the management of status epilepticus is dependent on whether there is established vascular access (Table 115.1).
- *Diazepam*: most commonly given rectally.
- *Lorazepam*: given intravenously, usually in hospital.
- *Midazolam*: increasingly being given via the buccal route, as this is preferred by carers and the person with epilepsy alike because of the less invasive nature of administration.

Although epilepsy is a chronic condition (meaning that people live with it all their lives and do not 'get better'), some children appear to grow out of it, in that their brains develop their own defences. Even if a child does not, there are a wide range of treatment options available and 70% of people with epilepsy have their seizures controlled with medication. Most children with epilepsy live a full and happy life.

Table 115.1	Medication for status epilepticus.	
Time frame	**Intravenous or intraosseous vascular access**	**No vascular access**
Step 1: 5 min after start of convulsion	Lorazepam	Buccal midazolam or rectal diazepam
Step 2: usually 10 min after start or step 1	Lorazepam Prepare phenytoin. If already on phenytoin, prepare phenobarbitone	Paraldehyde – rectal administration as an option
Step 3: 10 min after step 2	Prepare phenytoin. If already on phenytoin, prepare phenobarbitone. Administer as an infusion over 20 min	
Step 4: 20 min after step 3	If still fitting, anaesthetist must be present as may need advanced airway protection – rapid sequence intubation (RSI)	

Key points
- Epilepsy is classified into generalized seizures and focal seizures.
- The majority of children with epilepsy will be idiopathic; that is, the epilepsy is of unknown cause.
- Epilepsy is generally diagnosed on history alone.
- Knowing the function of the different lobes of the brain will indicate the altered behavior of the child during their seizure.

116 Childhood cancer

Figure 116.1 Childhood cancer.

> Cancer is a group of diseases that share common characteristics: uncontrolled cell growth following a genetic mutation

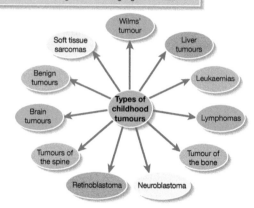

Types of childhood tumours:
- Wilms' tumour
- Liver tumours
- Leukaemias
- Lymphomas
- Tumour of the bone
- Neuroblastoma
- Retinoblastoma
- Tumours of the spine
- Brain tumours
- Benign tumours
- Soft tissue sarcomas

Childhood cancer: the facts

- Cancer in childhood is rare
- Approximately 1700 children in the UK are diagnosed with cancer each year
- Survival has improved from less than 30% in 1962–1971 to about 75%
- Cancer is the leading cause of death from disease in children and the second cause of death from all causes
- Leukaemia is the most common form of childhood cancer, followed by brain tumours
- Improved survival rates have been attributed to multimodal treatments, a centralized approach to treatment, and involvement in clinical trials

Treating childhood cancer

Treatments involve one or more of the following:

- **Surgery:** to excise solid tumour
- **Chemotherapy:** use of cytotoxic agents to eradicate cancer cells, shrink tumour before surgery, or for palliative control
- **Radiotherapy:** uses radiation to target tumour cells, or total body irradiation before transplantation
- Children in the UK are treated in specialized regional cancer centres
- Care is often shared with local hospitals
- Protocols are standardized through the Children's Cancer and Leukaemia Group (CCLG)
- Duration and combination of treatment modalities are dependent on the child's diagnosis
- **Proton therapy:** proton beam therapy is a type of radiotherapy that uses protons to target cancer cells. It targets the tumour precisely and minimizes damage to the surrounding tissues
- **Immunotherapy:** immunotherapy comes in many different forms and harnesses the body's own immune system to fight cancer

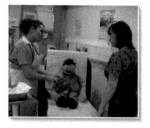

Adverse effects of systemic anti-cancer therapy

Immediate: nausea/vomiting, fatigue, allergic reactions, haemorrhagic cystitis

Short term: alopecia, stomatitis, myelosuppression, immunosuppression, gastrointestinal disturbances

Long term: infertility, growth retardation, secondary cancers, cardiomyopathy

Principles of care

- Centralized approach through CCLG
- Holistic care – biological, psychosocial, and spiritual
- Evidence-based care
- Child- and famil-centred approach to care
- Interdisciplinary approach
- Integrated model of care
- Cure with least cost to child
- Long-term follow-up

Assessing and addressing the needs of the child and family

Assessment of need is an ongoing process for the nurse caring for the child with cancer and their family, occurring throughout each stage of the illness trajectory. Such need centres on the following areas:

- Physical
- Emotional
- Cognitive
- Social
- Spiritual

Care of the child receiving systemic anti-cancer therapy

- Information regarding drugs and adverse effects
- Administration of chemotherapy usually via central line
- Minimizing and monitoring adverse effects
- Treatment of adverse effects
- Educating the child and family about minimizing and monitoring adverse effects, safe handling of bodily waste
- Preparation of the child for care during and after investigations (e.g. biopsy, lumbar puncture, MRI/CT scan)
- Supportive care for child (e.g. treating neutropenia, thrombocytopenia, and anaemia, with intravenous antibiotics), mouth care, blood or platelet transfusions

Team players – the child with cancer and their family

Quality care for the child or young person with cancer must be multidisciplinary:

- Oncologist/haematologist
- Psychologist
- Teacher
- Play specialist
- Nurse (CCN, specialist, clinic, ward)
- Radiologist
- Dietitian
- Physiotherapist/occupational therapist
- Dentist
- Doctor
- Laboratory staff
- Pharmacist
- Other families, children
- Voluntary organization
- Social worker
- Hospital chaplain
- Paediatric surgeon

CCN, critical care nurse; CT, computerized tomography; MRI, magnetic resonance imaging

Children and Young People's Nursing at a Glance, Second Edition. Edited by Elizabeth Gormley-Fleming and Sheila Roberts.
© 2023 John Wiley & Sons Ltd. Published 2023 by John Wiley & Sons Ltd.

Despite improved survival over the last few decades, the diagnosis of a childhood cancer is a life-altering experience for the child and their family. As the child and family adapt their daily life around the child's condition and necessary treatment, they find themselves in a period of sustained uncertainty in which they hope for cure, but are also conscious of the ever-present threat of death. Therefore, child- and family-centred care from the point of diagnosis of a childhood cancer is paramount and requires a skilled multidisciplinary team, which involves both statutory and voluntary services. The children's nurse has a crucial multifaceted role within this multidisciplinary team (Figure 116.1).

Nurse as supporter

On diagnosis, parents can experience a multitude of emotions: devastation, grief, fear, disbelief, and denial. The child or young person also faces a number of feelings: lack of understanding, uncertainty, fear, and anger. Emotional support from the nurse is imperative during this time in order to help the patient and family members develop coping strategies to manage the impact that a diagnosis of cancer and its subsequent treatment will have. This impact can be overwhelming and have an effect upon their psychological, social, financial, and relationship issues. The nurse is often present while the child and family initially hear of the diagnosis. Therefore, the nurse has an integral role in ensuring information is given in a way that is easily comprehended by everyone involved. Such information provides a platform for decision making and may help to combat some of the stress, anxiety, and feelings of helplessness often experienced by parents.

Play, as a communication tool, can help the child and siblings express fear and anxieties. It is also a useful mode for imparting information about treatment and care. Play therapists/specialists can facilitate this communication and play a vital role by voicing the child's concerns and wishes to the rest of the multidisciplinary team.

By assessing on an ongoing basis and recognizing key periods within the illness trajectory, the nurse can establish how the child and family is coping, subsequently providing the required care or referral to specialist support as necessary (e.g. psychologist).

Nurse as physical care provider

Nursing roles have expanded significantly during the last few decades and the administration of systemic anti-cancer therapy has become a central tenet of the children's cancer nurse's role. In order to administer this treatment, nurses must follow the appropriate specialized training. Alongside this, the nurse is responsible for the assessment, recording, and reporting of the child's physical condition to the medical team, thus enabling an appropriate plan of care. Assessment involves regular recording of temperature, pulse, respirations, blood pressure, fluid balance, weight, urinalysis, elimination, and skin assessment. These are all of paramount importance to the care of the child and requires the nurse to possess a comprehensive understanding of children's cancer, the drug-specific adverse effects that may be encountered, and how to act accordingly to these.

The prompt identification of untoward symptoms and subsequent implementation of appropriate care are vital to the success of supportive treatment. Supportive treatment is necessary as the chemotherapy not only affects fast-growing tumour cells, but the body's normally occurring fast-growing cells: healthy blood cells made within the bone marrow; haemoglobin; white blood cells; and platelets. Deficiency of these cells within the body contributes to major adverse effects for the child, including haemorrhage, lethargy, and fatal sepsis due to lack of infection-fighting cells. During neutropenic (very low neutrophils) sepsis episodes, prompt administration of intravenous antibiotics is required. Antipyretics, blood product transfusions, and nutritional support are also essential elements of care to prevent a catastrophic adverse event for the child and family.

In some patients granulocyte colony-stimulating factor (GCSF, a growth hormone used to help the body produce white blood cells and therefore fight infection) may be used; however, this is contraindicated in leukaemia patients due to their disease originating from these cells within the bone marrow. Fast-growing cells also include mucosal epithelial cells, which line the mouth through the gastrointestinal tract to the anus. Destruction of these cells by systemic anti-cancer therapy commonly leads to electrolyte imbalances and gastrointestinal disturbances, alongside increasing the risk of localizing infections. Furthermore, the control of symptoms due to drug administration or disease is also a focus of care for the children's nurse. The administration of antiemetics, analgesia, and other supportive interventions including parental and total parental nutrition helps to control these adverse effects, promoting optimum comfort for the child.

Nurse as teacher and educator

The children's nurse must ensure that any teaching carried out is family centred, considering any factors that would influence the family's ability to learn and understand the condition prior to discharge. Teaching involves identifying the signs and symptoms of anaemia and thrombocytopenia and how to act appropriately, identifying the signs of infection and how to act upon these appropriately, the safe handling of bodily fluids post systemic anti-cancer therapy; mouth care and assessing the mucosal membrane; safety in the sun; and the importance of reducing exposure to infection by limiting contact with crowds. Families must also fully understand the child's medications and their side effects.

Given the family-centred approach to care, families may choose to participate in technical aspects of care (e.g. care of their child's central line or nasogastric tube). A nurse-led teaching programme may be carried out where parents are supported in the attainment of necessary skills if it is deemed appropriate. The nurse educates parents and assesses their ability to learn new skills to care for their child. Teaching and education are a continuous process rather than a one-off activity. A parent's ability to retain the knowledge and skills should be reassessed as appropriate.

Nurse as team player

A diverse multidisciplinary team of professionals, each with their own specific expertise, provides care to the child with cancer and their family. The composition of the team for each individual child differs according to their diagnosis, condition at any given particular time, location, and specific family needs. Members of the multidisciplinary team include professionals from both statutory and voluntary organizations. Voluntary organizations have an invaluable role in supporting the child with cancer and their family. Given the amount of time spent with the child and family, nurses often have an in-depth insight into the child's and family's situation at a given time. Nurses must share their knowledge and maintain good levels of communication with the team to ensure the best possible care is provided.

Key points

- Children's nurses caring for children with cancer and their families must utilize a wide range of skills.
- Compassionate, holistic care must be tailored to the unique needs of each child and their family.
- A broad range of interpersonal skills is crucial, including the ability to build a therapeutic relationship with the child and family, to use age-appropriate language with the child and siblings, and to promote communication within families and among the whole multidisciplinary team.

117 Cleft lip and palate

Figure 117.1 Cleft lip and palate.

Cleft lip and palate can occur as a single abnormality or in association with other congenital abnormalities as part of a syndrome

Incidence
Approximately 1000 babies are born in the UK each year affected by a cleft lip and/or palate, an incidence of about 1 in 700 live births

Aetiology
- The fusion of the lip and palate happens early in pregnancy (4–11 weeks)
- A cleft lip or palate occurs as failure of this fusion
- A cleft lip can be detected on the 20-week antenatal scan

Causes and contributing factors
- Not known in most cases
- Can happen when a number of genetic and environmental factors occur together
- Smoking
- Alcohol intake during pregnancy
- Medicines taken during pregnancy
- Family history of cleft
- Use of recreational drugs during pregnancy

Associated problems
- Over 400 syndromes associated with cleft
- More likely to occur with an isolated cleft palate (50%)

Most common
- Pierre Robin sequence
- 22q deletion
- Stickler syndrome
- Van der Woude syndrome

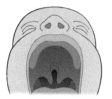

Cleft of the soft palate

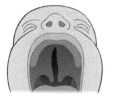

Cleft of the soft and hard palate

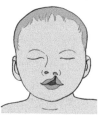

Incomplete cleft

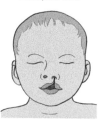

Complete cleft lip

Types of cleft

Types of cleft palate
- Hard palate
- Soft palate
- Hard and soft palate
- Submucous cleft palate

Cleft palate
- Up to 50% of births will be an isolated cleft palate, which can involve the hard palate, soft palate, or both
- This type of cleft is more common in girls

Submucous cleft palate
Occurs when the skin of the palate is intact but there is a cleft of the underlying muscle

Types of cleft lip
- **Complete:** up into the nose
- **Incomplete:** part of the lip
- **Unilateral:** one side
- **Bilateral:** both sides

Cleft lip
Approximately 20% of referrals will be an isolated cleft lip with or without a cleft of the alveolus (gum)

Cleft lip and palate
- Accounts for approximately 35% of births
- More common in boys
- 25% unilateral
- 10% bilateral

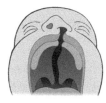

Unilateral cleft lip and palate

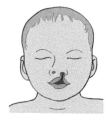

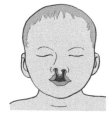

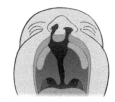

Bilateral cleft lip and palette

Orofacial cleft anomalies comprise a range of clefts, including the more common types of clefts, cleft lip, cleft palate, and combined cleft lip and palate (Figure 117.1). Atypical clefts are also part of this group and these include median, transverse, and oblique clefts. Cleft lip and palate is the most common facial anomaly in babies, and varies in frequency according to racial or ethnic group. The prevalence of cleft lip and palate is highest in native Indians, followed by Chinese and Japanese communities. It is lowest in those from the Afro-Caribbean and the Māori.

Cleft lip may be unilateral or bilateral. The line of the cleft always commences from the lateral aspect of the upper lip and continues through the philtrum to the alveolus between the second incisor and the canine tooth, up to the incisive foramen. A cleft anterior to the incisive foramen is a cleft of primary palate. There is a wide range in severity of a cleft lip.

Cleft palate is etiologically and embryologically different from cleft lip. Both the soft and hard palate and the uvula may be involved in the most severe cases. In the majority of cases, the cleft

Children and Young People's Nursing at a Glance, Second Edition. Edited by Elizabeth Gormley-Fleming and Sheila Roberts.
© 2023 John Wiley & Sons Ltd. Published 2023 by John Wiley & Sons Ltd.

of the hard palate is covered by a mucosal layer, and this continues through to the soft palate. This is referred to as a submucosal cleft. Careful examination of the newborn is required to correctly diagnose cleft palate and early referral to specialist services is required.

Cleft services

Cleft lip and palate is managed by a multidisciplinary team, including clinical nurse specialists, paediatricians, surgeons, speech and language therapists, physiologists, and orthodontists. Nine regional networks exist in the UK to facilitate high standards of care based on a hub-and-spoke principle.

Support and management

Patients with cleft and their families are seen according to nationally agreed standards and care pathways from birth until adulthood. Treatment includes surgical repair of the lip and/or palate, usually in the first year of life. Further treatment includes speech and language therapy, and hearing and dental interventions.

Common problems and their management

Feeding management

In an infant without cleft, the uvula and epiglottis lie adjacent to each other, which allows fluid to pool safely in the hyperpharynx or oropharynx until the swallowing reflex is triggered. In infants with cleft, the anatomical differences prevent this safety mechanism, resulting in the risk of aspiration if inappropriately fed.

Babies born with a cleft present with a range of feeding difficulties. Poor feeding and growth can lead to increased parental anxiety. The most notable difficulties are insufficient suction, excessive air intake, choking, nasal regurgitation, fatigue, inadequate milk intake, and extended feeding duration. The use of soft bottles allows the delivery of milk to the infant who is unable to generate suction to gain adequate nutrition (assisted feeding). Exclusive breastfeeding of these infants may not be possible and many mothers choose to give expressed breast milk.

Although the Department of Health guidelines state that milk alone is a sufficient food for babies up to 6 months of age, babies with cleft may be ready for weaning foods before this age. While weaning foods are not recommended for infants under 17 weeks, most babies enjoy a variety of consistencies prior to the repair of the cleft palate.

Missed diagnosis

There is a 23% incidence of missed diagnosis of a cleft palate in the first 24 hours of birth. This highlights the inadequacy of digital examination of the palate and identifies the importance of visualizing the palate with a spatula and light through to a single uvula. Late diagnosis can result in dehydration, readmission to hospital, faltering growth, increased parental anxiety, early cessation of breastfeeding, and litigation.

Otitis media with effusion

Otis media with effusion is almost universal in children with a cleft palate. This high incidence is attributed to eustachian tube dysfunction associated with anatomical and physiological variations of the tensor veli palatini muscle. This results in an accumulation of fluid in the middle ear causing a conductive hearing loss. The treatment includes the insertion of grommets and the use of hearing aids.

Speech

It is recognized that children with a cleft palate are at high risk of both speech disorders and language delay. Approximately 40% of children will require speech and language therapy.

Syndromes

There are over 400 syndromes associated with cleft lip and palate, with approximately 15% of cases affected. The most frequent are associated with an isolated cleft palate, with up to 50% having a congenital abnormality or syndrome.

Pierre robin sequence

Pierre Robin sequence (PRS) is the most common anomaly associated with cleft palate. It may occur on its own or part of a syndrome, with Stickler syndrome and 22q deletion being the most common. PRS includes the presence of a cleft palate, micrognathia (small jaw), and glossoptosis (a retroverted retroplaced tongue), resulting in respiratory obstruction, which presents on a continuum of severity. The treatment of the obstruction includes positioning, nasopharyngeal airways, and continuous positive airway pressure (CPAP).

Reparative surgery for lip and palate

Surgical repair of the lip is undertaken at 3–6 months and repair of the palate at 6–9 months of age. The displaced muscles of the lip and palate are surgically repositioned and joined together. In clefts of or including the hard palate, the palatal shelves are brought together. Further surgery on the palate may be undertaken at 3–9 years of age to improve speech outcomes.

Alveolar bone graft

For clefts involving the alveolus (gum), a bone graft is undertaken at approximately 7–9 years of age.

Postoperative care

The main issues following surgery are breathing, feeding, and pain relief. The main emphasis is directed towards protecting the repair, monitoring for excessive bleeding, ensuring adequate hydration, and maintaining the airway.

Airway management

Postoperative swelling can result from oedema and the presence of blood or exudate in the respiratory tract. Problems can be caused by an infant used to a large airway coping with a smaller one. Signs of airway difficulties are 'sucking in' of the lower lip on inspiration and sternal, intercostal, or subcostal recession. Distress should be acted on promptly, as these infants can deteriorate rapidly. Some will benefit from the insertion of nasal airways.

Adequate pain relief is important for both pain management and to facilitate feeding and adequate hydration.

Key points
- Maintaining normal growth in an infant with cleft lip and palate is an essential part of their management, so parents will need teaching on positioning and the use of feeding tools to achieve adequate nutrition and hydration.
- Parental support is an essential aspect of the children's nurse's role, as the family need to be able to verbalize their emotions and fears.
- Good pain management is essential after repair of cleft lip and palate.

118 Diabetes

Figure 118.1 Type 1 diabetes.

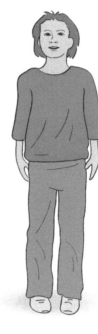

Type 1 diabetes

- Acute presentation due to rapid onset of symptoms over several days or weeks
- Prevalence in children is 1 in 700–1000
- Peak age for diagnosis is 10–14 years; 4% increase in incidence annually, particularly in under-5-year-olds

Diagnosis

- Fasting plasma glucose ≥7 mmol
- 2-hour post-prandial level ≥11.1 mmol
- Polyuria
- Polydipsia
- Weight loss
- Tiredness

Diabetic ketoacidosis (DKA)

- Serious life-threatening complication
- Presence of ketones
- Hyperglycaemia
- Vomiting and dehydration
- Abdominal pain
- Polydipsia, polyuria
- Kussmaul respiration
- Weight loss

Complications

- DKA
- Hyperglycaemia/hypoglycaemia
- Nephropathy
- Neuropathy
- Retinopathy
- Hyperlipidaemia

Hypoglycaemia

- Blood glucose ≤3.9 mmol or below; '4 is the floor'
- Possible causes: missed meals, exercise, alcohol, and too much insulin
- Confirmed by blood glucose testing
- Symptom awareness important and prompt treatment is needed
- *Neuroglycopenic*: confusion, irritability, headache, slurred speech, dizziness
- *Adrenergic*: sweating, shakiness, paleness, anxiety, palpitations, hunger
- *Mild:* symptoms recognized and successfully treated with fast-acting and starchy carbohydrate
- *Moderate:* assistance required, consider Glucogel if conscious, but airway concerns
- *Severe:* loss of consciousness, risk of seizure, coma, and death, give intramuscular glucagon
- Over-treating can result in rebound hyperglycaemia
- Fear can develop, especially regarding nocturnal episodes
- If glycaemic control is good, loss of hypoglycaemia awareness can occur
- Symptoms can occur ≥4 mmol or above if glycaemic control is poor or blood glucose level is falling quickly

Hyperglycaemia

- Fasting blood glucose >7 mmol or 2-hour post-prandial level of ≥11.1 mmol
- Symptoms include polyuria, polydipsia, tiredness, abdominal pain, behaviour change, lack of concentration
- Causes include insufficient insulin, growth spurts, omitted doses, snacking, interaction from other medications, illness, infection, reduced exercise, stress, unhealthy injection sites, if an insulin pump is used there can be problems with insulin delivery
- Increased frequency of blood glucose testing advised
- Test for blood ketones if blood glucose ≥14 mmol; frequency of testing level dependent
- Utilize correction factor
- Use sick day rules advice if concurrent illness, never stop insulin
- Management different if using insulin pump

Children and Young People's Nursing at a Glance, Second Edition. Edited by Elizabeth Gormley-Fleming and Sheila Roberts.
© 2023 John Wiley & Sons Ltd. Published 2023 by John Wiley & Sons Ltd.

Type 1 diabetes mellitus is a chronic irreversible condition resulting from a lack of insulin caused by autoimmune destruction of pancreatic beta cells; underlying triggers for this are not yet identified. Early recognition of signs and symptoms is essential (Figure 118.1), as insulin insufficiency results in hyperglycaemia and, if undiagnosed, the life-threatening complication of diabetic ketoacidosis (DKA) occurs. There is a short-term impact on and long-term implications for health, due to associated complications.

Type 2 diabetes occurs because of insufficient insulin production or resistance by the body's cells to insulin. Treatment options are determined by the severity and progression of the condition. Management options include diet and physical activity, oral medication, and insulin. Incidence within children and adolescents is increasing; the rationale for this includes changes in lifestyle, reduction in exercise, and obesity.

Other types of diabetes can occur as a result of underlying medical conditions or treatment, and they can also be attributable to genetic factors.

Complications and associated conditions

Hypoglycaemia

Regulation of blood glucose is primarily achieved by the hormones insulin and glucagon. Insulin facilitates absorption of glucose from the blood, allowing its utilization by the body for energy. Glucagon produced by pancreatic alpha cells stimulates glycogen to be released from the liver and muscles, preventing hypoglycaemia. The effectiveness of this glucagon response in type 1 diabetes is suppressed by artificial insulin and it is common for the production of glucagon to become insufficient; consequently episodes of hypoglycaemia will always require treatment according to their severity.

The classification of hypoglycaemia, of which there are three categories, is dependent on the level of impairment to cognitive functioning, because the brain is unable to store glucose and is reliant on a continual supply. The symptoms experienced and signs exhibited are unique to the individual and it is important they are able to recognize and treat the episode promptly before it escalates in severity; concentration can be affected for several hours. Frequent hypoglycaemia could indicate that insulin adjustments are necessary; wearing medical identity jewellery is advisable. The signs and symptoms of hypoglycaemia can be categorized into neuro-glycopenic (brain or central nervous system response to reduced glucose) and adrenergic (the body's response to the lack of glucose).

Hyperglycaemia

Elevated blood glucose levels can occur and are considered significant if >14 mmol because of the potential for ketone production and development of DKA. There are various causes of raised levels and the degree of insulin sensitivity (how much 1 unit of rapid-acting insulin returns the blood glucose by) is utilized to return the blood glucose to the target level. If ketones are present, corrections might not be as effective; more insulin will be needed. Rapid-acting insulin can accumulate, causing a stacking effect; caution should be applied to frequency of corrections. Insulin pump users should consider infusion set problems or insufficient insulin as potential explanations for hyperglycaemia.

Diabetic ketoacidosis and long-term health

Patients with newly diagnosed type 1 diabetes mellitus can present with DKA and there is the potential for those with an existing diagnosis also to develop this condition. As a result of the lack of insulin, the body requires an alternate energy source and produces ketones by utilizing fat and protein. Excessive ketone production causes the pH of the body to become acidic and, accompanied by hyperglycaemia and dehydration, DKA results; cerebral oedema can occur. DKA is a serious preventable medical condition that requires hospitalization and national guidelines dictate its management. There is a high mortality and morbidity rate associated with this complication.

Long-term health complications encompass renal failure, blindness, and foot problems, with the risk of amputation, heart disease, and stroke. Achieving the recommendation for glycaemic control reduces the risk of developing these and screening is undertaken as part of the annual review.

Treatment

Insulin is given using pen devices or infusion pumps and attempts to replicate the body's natural insulin secretion. Regimens are chosen based on their suitability and individual appropriateness to optimize glycaemic control. The frequency of insulin administration is dependent on the regimen used.

Psychological and social issues

Appropriate education should be given to staff involved in supporting the individual within the educational setting and care plans should be implemented. The level of support needed will correlate to age and cognitive ability, but will also be dependent on the individual's involvement in their practical diabetes care. Attending to health needs during school hours is imperative and must be accommodated.

Many families manage well; however, the diagnosis can be devastating, triggering a grief response because of the perceived loss of their healthy child. The incidence of chronic sorrow among parents has been identified. Although they are not responsible, since type 1 diabetes is not preventable, parental guilt is common. The whole family is affected and life changes dramatically for the individual diagnosed. Diabetes intrudes and practical management causes discomfort. Acceptance of the condition can be problematic and resentment can result in concordance issues. Understanding is influenced by cognitive age, and challenges occur at each stage of development, producing added stress. Parents worry about the long-term health implications of suboptimal control. This can potentially cause conflict, but concern can be interpreted as nagging.

Adolescence is a notoriously difficult period, presenting its own unique obstacles, particularly the desire for greater independence and the introduction of risk-taking behaviour. Parents can be reluctant to relinquish control; independence regarding diabetes self-care is not always successful, manipulation is common, and diabetes management is often negatively affected during this stage of development.

Key points

- Normal blood glucose level is 3.5–6.5 mmol/L.
- A type 1 diabetes diagnosis will have a major impact on the child and their family in terms of their normal daily activities.
- Other autoimmune disorders are more common in the child with diabetes, e.g. coeliac disease.

119 Diabetes management

Figure 119.1 Diabetes management.

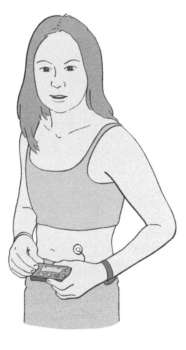

Management

- Secondary healthcare multidisciplinary team approach
- Achieves best practice tariff requirements
- Identifies a suitable insulin regimen
- Delivers comprehensive education
- Aims to reduce development of the associated complications
- Monitors and reviews glycaemic control
- Prepares young person for transition into adult services. Equips schools/education establishments with the training required to support children and young people with diabetes

Illness management

- Always give insulin
- Insulin adjustments might be required
- Increase frequency of blood glucose testing
- Test for ketones
- Monitor hydration
- If not eating an alternative source of energy is required
- Early contact with diabetes team for support

Education

- Continual structured programme
- Identified aims and learning objectives
- Considers learning needs and styles
- Provision of supportive literature or written information

Blood glucose testing

- Testing should occur before meals and bed, is advised if participating in physical activity or at any other time if unwell
- Greater frequency of testing if using an insulin pump
- Wash hands with soap and water, dry properly
- Prepare lancet device using a new needle each time
- Prepare blood glucose meter for use
- Obtain blood sample
- Apply to strip
- Result obtained
- Depending on rationale for testing, implement action accordingly

Insulin administration – basic rules

Injection pens

- Ensure correct insulin and is fit for use
- Use new needle every time and prime before use
- Check correct insulin, correct dose, correct time, correct way
- Dial up required amount and administer into a healthy injection site
- Once plunger depressed, fully count for 10 seconds before removing the device
- Dispose of needle in sharps container

Insulin pumps

- Delivered by an indwelling subcutaneous cannula
- Difficulties can be experienced with insulin delivery; troubleshooting required
- Cannulae should be inserted into healthy sites, and are usually changed every 2 days or earlier if problems with insulin delivery are experienced

Insulin regimens

- **BD:** twice-daily insulin administration, using a mixed insulin (combination of short and intermediate acting)
- **TDS:** three insulin injections a day, utilizing a combination of rapid, intermediate, and long-acting insulin
- **MDI:** multiple daily injections, minimum of four a day. Combines rapid-acting insulin with food and long-acting insulin usually given once a day
- **CSII:** continuous subcutaneous insulin infusion of rapid-acting insulin. No basal insulin used. Boluses given with food

Different insulin regimes require different eating advice. However, nutritional intake should be healthy and well balanced

Management of diabetes in children and young people (Figure 119.1) is provided by secondary health care using a multidisciplinary approach. The introduction of the best practice diabetes tariff aims to standardize diabetes care nationally to ensure all service provision is equitable. The objective is to equip the individual and their family with the essential practical skills required and the underlying knowledge needed to understand and make informed decisions regarding their diabetes management.

Health education includes developing the motivation to succeed, through a programme of structured education addressing self-care, crisis management, and lifestyle. Delivery must accommodate cognitive abilities and preferred learning styles. Challenges are encountered, and families are asked to question their existing health beliefs and accomplish behavioural changes that are difficult to implement consistently. Specific stages of childhood development present their own management issues.

Children and Young People's Nursing at a Glance, Second Edition. Edited by Elizabeth Gormley-Fleming and Sheila Roberts.
© 2023 John Wiley & Sons Ltd. Published 2023 by John Wiley & Sons Ltd.

Glycaemic control is determined by the haemoglobin (Hb)Alc. The target is less than 58 mmol/L (7.5%), achieved without frequent or disabling hypoglycaemia. This level reduces the risk of developing the associated complications. Testing for concurrent medical conditions and screening for the associated complications resulting from micro- and macrovascular disease occur as part of the annual review. Blood glucose testing identifies blood glucose levels and these are recorded in a diary and reviewed regularly by the paediatric diabetes specialist nursing team.

Insulin regimens

Insulin therapy endeavours to replicate the natural insulin secretion by the body; however, the endocrine system is incredibly complex and many factors impact on achieving this. A common adverse effect of artificial insulin is hypoglycaemia. The aim is to achieve a pre-prandial blood glucose level of 4–8 mmol/L and two-hour post-prandial levels of no greater than 10 mmol/L. Insulin regimens are chosen for their suitability for each individual child and NICE guidance is provided. Intensive insulin regimens reduce the risk of developing the associated long-term health complications.

Insulin types

Rapid-acting insulin is given immediately before a meal or snack. The dose is calculated by counting the content of the carbohydrate of the food to be consumed and starts working within 15 minutes of being administered, peaks at 30–90 minutes, and lasts for 3–5 hours.

Short-acting insulin is also given with meals and starts working within 30–60 minutes, peaks at 2–4 hours, and lasts for 5–8 hours. *Intermediate-acting insulin* onset occurs after 1–3 hours, peaks at 8 hours, and lasts for 12–16 hours.

Long-acting insulin starts working after 1 hour and does not have a peak; its duration is 20–24 hours. This is usually given in the evening; however, it can be necessary to halve the dose and also administer it in the morning.

Insulin administration

Insulin is given subcutaneously by insulin pens (pre-filled or cartridge) or delivered by an insulin pump. It is absorbed through the underlying fat cells in the skin. Areas for administration include buttocks, thighs, upper arm, and stomach; insulin absorption rates are influenced by injection site choice. Injection site rotation is imperative, as repeated administration of insulin in specific areas results in lipohypertrophy, a common problem causing erratic insulin absorption. Desensitization to injections in these areas occurs, impacting on willingness to rotate injection sites appropriately. A dose of insulin should never be repeated; additional blood glucose testing is advised if it is unclear whether the correct dose or full dose was given.

Nutrition

A healthy, well-balanced diet is advocated to optimize growth and maintain a healthy weight. Carbohydrate counting is used with continuous subcutaneous insulin infusion (CSII) and multiple daily injection (MDI) regimens to calculate the insulin to food ratio; a diary is kept and ratios assigned to meal times. Twice (BD) and three times daily (TDS) regimens require regular snacks to prevent hypoglycaemia. Issues can develop regarding attitudes towards food: binging and restricted eating can occur and will impact on blood glucose stability and glycaemic control; intentional hyperglycaemia assists with weight loss. All of these issues will require additional management support by the multidisciplinary team.

Physical activity

Aerobic (low-intensity) or anaerobic (high-intensity) exercise affects blood glucose. Counter-regulatory hormones released during anaerobic activity can cause a temporary glucose elevation, but this can be followed by hypoglycaemia several hours later. Aerobic activity lowers the blood glucose during exercise and afterwards. Prior to the activity, additional carbohydrate and increased testing, possibly in conjunction with insulin reductions, can be utilized to prevent hypoglycaemia. If hyperglycaemia is present this could be exacerbated if there is a lack of insulin within the body, so it is advisable to check that the blood glucose is within target before commencing exercise.

Illness management

A diagnosis of diabetes does not increase the risk of developing illnesses or infections unless blood glucose control is suboptimal. During episodes of illness, control can be affected by insulin resistance because of counter-regulatory hormones increasing, requiring additional insulin doses. However, not all illnesses will result in hyperglycaemia. It is not uncommon for episodes of diarrhoea and vomiting to cause hypoglycaemia due to reduced food intake and increased gut motility resulting in poor absorption, therefore a reduced amount of insulin will be needed.

Irrespective of how the blood glucose is affected during times of illness, insulin should always be given, the frequency of blood glucose and ketone testing should be increased, and hydration should be maintained. It is advisable to test for blood ketones if the blood glucose level is 14 mmol or above. Blood ketone testing is more accurate; ketone excretion in the urine is delayed, potentially impacting on management. If appetite is decreased, carbohydrate will need to be given in the form of drinks. If this is not tolerated and vomiting occurs, medical assessment is advised because of the risk of diabetic ketoacidosis (DKA). Encouraging the individual or their family to contact their healthcare provider for support at the start of illness could prevent hospital admission and reduce the incidence of DKA.

Key points
- The main goal of treatment is to maintain good metabolic control.
- The child should be supported to enable them to take maximum responsibility for their diabetes as appropriate for their age.
- Prompt treatment of any illness is required in order to prevent either hypoglycaemia or diabetic ketoacidosis from occurring.

120 Childhood obesity

Figure 120.1 Childhood obesity – health implications.

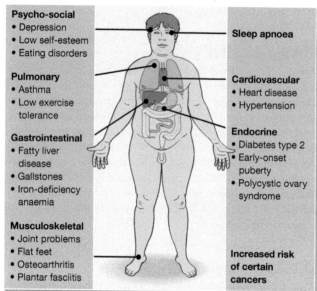

Psycho-social
- Depression
- Low self-esteem
- Eating disorders

Pulmonary
- Asthma
- Low exercise tolerance

Gastrointestinal
- Fatty liver disease
- Gallstones
- Iron-deficiency anaemia

Musculoskeletal
- Joint problems
- Flat feet
- Osteoarthritis
- Plantar fasciitis

Sleep apnoea

Cardiovascular
- Heart disease
- Hypertension

Endocrine
- Diabetes type 2
- Early-onset puberty
- Polycystic ovary syndrome

Increased risk of certain cancers

Figure 120.2 Anthropometry parameters.

Age-dependent factors:
- Weight
- Height
- Head circumference
- Chest circumference

Age-independent factors:
- Mid-arm circumference 1–5 years
- Weight to height
- Skin-fold thickness
- Mid to upper arm/height ratio

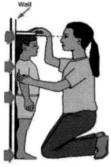
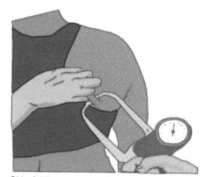

Height measurement

Skin-fold measurement

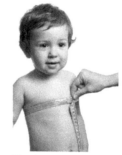
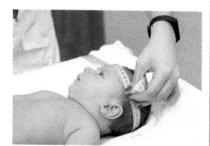

Chest measurement. Source: ia_64 / Adobe Stock.

Head circumference. Source: Dmitry Naumov/Adobe Stock.

Childhood obesity is a global concern. Generally, it begins in early childhood and continues into adolescence and then adulthood. Once established, obesity is difficult to reverse. Poor health outcomes are associated with obesity, so early intervention is required to reduce risk and promote good health.

Causes of childhood obesity

Lifestyle is a key consideration when seeking to identify the causes of childhood obesity. Many children are overweight because they simply eat more calories than they need, resulting in an energy imbalance. Many foods liked by children are high in fat, salt, and sugar. From an early age children also pick up poor dietary habits from their parents and family. Excessive portion sizes and insufficient physical activity only serve to compound the issue.

A lack of sleep has also been suggested as a contributory factor. Children going to bed later and getting less sleep has been shown in some cases to increase the levels of the hormones leptin and ghrelin, which monitor and act on body fat stores. Other hormone imbalances such as hypothyroidism can have an effect on appetite and body fat, as can some medications.

Indication of a strong genetic tendency is possible when other family members are also obese.

Current statistics

In the UK more than 1 in 4 children is now overweight when they start their primary school education. Obesity is more prevalent in boys than in girls. It is more prevalent in children who live in areas of deprivation and this is increasing. It is estimated that obesity and its health consequences cost the NHS approximately £4 billion a year; this is set to rise as long-term health implications manifest for the increasing numbers of overweight and obese children in future years (Figure 120.1). The current state of affairs in the UK, and indeed globally, is referred to as the 'obesity epidemic'.

National child measurement programme

The National Child Measurement Programme (NCMP) measures the height and weight of children at primary school in Reception (age 4–5 years) and Year 6 (age 10–11 years). From these measurements the body mass index (BMI) can be calculated using a simple equation:

$$BMI = \frac{weight(kg)}{height(m)^2}$$

The NCMP is dependent upon parental consent; thus, it could be argued that the results are not representative of the population as a whole, as some families do not participate. It is also suggested that there is a higher than average representation of overweight and obese children within those families that refuse consent, and in reality overweight and obesity rates are significantly higher than current figures indicate.

There is further evidence to suggest that parents will consistently under-estimate their child's weight. We are becoming so used to seeing morbidly obese people in the media that we naturally adjust what we think is 'normal' and do not recognize overweight children in many cases.

It is important to be aware that BMI should not be calculated for children in the same way as an adult's BMI. There are specific growth charts for children (World Health Organization centile charts) that indicate a normal BMI range for children of a similar height, age, sex, and ethnic background.

Anthropometry

The core element of anthropometry are measurement of height/length; head circumference; BMI; body circumference to assess for adiposity on the waist, hips, and limbs; and skin-fold thickness (Figure 120.2). This is a non-invasive quantifiable measure of the human body and can be used to estimate total body fat. It is important that these measurements are calculated as part of the screening process for the child who is obese and who is commencing a weight reduction programme.

Health risks

There are increased intermediate and long-term health risks clearly associated with childhood overweight and obesity. Of mounting concern is the growing body of evidence that many overweight and obese children become overweight or obese adults. Morbidities linked with obesity include heart disease, type 2 diabetes, hypertension, fatty liver disease, gallstones, osteoarthritis, early puberty, asthma, sleep apnoea, and musculoskeletal problems. Lack of self-esteem is reported in young people who are obese.

What can be done?

Of key importance to the progress of any weight management programme has to be a wide approach that involves all the family, with gradual changes more likely to be successful. Children's nurses are ideally placed to offer healthy eating advice on an opportunistic basis when working with children and families, but will require further training in order to give up-to-date and effective advice at an appropriate time.

The following suggestions have some merit:
- Avoid snacking – have three regular meals instead.
- Eating together at a table instead of in front of the TV.
- Reduce the intake of fizzy drinks.
- Eat a balanced and varied diet, high in fibre and starchy foods.
- Have five portions of fruit and vegetables a day.
- Take care with portion sizes.
- Eat healthy snacks if needed.
- Avoid fried food.

It is recognized that dietary intake is only a part of the solution, as increasing physical activity is crucial to any weight management plan. Children need to be more physically active and spend less time on sedentary behaviours such as computers, video games, and television.

Obesity in childhood can also lead to psychological issues and poor self-esteem. Confidentiality and building confidence are important, in particular when working in schools with individual children. Strategies must be discreetly employed and sensitive to the needs and feelings of these vulnerable children. This is also applicable to the implementation of the NCMP.

Change4Life

The Change4Life programme is a government-led initiative aimed at supporting people with healthier choices. It was advised that children over 5 years old should be engaging in physical activity for at least 60 minutes each day, while children under 5 years should be engaged on a daily basis in active play for 180 minutes. Other Change4Life initiatives include information about healthy snacks, portion control, and hidden fats and sugars in everyday foods.

Lifestyle, eating and activity for families (LEAF) programme

The Lifestyle, Eating and Activity for Families (LEAF) programme was designed to treat childhood obesity in accordance with NICE guideline CG189. It sought to empower families to take control of their lives and become healthier. As a community-based programme, families in areas of high deprivation were the initial targets. Three-monthly reviews followed an initial workshop. This workshop was facilitated by a dietician and a physical activity adviser. Families who achieved weight loss, as evidenced by a reduction in BMI and a healthier lifestyle, were referred back to the primary care setting for ongoing support and monitoring. Multi-component strategies have been shown to be effective in managing childhood obesity.

Key points
- Reducing the number of calories eaten is crucial to a successful reduction in weight.
- Successful weight loss programmes must include a range of strategies and an increase in physical activity.
- Changes must be made gradually and sustained to increase the chances of success.
- All health professionals have an important role in childhood weight management and should receive appropriate training and support to implement this.

121 Eating disorders

Figure 121.1 Eating issues.

Common eating disorders	
Anorexia nervosa (AN)	Inability to eat and maintain body weight. Fixation and anxiety related to body shape, weight, and food. Usually affects young girls aged 12–17 years, but approximately 1 boy in 100 of the same age
Bulimia nervosa (BN)	A range of behaviours related to periods of excessive overeating followed by purging and accompanying feelings of anxiety and self-loathing
Binge eating disorder (BED)	Over-eating to compensate, reduce feelings of poor self-esteem, or as a comforting ritual

Risk factors (AN and BN)

- Family history of eating disorders and depression
- Bullying and perceived criticism over eating behaviours, body shape, and weight
- Anxiety and desire to be thin due to peer pressure, media, or sport needs (e.g. athletics, modelling, dancing, ballet)
- Poor self-esteem, anxiety-provoking triggers such as social situations, obsessive personal and family traits
- Critical parents, a need to please and always achieve perfection
- Past traumatic experiences including emotional, sexual abuse, and neglect
- Fear of failure, adaptation, change

Physical symptoms (AN)

The symptoms of AN are those of chronic starvation. In recovery, young people also experience periods of obsessive and checking rituals, self-harm, devious and distracting behaviours (including purging, water loading, hiding food, excessive exercise) in an attempt to reduce feelings of anxiety

Starvation symptoms include amenorrhoea, diarrhoea, pellagra, lanugo (fine hair), muscle and brain atrophy, poor dental hygiene, oedema, kidney failure, osteoporosis, constipation, acne, cardiac arrest, reduced cognitive ability, electrolyte abnormalities, delayed gastric emptying, endocrine disorders, cold extremities

Summary of recovery treatment for AN and BN

Recovery takes the form of redeveloping a sustainable relationship with food, body image, and identity, including self-esteem and self-worth

Cognitive behavioural therapy (CBT) aims to help young people rationalize, think, and perceive differently. It aims to provide awareness of coping strategies, cognitive drills, and new ways of acting

Family therapy aims to explore the nature of dynamics and ways family members can begin to support one another

Individual therapy provides a safe space to build authentic relationships and explore personal issues

Body image work explores personal and wider expectations made about appearance and notions of beauty

Warning signs

- Ritual and routine related to eating in certain places and time
- Wearing oversized and concealing clothing
- Missing meals, claiming to have already eaten
- A denial of sexual development, libido, and sexual maturity
- Gives a feeling of mastery, power, and control
- Feeling physically defective, socially judged
- Symbolic of becoming invisible, not existing, having low self-esteem

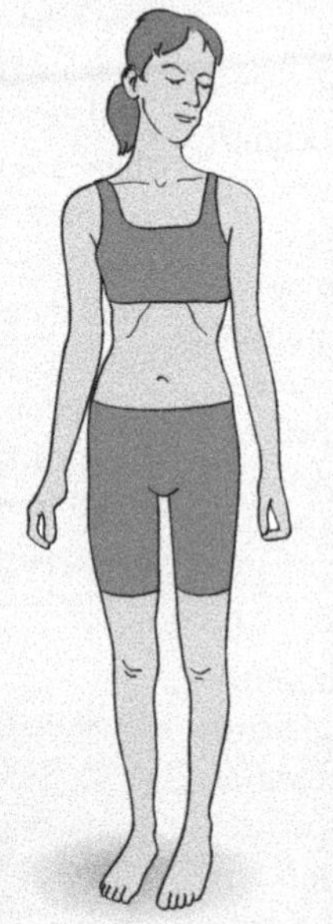

- Ritual and routine related to eating in certain places and at certain times
- Purging, water loading, vomiting, daily/hourly weighing
- Excessive exercising, preoccupation with body image
- A false and distorted sense of confidence
- Eating disorder gives feelings of control, self-respect, and success
- Consumption of only low-calorie foods

Children and Young People's Nursing at a Glance, Second Edition. Edited by Elizabeth Gormley-Fleming and Sheila Roberts.
© 2023 John Wiley & Sons Ltd. Published 2023 by John Wiley & Sons Ltd.

What are eating disorders?

An eating disorders is an abnormal attitude towards food, body image, and body weight, which transpires in a number of disorder classifications. The primary three conditions are anorexia nervosa (AN), bulimia nervosa (BN), and binge eating disorder (BED); see Figure 121.1. Other specified feeding or eating disorders (OSFED) may be diagnosed if the child or young person does not 'fit' one of the other three types.

Anorexia nervosa is when someone attempts to maintain a chronically dangerously low weight by purposefully starving themselves, exercising excessively, and purging. It is characterized by an anxious preoccupation with food and body image, with corresponding secretive, ritualistic, and manipulative behaviours.

Bulimia is a chronic condition that for some people may be constant in their lives. For others it is reactive to stressful events. Bulimia, like binge eating, is the attempt to control weight and emotional aspects of life by overeating and then deliberately being sick or using laxatives (medication to help empty the bowels). Binging is a response to emotional distress, over-compensating, self-esteem issues, and difficulty recognizing bodily sensations.

Binge eating disorder is classified as being more spasmodic than bulimia, but no less serious. It is characterized by control and compulsion to overeat.

These eating disorders have a significant impact on the developmental needs of young people, usually during their most significant developmental period (puberty). The direct causes are unknown, but it is known that eating disorders impact not only physically, but also psychologically and on social developmental needs.

Who is affected by eating disorders?

Around 1 in 250 girls and 1 in 2000 boys will experience AN at some point. The condition usually develops around the age of 13–17 years. Based on these figures, it can be estimated that 5–10 million people in the UK will at some time experience some type of eating disorder, ranging from full-blown AN to picky and finicky eating patterns. BN is around five times more common than AN and 90% of patients are female. It is often the case that boys are diagnosed with depression or associated appetite disorders rather than AN or BN.

Causes of eating disorders

The causes of eating disorders are unknown, but there is consensus that there are a number of probable causes, which include biological, genetic, attachment issues, bullying, media, environmental abnormalities, sexualized trauma, and idealized and irrational beliefs about shape, weight, and health. These appear to be influencing factors in eating disorders combined with an ever-increasing concern with celebrity, image, and issues of thinness. Food is used as a coping mechanism or as a means to retain control.

Treatment

The aim of treatment for AN is to help the child/young person reach a healthy body weight for their age and to be aware that weight gain is essential in supporting their psychological wellbeing, which will impact positively on their quality of life and therefore improve their chances of recovery. Therapeutic strategies to manage AN typically involve psychological approaches to help understand beliefs and behaviours along with interventions to increase the child/young person's body weight.

Psychological interventions may include cognitive behavioural therapy (CBT), individual psychotherapy, family therapy, self-help, and psychodynamic therapy. This will be long term.

Refeeding programme (AN)

It is usual that when a young person's body weight has dropped below a body mass index (BMI) of 13–15 and they are a seriously low weight (e.g. 35–40 kg), they will be admitted for inpatient treatment to local Child and Adolescent Mental Health Services (CAMHS). There is no hard-and-fast rule regarding these criteria, but a safeguarding decision by professionals regarding the welfare of the young person who is suffering the effects of chronic starvation is the high priority at this point. It might be the case that a young person is admitted against their will on a section of the Mental Health Act (1983), because they are cognitively unable or unwilling to consent to necessary life-saving treatment. Treatment usually takes the form of a two-phase programme: refeeding and recovery. The two phases are often blurred because of the long-term and chronic nature of eating disorders (young people can have both AN and BN for a number of years, sometimes past their teenage years). In the first instance, the refeeding programme can take months, with the aim of gaining 1 kg/week.

This first refeeding stage involves the establishment of strict mealtime routines, restriction of exercise, a response to increased anxiety and subsequent self-harm, close monitoring at meal times, and daily structure. Young people will have increased anxiety because they are either gaining weight as in the case of AN, or being prevented from the stress-reducing behaviour of binging, overeating, and purging in the case of BN. This often creates complex multiple dimensions to diagnosis (sometimes referred to as dual diagnosis). In practice, it means that young people will experience high levels of anxiety, depression, self-harm urges, and obsessive compulsive disorder (OCD)-type symptoms over a period of weeks and months. These vary between individuals, especially in the initial stages of reducing the effects of starvation and gaining weight.

Treatment regimens will vary, some units may focus on weight, others may consider general health and implications of change. Young people may also be prescribed medication for anxiety or depression.

Recovery programme (AN, BN, and BED)

The recovery phases of treatment vary according to the type and acuteness of the eating disorder. However, it is nearly always the case that a number of interventions are used in combination. When engaging in supportive, psychotherapeutic, and self-esteem–building interventions, the young person and their family are also being instructed in new ways of relating to food and each other. Some units have facilities that allow for planned meals, where the family can eat and plan meals prior to slowly increasing the number of meals expected to be eaten away from the unit. Thus, the mechanics of food preparation and consumption remain at the forefront of treatment, but during the recovery phase there is an expectation of reduced monitoring and surveillance as the young person and family improve and adapt to the disorder. Other interventions that occur during the recovery phase are intended to support and provide skills in maintaining and confronting the triggers that can lead to relapse. They include attendance at body image–type therapy, CBT, family therapy, and more expressive and creative therapies such as music and art therapy.

Key points

- Eating disorders may develop at any stage of life.
- The causes of eating disorders are unknown, but there is consensus that there are a number of probable causes, which include biological and genetic causes and attachment issues.
- Recovery is possible and can be achieved by repositioning food in the life of the child/young person.

122 Mental health problems

Figure 122.1 Mental health problems.

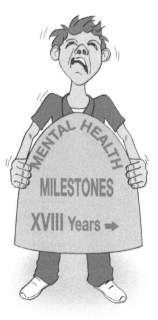

Predisposing influences on mental health

Genetics

Some characteristics such as temperament and intelligence are influenced by genetics. Specific conditions such as autism, Down's syndrome, and language disorders

Prenatal and perinatal complications

Maternal impact such as age, smoking, malnutrition, blood type, and drug use

Physiological dysfunction

Poorly functioning bodily systems indicative of anxiety, acute psychosis

Parent, family, and social factors

Attachment difficulties, neglect, poor parenting, stress, abuse, social disadvantage, chaotic family circumstances, domestic violence, criminality, poor parental mental health, poverty, inadequate role models

Psychological factors

Poor and low self-esteem, deficient cognitive ability, immature defence and coping mechanisms

Developmental milestones

Parenting roles

Safety, care, control, intellectual stimulation, able to take instruction, moral development

Physical

Appropriate physical growth, puberty, sexual maturity

Cognitive

Psychometric intelligence, Piagetian cognitive development, skill acquisition, problem solving, information processing

Emotional

Self-soothing skills, expression and appropriate response to stimuli, curiosity, rudimentary empathy, recognition and anticipation of others, development of temperament

Social

Able to engage in creative play, responsive arousal, identity development, autobiographical memory, appropriate adaption to life transitions, language development, ability to self-evaluate and self-regulate, commitment to social values

What is a mental health problem?

There are many factors that contribute to mental health problems for young people and children (see Figure 122.1). Typical statistics suggest that 1 in 10 children and young people will require professional help at some time in their lives regarding their mental health before the age of 18.

Typically, mental health problems show themselves in two distinct age periods: first, for children aged from 5 to about 12 years; and second, for young people aged 12–18 years. Mental health problems for both groups affect the child or young person's emotional, cognitive, educational, and behavioural capacity. The most common mental health problems for children are those associated with inattentiveness and poor social behavior, such as attention deficit hyperactivity disorder (ADHD), disruptive behavior such as conduct disorders, and language and emotion-type disorders such as Asperger's syndrome.

For teenagers, mental health problems include depression, self-harm, anxiety disorders, social disorders focused on an inability to cope (including para-suicide), obsessive compulsive disorders (OCD), bipolar disorders, psychosis, and eating disorders such as anorexia nervosa. Unlike adult psychiatry, young people often have a complex or dual diagnosis, which means a combination of the above, on their path to achieving their key maturational milestones. According to the World Health Organization (WHO), mental health is 'a state of well-being in which the individual realizes his or her own abilities, can cope with the normal stresses of life, can work productively and fruitfully'. For young people and their families, mental health is not only the absence of mental health problems, but also the accomplishment of developmental milestones that impact and compound difficulties in this life stage.

Types of services

In the UK, children and young people come under the care of Child and Adolescent Mental Health Services (CAMHS). Every region has access to Tier 3 (community-based specialist teams)

Children and Young People's Nursing at a Glance, Second Edition. Edited by Elizabeth Gormley-Fleming and Sheila Roberts.
© 2023 John Wiley & Sons Ltd. Published 2023 by John Wiley & Sons Ltd.

and Tier 4 (specialist adolescent inpatient facilities). Both of these tiers have multi-agency specialist professionals (including mental health nurses, social workers, occupational therapists, consultant psychiatrists, teachers, psychologists, family therapists, art therapists, and other therapists) who assess, treat, and follow up young people and families in their care.

Most mental health problems take a long time to recover and the need for ongoing support is provided by seamless service delivery and interdisciplinary teamwork. The liaison of Tier 3 CAMHS teams with other healthcare professionals such as children's nurses usually shows itself in the assessment of risk and evaluation of young people admitted to emergency settings for self-harm, parasuicide attempts, and distorted body image issues. It is not uncommon for these young people to be repeat service users, as they often come from chaotic and unsettled backgrounds and show their distress through their behaviour.

The role of CAMHS is to respond quickly, provide specialist assessment of mental health status and treatment as necessary, create conditions for seamless service provision between multi-agency teams, provide specialist knowledge (including that related to the Mental Health Act 1983), and specify follow-up, appropriate monitoring, and referral.

Types of mental health problems

Mental health problems in childhood very rarely manifest as a simple single diagnosis as they might in adulthood. Diagnosis is more often dual or complex. What this means is that a child will never present as simply having depression, but rather depression as a symptom of some other conflicting social dilemma confronting the child. Thus, it is common for children with ADHD to show classic signs of inattentiveness, spontaneous outbursts, and inability to control their temper, as well as having feelings of despair, low mood, and anxiety as they get older. Likewise, teenagers with anorexia nervosa will more than likely have periods of anxiety, extreme agitation, low mood, and depression as they work through their recovery.

Anxiety disorders (including panic disorders, phobias, and post-traumatic stress disorder)

These types of mental health problems for children and young people manifest as severe to moderate fear of social situations, objects, people, and places. They result in maladaptive coping strategies and triggers including avoidance, and physiological responses including panic. Most patients will complain of persistent and constant intrusive thoughts and sometimes the obsessive and compulsive repetition of comforting acts. If the young person is suffering from the effects of past trauma, they may be experiencing symptoms of post-traumatic stress disorder (PTSD), which include flashbacks, self-harm, fear of losing control, and disruption to everyday self-care activities.

Mood disorders

These are sometimes referred to as affective or depressive disorders and relate to a young person feeling either elated (manic) or low (depressed). Most patients recover given time with the use of anti-depressant medication. Major depressive episodes have symptoms of withdrawal, suicidal ideation, poor self-care, and slowed cognition. Some mood disorders such as bipolar disorder may have a physiological and genetic cause that affects the regulation of mood-balancing neurotransmitters. Seasonal affective disorder (SAD) is thought to be triggered by a response to a lack of daylight.

Psychosis

It is rare for children to have psychotic-type disorders, including schizophrenia. However, a few young people in their teenage years experience psychotic symptoms associated with distorted delusional thinking, hallucinations (which can be visual, auditory, olfactory, or sensory), or negative symptoms such as social withdrawal, poor self-care, disrupted thinking patterns, and flatness of mood. Psychosis-type disorders can be acute and a one-off as a result of physical or emotional trauma or induced by the use of drugs. For some young people, psychosis can be chronic and need treating with medication or depot injections for a number of years.

Language and learning disorders

There are a number of categories of ADHD, but they all share symptoms of hyperactivity, inattentiveness, and impulsiveness. Disruptive behavior makes it difficult for the child to fit in with their peer group because they are often fidgeting, easily distracted, unable to complete tasks, loud, and disruptive. The cause is uncertain, but may be related to anxiety, depression, undetected seizures, emotional trauma, or genetics.

Autism and Asperger's syndrome

Autism and Asperger's syndrome are developmental disorders that impact on the ability of the child or teenager to form relationships, emotionally connect, relate to reality, have imagination, and socialize. There are different degrees and characteristics, so the disorders are often considered as a spectrum.

Conduct disorders

Children and young people who over a long period of time show an inability to follow rules, or display aggressive and violent behavior out of context, may be diagnosed as having conduct disorders.

Recognizing problems

The following are behaviours that most young people experience at some time in their lives. However, in their chronic state they often accompany a number of mental health problems in childhood and adolescence:

- *Acting out*: expressing distress and over-arousal in inappropriate ways, such as tantrums, screaming, running away, self-harm and physical threats, somatic problems, dangerous risk-taking, parasuicide.
- *Withdrawal*: a persistent rejection of company, isolation in bedroom and solitary comfort, elective mutism, phobias, chaotic family systems, special education issues, psychosis, abuse, neglect.
- *Emotional avoidance*: procrastination, seeking risk, desire to question reasonable requests, low self-esteem and pessimistic outlook, seeking destructive relationships, dogged denial, drug and alcohol abuse, engaging in distracting activities, mental and social disengagement, generalized anxiety disorder, PTSD, repetition problems such as OCD, mood disorders, suicide.
- *Attachments and bonding*: affected by neglect, failure to thrive, inconsistent discipline, confused communication patterns, poor protective systems.
- *Physical*: anorexia nervosa, bulimia nervosa, eating disorders, self-harm.

Key points

- Childhood mental health problems are increasing in number year on year, with an estimated 1 in 8 children having a mental health disorder at any one time.
- There is an association between sleep–wake problems in childhood and longer-term mental health in young people.
- Childhood mental health problems will often continue into adulthood.

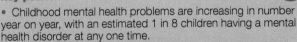

123 Self-harm in childhood

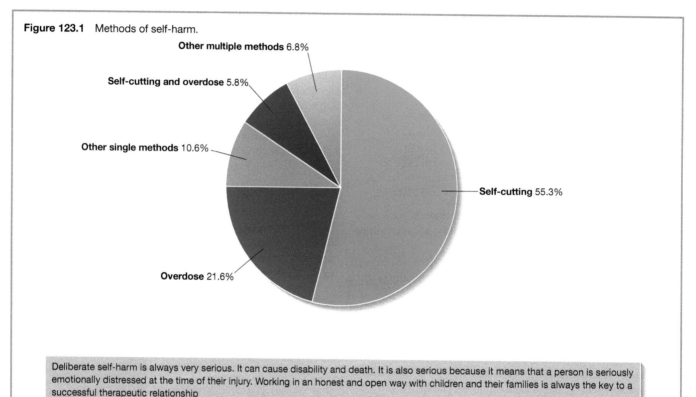

Figure 123.1 Methods of self-harm.

Other multiple methods 6.8%

Self-cutting and overdose 5.8%

Other single methods 10.6%

Self-cutting 55.3%

Overdose 21.6%

Deliberate self-harm is always very serious. It can cause disability and death. It is also serious because it means that a person is seriously emotionally distressed at the time of their injury. Working in an honest and open way with children and their families is always the key to a successful therapeutic relationship

What is self-harm?

While the term self-harm may at first seem self-explanatory, a universally accepted definition of this phenomenon is not easy to find. Professionals and organizations within which these disciplines work use a range of words to describe this behaviour. Various terminologies have frequently been used in the literature:

- Deliberate self-harm
- Self-injurious behaviour
- Repeated self-injury
- Self-wounding
- Parasuicide
- Self-mutilation
- Self-wounding
- Episodic and repetitive self-injury
- Auto-destructive behaviour

Furthermore, definitions can vary from short explanations such as the one offered by the NICE guidelines on self-harm, 'Self-poisoning or injury, irrespective of the apparent purpose of the act', to longer definitions, for example the one used by the World Health Organization:

An act with a non-fatal outcome in which an individual deliberately initiates a non-habitual behaviour that, without intervention from others will cause self-harm, or deliberately ingests a substance in excess of the prescribed or generally recognised therapeutic dosage and which is aimed at realising changes which the subject desired via the actual or expected physical consequences.

However, the International Child and Adolescent Self-Harm in Europe (CASE) study group utilizes a working definition whereby self-harm is seen as an act with a non-fatal outcome in which one or more of the following behaviours are present:

- Ingesting a substance in excess of the prescribed or generally recognized therapeutic dose.
- Ingesting a recreational or illicit drug that was an act that the person regarded as self-harm.
- Ingesting a non-ingestible substance or object.
- Any initiated behaviour that an individual intends to cause harm to self. For example, deliberately cutting oneself, jumping from a height, self-inflicted cigarette burning, wound excoriation, and mutilation of the face or other body parts.

There are variable methods of methods of self-harm among school-based adolescents (Figure 123.1).

Prevalence of self-harming behavior

Self-harm is a serious public health problem and has become increasingly more common among young people. Self-harm behaviour has been described as a morbid form of self-help that is antithetical to suicide. People who deliberately hurt themselves contravene the most basic of human drives – self-preservation. The consequent shaming experience and diminished self-efficacy that may emerge can lead a child's motivation from being self-harming to suicidal. Subsequently, deliberate self-harm is indirectly related to suicide, as people who deliberately self-harm are 18 times more likely than the rest of the population to eventually complete suicide. There is a 30-fold increase in the risk of suicide for those who self-harm compared with non-self-harmers. In addition, suicide may be an unintended consequence of deliberate self-harm, and therefore self-harming behaviours are an ominous sign of the potential to complete suicide.

Research findings show that self-harm is more common in females (13.9%) than in males (4.3%). Young women aged 15–18 years had the highest incidence of deliberate self-harm based on hospital presentations to Accident and Emergency in 2011, at 589 per 100 000. These rates imply that 1 in every 171 girls presented to hospital with a presentation of self-harm. In the UK, self-harm is one of the top five reasons for acute medical admissions.

What causes self-harming behavior?

There is no single cause for self-harming activity. However, research suggests that some children may be at more risk of this behaviour than others:
- Young people who are involved in risk-taking behaviours such as alcohol and substance misuse or have addictions.
- Those with mental health disorders (e.g. depression, anxiety, eating disorder, or schizophrenia).
- Individuals at crisis point or under severe stress (e.g. ongoing family relationship problems).
- Those who have a debilitating or chronic illness.
- People who have had experiences of childhood trauma and/or abuse.

Is it just 'attention seeking'?

Some people view self-harming behavior as 'attention seeking'. This negative attitude is unhelpful to the child, as it can leave them feeling as though their distress and feelings are trivial. Research has shown that children who harm themselves often have great difficulty with asking for help and generally have very poor problem-solving skills. They tend to have memories that over-generalize their experience and may forget how they solved a similar problem in the past. They can get stuck when trying to solve a current problem. This can lead to feelings of frustration and being out of control. For other young people, self-harm may indicate that they are experiencing symptoms of a mental disorder.

Management and treatment

The primary purpose of intervention is to prevent suicide, prevent any repetition of self-harm, and address the worries and issues that are causing this behaviour.

Screening instruments for at-risk individuals include the following:
- Beck Hopeless Scale (BHS)
- Child Suicide Assessment (CSA)

- Expendable Child Measure
- Firestone Assessment of Self-destructive Thoughts (FAST)
- Hopeless Scale for Children (HPLS)
- Inventory of Suicidal Orientation 30 (ISO-30)
- Life Attitudes Schedule (LAS)
- Measure of Adolescent Potential for Suicide (MAPS)
- Millon Adolescent Clinical Inventory (MACI)
- Multi-Attitude Suicide Tendency Scale (MAST)
- PATHOS
- Reasons for Living (RLF)
- Suicide Probability Scale (SPS).

Treatment options available for this group include:
- Psychological interventions (e.g. cognitive behavioural therapy, dialectical behaviour therapy, problem-solving therapy).
- Behavioural techniques.
- Family therapy.
- Psychopharmacological interventions.
- Group psychotherapy.

Management of self-harm in the paediatric setting

Environmental

Ensure all sharps, ligatures, and dangerously ingestible substances are removed from the immediate area. Observe the young person regularly at 15- or 30-minute intervals.

Interpersonal

Provide support to the young person to discuss their concerns, anxieties, and low mood.

Behavioural

Consider a behavioural support strategy like a first aid distraction kit. This can consist of a shoe box containing items for soothing or distraction, such as a music device, stress ball, and writing materials.

Consider a behavioural contract in conjunction with the multidisciplinary team, which will incorporate a commitment to approach staff when the young person experiences the urge to self-harm.

Family

Liaise with the family to assist them to understand self-harm and help them to source community services for ongoing care.

Key points
- There is a strong link between early childhood adversity and self-harm.
- Self-harm is a growing global concern.
- There is a proven link between self-harm/injury and suicide in later life.
- The family must be involved in the management plan, as they need to understand self-harm if they are to support their child effectively.

124 What is a learning disability?

Figure 124.1 Types of learning disability.

It is estimated 1% of the population has a learning disability

'A complex way of being'

What a learning disability is	What a learning disability is not
• A significantly reduced ability to understand new or complex information (impaired intelligence) • A reduced ability to cope independently (impaired social functioning) • That has started before adulthood (age 18 years) and has a lasting effect on a person's development	• A learning difficulty – an educational need that does not affect intellect – dyslexia/dyspraxia/dyscalculia • Mental illness • Autism – approximately 44–52% of people will have an additional learning disability • Physical disabilities – cerebral palsy/spinal muscular atrophy (SMA) • Acquired brain injury – consequence of stroke/dementia/road traffic injury/etc. post 18

Degree of intellectual disability	IQ range	Possible presentation
Mild (85% cases)	50–70	Conversational language. Struggle academically but usually able to read, write, count. Usually live independently and may work. Require support with more complex demands and at times of stress
Moderate (10% cases)	35–49	Language ability varies and understanding may be over-estimated. Limited achievement in school. Likely to need support in activities of daily living Supervised practical work may be possible
Severe (4% cases)	20–35	Single words or no speech. May communicate with 'objects of reference', by gesture or expression. Can learn routines. Require assistance for basic tasks and self care. Highly supported accommodation
Profound (1% cases)	<20	Require intensive support. High rates of medical comorbidity (e.g. epilepsy) and physical disability that need ongoing nursing and therapy

Figure 124.2 Classification of learning disabilities.

Idiopathic
• Unknown cause, may cluster in families

Genetic/chromosomal
• Chromosomal abnormalities – e.g. Down's syndrome
• Gene mutations – e.g. Fragile X syndrome

Antenatal
• Maternal TORCH infection (toxoplasmosis, other, rubella, cytomegalovirus, herpes)
• Tertogens (alcohol, illicit drugs, valproate)

Perinatal
• Hypoxia
• Metabolic – hypoglycaemia, severe jaundice

Infancy/childhood
• Biological – central nervous system infection or injury
• Psychosocial – abuse and neglect

Figure 124.3 Examples of reasonable adjustment actions.

First or last appointment of the day	Longer appointment times	Speak slowly, use short simple sentences, no jargon
Involve family and carers	Contact the Learning Disability team for support	Use hospital communication book
Read the patient's hospital passport	Identify sensory needs	

Figure 124.4 Reasonable adjustments for accessibility and communication. Credit: National Institute for Health and Care Research (NIHR).

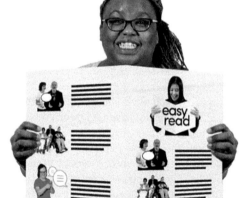

Figure 124.5 Reasonable adjustment mnemonic to assist children and young people with a learning disability to promote patient safety.

GREAT
- Give me more time
- Repeat yourself
- Effective communication
- Accompanied?
- Think Team

A learning disability is a reduction in intellectual ability that affects the child or young person in their everyday life. A learning disability will impact a child's development and significantly reduce their ability to understand information or learn new skills. This in turn will reduce the child's/young person's ability to live independently. A learning disability is defined as a condition that starts during childhood and has a lasting impact on development, and should not be confused with a learning difficulty such as dyslexia. Life for children or young people (and their families) is challenging and additional support may be required to ensure the individual can reach their personal potential (Figures 124.1 and 124.2).

Barriers to accessing health services

Children with a learning disability may have multiple health needs. A number of reports have highlighted the correlation between services and mortality rates for people with a learning disability. As a

Children and Young People's Nursing at a Glance, Second Edition. Edited by Elizabeth Gormley-Fleming and Sheila Roberts.
© 2023 John Wiley & Sons Ltd. Published 2023 by John Wiley & Sons Ltd.

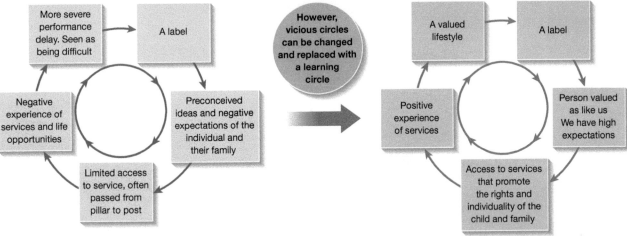

Figure 124.6 Key terms.

How do we label a person? Or indeed a family?

Consider what you know about children who have a learning disability and treat this as a reflection or portfolio exercise
- When did you first become aware of people with a learning disability?
- What was the nature of the contact?
- What was the position of your community about these people?
- How much did that influence you?

The right to be yourself!

How do we devalue people who are different? By the imposition of a vicious circle that can reinforce a label and prove to us we were right to have such thoughts

The vicious circle

However, vicious circles can be changed and replaced with a learning circle

How to reverse the trend?

By measuring people by what they can do, rather than by what they cannot, and using the normalization philosophy in a productive therapeutic way. The concept of being 'ordinary' within your own social sphere is inextricably linked with the **philosophies of normalization,** which were developed across Europe and Canada over the last 30 years. Essentially, normalization is a set of guidelines that should ensure that people who are labelled as different get what the rest of us take for granted – a valued social role, and their place in society

Remember!
- A set of values
- A moral code
- Something in which you believe
- It influences how you view people and what you do with them

result of these inequalities in the care provided for people with a learning disability, Mencap has launched a 'Treat me well' campaign, which seeks an adjustment in the way services for people with a learning disability are currently configured and delivered. Several barriers have been identified that prevent children with a learning disability and their families from getting the care and services they need to meet their needs. These include:
- Lack of accessible transport links.
- Lack of staff knowledge, awareness, and understanding.
- Lack of recognition of deteriorating health in the child with a learning disability.
- Failure to correctly diagnose.
- Lack of staff confidence and anxiety.
- Lack of joint working.
- Not listening to family/carer.
- Lack of follow-up care.

Reasonable adjustments

By law, the Equality Act 2010 says that there is a duty to make reasonable adjustments in order to achieve equality (Figures 124.3–124.5). This duty requires all healthcare providers to take positive

steps to ensure that services are accessible to the child with a learning disability and their families. A reasonable adjustment to the planned care that a child and family require can make a significant difference in their overall experience of their healthcare experience. Reasonable adjustments should be reviewed to see whether they are appropriate and helpful.

Key points
- The child with a learning disability needs to be seen in the context of their family and appropriate support provided for all.
- The life goals for a child with a learning disability can be achieved if the correct adjustments are made to facilitate their needs.
- Some children with a learning disability are at increased risk of certain health conditions.
- The children and young person's nurse needs to be aware of the significant key terms (Figure 124.6) and key stages in the life of the child/young person with a learning disability, e.g. starting school, transition to adult services, and plan well in advance.

125 Autistic spectrum disorder

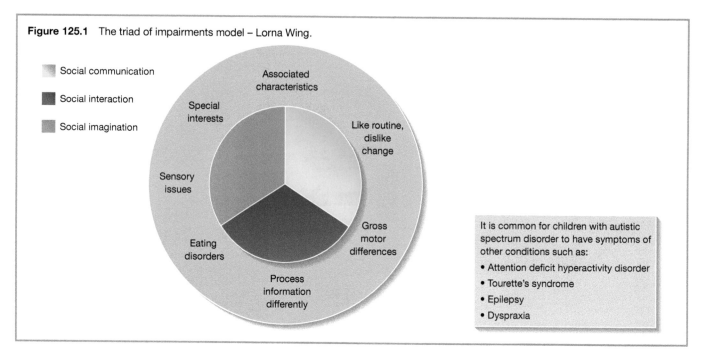

Figure 125.1 The triad of impairments model – Lorna Wing.

- Social communication
- Social interaction
- Social imagination

Associated characteristics

Special interests

Sensory issues

Eating disorders

Like routine, dislike change

Gross motor differences

Process information differently

It is common for children with autistic spectrum disorder to have symptoms of other conditions such as:
- Attention deficit hyperactivity disorder
- Tourette's syndrome
- Epilepsy
- Dyspraxia

What is autistic spectrum disorder?

Autistic spectrum disorder (ASD) is a neurobiological disorder of development. It is a lifelong condition; people do not get better from ASD. It is a 'spectrum', which means that while all people with autism share certain difficulties or characteristics, their condition will affect them in different ways and can vary hugely. It includes Asperger's syndrome as well as autism with learning disabilities. It affects how a person communicates with, and relates to, other people. It also affects how they make sense of the world around them. Many people with ASD experience over-sensitivity or under-sensitivity to sounds, touch, tastes, smells, and light; this is called sensory hypersensitivity or hyposensitivity.

Autism

The three main areas of difficulty that all people with autism share are sometimes known as the 'triad of impairments':
- Difficulty with social communication.
- Difficulty with social interaction.
- Difficulty with social imagination.

Children with ASD do not 'look' disabled. Parents of children with autism often say that other people simply think their child is poorly behaved, but this is not the case.

Autism is a common condition, with over half a million people with autism in the UK; that is around 1 in 100 people. People from all nationalities and cultural, religious, and social backgrounds can have autism, although it appears to affect more boys than girls.

Causes

The cause of autism is still not known. However, research suggests that a combination of factors, particularly genetic and environmental, lead to changes in brain development. There is some thought that men over the age of 40 years are more likely to father children who may be autistic. Autism is not caused by the child's upbringing or their social circumstances, and is not the fault of the child with the condition or their parents. It is not linked to 'bad parenting' and it is not caused by the measles, mumps, and rubella (MMR) vaccination.

Brain differences

Studies have shown that the brains of people with ASD are different in the:
- Frontal lobes
- Limbic system
- Brain stem and fourth ventricle

Between 30% and 50% of people with autism have been found to have abnormally high levels of serotonin (a chemical responsible for transmitting signals in nerve cells). Autistic brains have been shown to have additional neurons to neurotypical (non-autistic) brains. There are differences in the location of electrical activity in the brain in people with ASD, as well as differences in the time course of electrical activity in the brain. Communication between different parts of the brain is reduced in people with ASD. The brain receives a lot of information from the world and people with ASD take more time to process this information.

Children and Young People's Nursing at a Glance, Second Edition. Edited by Elizabeth Gormley-Fleming and Sheila Roberts.
© 2023 John Wiley & Sons Ltd. Published 2023 by John Wiley & Sons Ltd.

Triad of impairment

The areas of difficulty in the triad of impairment (Figure 125.1) manifest in different ways in each individual, but some of the ways it can affect them are outlined here.

Impairment of social communication

- Talk at you.
- Incessant communication.
- Not true communication (e.g. may not follow the usual rules).
- Have only a concrete understanding.
- Do not engage in social chat.
- Communication confined to own needs.
- Struggle to understand non-verbal communication.
- Echolalia.
- Repetition.
- Formal speech.

Impairment of social interaction

- Abnormal eye contact.
- Indifference to others.
- Aloofness.
- Pay little attention to responses.
- Preference for isolation.
- Impaired social behaviour.
- Empathy issues.
- Active but odd.
- Passive.

Impairment of social imagination

- Rigid, inflexible thinking.
- Restrictive, repetitive play.
- Abnormal play: spinning, flapping.
- Lack of imagination.
- Self-stimulatory behaviours.
- Difficulty in generalizing concepts.
- Circumscribed interests.

Supporting children with autistic spectrum disorder

To support the child who has an autistic spectrum disorder and their family, some of the difficulties encountered could be managed by considering the acronym SCRAMBLE:

Sensory management to reduce stimuli overload.
Communication should be kept simple and be direct.
Reduce or limit number of people in a setting at any one time.
Allow extra time always.
Medication review regularly.
Box of sensory toys/gadgets available for distraction.
Listen – active listening always.
Examination and treatment – child centred and modified to their needs.

Transition of care

There are many transitions that all children and young people will experience as they move into various education settings and then into employment. For the child and young person with an ASD, these transitions may often be more challenging and induce additional stress. National guidance to support the transition from children to adult healthcare settings should be followed. Relationships and a care pathway will need to be established in adult services to ease this transition.

Key points

- An autistic spectrum disorder affects different people in different ways, but they will share some characteristics or difficulties.
- There are three main areas of difficulty: social communication, social interaction, and social imagination.
- Autism has a strong genetic basis.

126 Communication with the parents of a child with learning disabilities

Figure 126.1 Parent experiences.

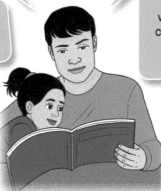

Don't say this	Say this
There is a risk...	There is a chance...
I am sorry, it's bad news	The results of the test indicate characteristics...
I will arrange the termination for this week	I am here to help you understand the diagnosis
Your baby will have multiple disabilities, here is a leaflet of all the common medical conditions common with Down's syndrome	Your baby has an extra chromosome that may affect development
You can terminate up to 39 weeks if you change your mind	I will connect you with the resources that can support you
But you wouldn't want another one like him/her, would you?	You have such a beautiful baby

Children and Young People's Nursing at a Glance, Second Edition. Edited by Elizabeth Gormley-Fleming and Sheila Roberts.
© 2023 John Wiley & Sons Ltd. Published 2023 by John Wiley & Sons Ltd.

All too often hospital staff rely on parents to provide information about their child, particularly when the child has a learning disability. Learning disabilities can range from mild to profound, with multiple disabilities in some individuals. Parents can feel 'a weight of responsibility' about their child's communication and overall safety that impacts on their willingness to leave them alone in hospital. A survey conducted by Mencap found the following:

- 70% of parents have felt unwelcome in public.
- 66% missed social engagements.
- 21% have been asked to leave a public space.
- 47% have visited their GP due to anxiety.
- 57% have been prescribed antidepressants.

Without the right support, parent carers may feel helpless and overwhelmed and may lack skills and understanding to support their young person. Families can become isolated, feeling that it is easier to manage life at home rather than go out into the community.

If a parent carer is struggling with their health, it may affect the consistency of care they can offer, and their child may become anxious and frustrated. Depression in mothers and fathers of children with learning disabilities is far higher than among those who do not have a child with an learning disability.

Children with learning disabilities are also known to have severe sleep problems and this will impact on parental sleep also. Parents may struggle to allocate enough time to all of their children.

Siblings may experience bullying, lack of privacy, disruption to home life and experience complex feelings about their situation.

Stress and coping are common early features in families who have a child with an learning disability, and this then shifts to a model of family adaptation once interventions have been identified and put in place.

Receiving a diagnosis

Getting a diagnosis that your child has an learning disability is often confirmation of existing parental suspicions. Most parents who receive this diagnosis will nevertheless experience strong emotions, including shock, despair, loss, confusion, and sadness. This experience shares similar emotions to grief and mourning.

Some diagnoses are possible during pregnancy, such as Down's syndrome (see Chapter 128). How these results are delivered creates a framework for patients and families and may eventually become imprinted as their stories (Figure 126.1). Research highlights that implicit biases or ideas about specific types of diagnoses, particularly those involving physical or learning disabilities, may influence how clinicians and allied healthcare professionals present this news to families. Numerous parents have reported being encouraged or pressured into terminating the pregnancy by medical professionals. In the UK, 92% of Down's syndrome pregnancies are terminated.

Syndrome without a name

'Syndrome without a name' is not a diagnosis, but a term used when a child or young adult is believed to have a genetic condition and testing has failed to identify a genetic cause. Not all children with a syndrome without a name will have learning disabilities.

Equally, not all children with a syndrome without a name will have physical disabilities.

Every year, approximately 6000 children are born in the UK with a syndrome that is so rare it cannot be diagnosed. Parents of these children will feel incredibly isolated. They are unable to receive peer support from other parents who have a child with the same syndrome. Lack of awareness and understanding means many parents are unaware that there are other children who also will never receive a diagnosis.

This results in the parents lacking a sense of identity. They are unable to compare what would be atypical/typical for their child. They are unable to prepare for any health conditions or complications. They are unable to gain information or prepare for their child's future:

- Will my child have a normal life expectancy?
- Is my child's syndrome life-limiting?
- Will they lose the abilities they have achieved – sight/hearing/ swallowing/mobility/communication/smile?
- Will they begin to regress tomorrow?

Person First Language

There is a shift towards Identity first language, particularly within the Neurodivergent (Autistic/ ADHD) community as the disability is who they are, not just a part of them, it affects every aspect of their lives.

It is important for health professionals not to make assumptions about a person based on their diagnosis, or discriminate due to disability. Ultimately it is the preference of the disabled person as to how they wish to be defined.

Person First Language refers to the person before the disability, i.e. a person with a disability. Identity first language refers to the condition, i.e. a disabled person.

Key points

- Support for the parents is essential, as parents of children with disabilities will need additional skills to meet their child's needs.
- Parents with children who have an unnamed syndrome often feel very isolated as there may be many unknowns about their child's condition.
- The impact on the siblings when a child with a disability is born into a family may further add to the parental stress.
- Person first communication is key. The child is a person with a learning disability – for example, 'Ravi has cerebral palsy' rather than 'Ravi is a cerebral palsy child'.

127 Positive behavioural support

Figure 127.1   Challenging behaviour.

Challenging behaviour is defined as 'Culturally abnormal behaviours of such intensity, frequency or duration that the physical safety of the person or others is placed in jeopardy, or behaviour that is likely to seriously limit the use of or delay access to ordinary community facilities'.

Examples include:

Self-harm

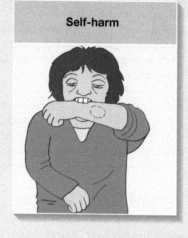

Violence and aggression

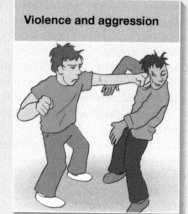

Unsociable behaviours

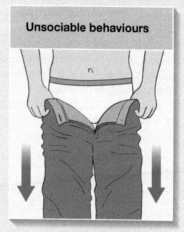

Damage or destruction of property or items

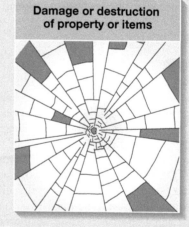

Antecedent

In this box you should write everything that is happening before the child displays the challenging behaviour:
• Who is there
• The date, day, and time
• What is happening
• Temperature, noise levels
• What activities are taking place
• Is anything being asked of the child?

Behaviour

In this box you should write a clear description of the behaviour. Try to avoid 'broad' words such as aggression. Different people have different ideas about what aggression is. So be really clear and describe the behaviour.

For example: 'Tom shouted at Rebecca. He called her a fat slob. He then knocked over a chair and walked out of the room slamming the door behind him.'

This way everyone gets a clear picture of what Tom did, which we would not get from 'Tom was aggressive'

Consequence

In this box write everything that happens after the behaviour. Include who says what? Who does what? What does the child do? What changes? What stays the same?

Children and Young People's Nursing at a Glance, Second Edition. Edited by Elizabeth Gormley-Fleming and Sheila Roberts.
© 2023 John Wiley & Sons Ltd. Published 2023 by John Wiley & Sons Ltd.

From time to time, children and adolescents may display behaviours that can be described as challenging. The term 'challenging behaviour' is used to represent the challenge the behaviour presents to the service providers and illustrates that it is not intrinsic to the person. Challenging behaviour is defined as 'culturally abnormal behaviours of such intensity, frequency or duration that the physical safety of the person or others is placed in jeopardy, or behaviour that is likely to seriously limit the use of or delay access to ordinary community facilities'. It is an umbrella term, which can include socially unacceptable behaviours, destruction of property, self-injurious behaviours, and violence and aggression to others.

Challenging behaviours can be life-threatening, such as in cases of extreme self-injury, but in most cases they are not, although they have a huge impact on the person's quality of life and the quality of life of those around them. The presence of challenging behaviour is often the reason cited for the breakdown of service provision, resulting in exclusion from services and isolation from families, friends, and society.

Children and adolescents do not just decide to suddenly display challenging behaviours. Any behaviour the child is displaying must be occurring for a reason and must be serving a purpose for them. The challenge to staff is to understand that behaviour and work out what purpose it is serving. Any new behaviour may be occurring as a result of many things, such as bullying, emotional disturbances, low self-esteem, mental health problems, physical pain, abuse and neglect, or grief, or be linked to a condition or environmental aspects.

What is positive behavioural support?

Positive behavioural support is about understanding why the behaviour occurs and what maintains it – why does the child continue to do it? Behaviours are 'functional'; that is, they serve a purpose for the child.

In order to understand why challenging behaviours are occurring, we need to study other aspects of the child's life. Causes of challenging behaviours are often divided into two main groups: non-biological and biological. Abuse, changes at home, and lack of understanding of social rules are non-biological causes. Biological causes could be associated with specific syndromes and mental health problems. Many conditions have a predisposition to the manifestation of challenging behaviours. For example, autism is an often-cited example of a condition associated with a wide range of behavioural manifestations, including self-injury, aggression, injury to others, and socially inappropriate behaviours. Gilles de la Tourette's syndrome is associated with verbal outbursts, obsessive–compulsive behaviour, aggression, and self-harm. Challenging behaviour is also associated with epilepsy in some people as part of their seizures. Phenylketonuria, mental illness, and physical pain are additional causes of challenging behaviour.

The first stage with a new behaviour is a full and detailed assessment in order to understand the behaviour. Without an assessment, any interventions attempted may be a waste of time, potentially adding to the problems, leading to frustration for the children's nurse, the child, staff, and families. Assessment may involve a combination of more than one assessment tool such as functional analysis and the Motivation Assessment Scale, as well as more detailed holistic assessments. These assessments are straightforward and easy to use. An example of functional analysis is shown in Figure 127.1.

When you have completed several of these it is important to analyse them. This means looking for trends and patterns in the behaviour:

• Does it occur at the same time or on the same day?
• Does it occur when the same task is being asked of the child?
• Does the behaviour always occur when a particular other person is around? This may be a sign that the child does not like that person, but it can also be a sign that they like the person very much and do not know how to express themselves.
• Does the behaviour always manifest in the same way or does the child display different types of behaviour?
• What are the outcomes? Do staff or parents always respond in the same way?

When you analyse the information you may see trends that are reinforcing or maintaining the behaviour that help us to understand it. Once we have a better understanding of why the behaviour is occurring, we can then introduce strategies to deal with it. Strategies include proactive (preventative) approaches to avoid the behaviours occurring and reactive approaches, how staff or parents will react when the behaviour occurs.

Positive behavioural **support does not include punishment.** Positive behavioural support needs to contain several key features:
• Values-led: delivers child-centred outcomes.
• Based on functional analysis – the why, when, and how of behavioural analysis.
• Focuses on triggers to reduce likelihood of behaviours reoccurring.
• Recognizes that lack of skills can maintain behaviours, so focuses on skills training, such as becoming better at expressing oneself.
• Changes in quality of life are used as an intervention and outcome measure.
• Has a long-term and multicomponent focus.
• Eliminates punishment approaches.
• Includes proactive and reactive strategies.

Key points
• Challenging behaviours can be life-threatening in cases of extreme self-harm.
• The behaviour serves a purpose for the child or young person.
• A full assessment is required prior to implementing intervention, as the behaviour needs to be understood.

128 Genetic conditions: Down's syndrome

Figure 128.1 Down's syndrome – dysmorphic features.

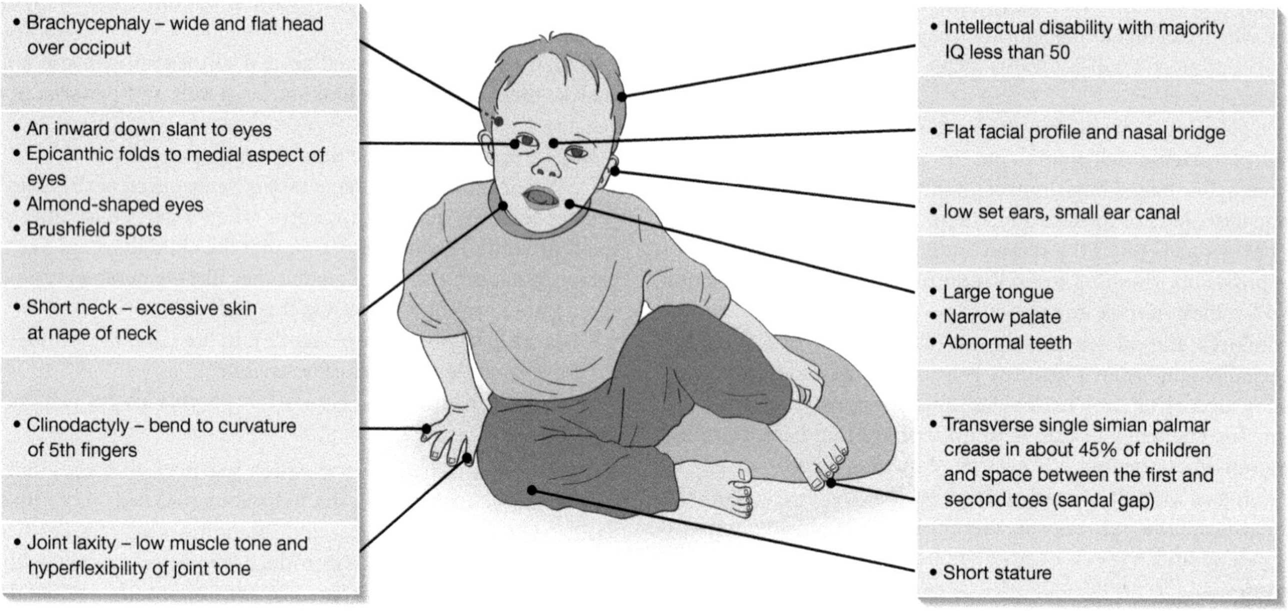

- Brachycephaly – wide and flat head over occiput

- An inward down slant to eyes
- Epicanthic folds to medial aspect of eyes
- Almond-shaped eyes
- Brushfield spots

- Short neck – excessive skin at nape of neck

- Clinodactyly – bend to curvature of 5th fingers

- Joint laxity – low muscle tone and hyperflexibility of joint tone

- Intellectual disability with majority IQ less than 50

- Flat facial profile and nasal bridge

- low set ears, small ear canal

- Large tongue
- Narrow palate
- Abnormal teeth

- Transverse single simian palmar crease in about 45% of children and space between the first and second toes (sandal gap)

- Short stature

Box 128.1 Specific medical problems that occur more frequently in people with Down's syndromeT.

Ear, nose, and throat

- Upper airway obstruction
- Chronic catarrh
- Conductive hearing loss
- Sensorineural hearing loss

Cardiac

- Congenital malformations
  - atrioventricular septal defects (AVSD)
  - pulmonary vascular disease (PVD)
- Cor pulmonale
- Acquired valvular dysfunction

Ophthalmic

- Nasolacrimal obstruction
- Cataracts
- Glaucoma
- Nystagmus
- Squint
- Keratoconus
- Refractive errors
- Blepharitis

Endocrine

- Growth restriction
- Diabetes hypothyroidism
- Hyperthyroidism

Immunological

- Immunodeficiency
- Autoimmune diseases, e.g. arthropathy, vitiligo, alopecia

Gastrointestinal

- Congenital malformations
- Feeding difficulties
- Gastro-oesophageal reflux
- Hirschsprung's disease
- Coeliac disease

Haematological

- Leukaemia
- Neonatal polycythaemia
- Transient neonatal myeloproliferative states
- Neonatal thrombocytopenia

Dermatological

- Alopecia
- Vitiligo
- Dry skin
- Folliculitis

Neuropyschiatric

- Depressive illness
- Autism
- Infantile spasms and other myoclonic epilepsies
- Dementia (adults only)

Orthopaedic

- Metatarsus varus
- Pes planus
- Hip subluxation/dislocation
- Cervical spine instability
- Scoliosis
- Patellar instability

Children and Young People's Nursing at a Glance, Second Edition. Edited by Elizabeth Gormley-Fleming and Sheila Roberts.
© 2023 John Wiley & Sons Ltd. Published 2023 by John Wiley & Sons Ltd.

Down's syndrome is a naturally occurring, congenital chromosomal disorder that has always been part of the human condition. It was first recognized as an entity in 1866, by Langdon Down (1828–1896), an English doctor working in Surrey, who first described the characteristic features of the syndrome. In most children with Down's syndrome, the condition is recognized at or shortly after birth, although it may also be suspected antenatally due to routine screening at 10–14 weeks of pregnancy. In most cases, the doctor will be quite certain of the diagnosis on the basis of the child's appearance alone (see Figure 128.1).

Genetics

Down's syndrome, also known as trisomy 21, is a common chromosome disorder that results from changes on chromosome 21. Almost 95% of cases are triggered by non-disjunction, meaning the chromosome 21 pair fails to separate during cellular division. The second chromosomal defect is translocations – when a chromosomal segment moves to a new position. The third chromosome defect is mosaicism, which arises when a mutation on chromosome 21 takes place later in cell division, and subsequently in affected and normal cells. This mosaic arrangement of Down's syndrome is thought to affect individuals less severely than non-disjunction or translocation. Down's syndrome occurs in all racial and ethnic groups, and becomes more predominant with advanced parental age. The incidence is approximately 1 in 800 live births.

Phenotype features

- *Face*: When looked at from the front the child with Down's syndrome typically has a rounded face. From the side, the face is apt to have a flat profile.
- *Head*: The occiput (back of the head) is slightly flattened in most children and adults with Down's syndrome. This is known as brachycephaly.
- *Eyes*: The eyes of nearly all children and adults with Down's syndrome slant upwards a little. In addition, they have a small fold of skin that runs vertically between the inner corner of the eye and the bridge of the nose. This is known as the epicanthic fold or epicanthus. The eyes may have white or light yellow speckling around the rim of the iris (the coloured part of the eye). These specks are called Brushfield spots.
- *Hair*: The hair of children with Down's syndrome is often soft and straight.
- *Neck*: Newborn babies with Down's syndrome might have extra skin over the back of the neck, usually taken up as they grow. Older children and adults tend to have a short, broad neck.
- *Mouth*: The mouth cavity is slightly smaller than average, and the tongue is slightly larger. This arrangement encourages the children to have the habit of putting their tongues out at all times.
- *Hands*: The hands of a child with Down's syndrome tend to be broad, with short fingers. The little finger sometimes has two joints, and tends to be incurved towards the fourth finger, known as 'clinodactyly'. The palm may have only one crease going across it, usually extending right across the hand.
- *Feet*: These incline to be stubby, and to have a wide space between the first and second toes known as 'sandal gap'. This may be associated with a short crease on the sole, which starts at this gap.

- *Muscle tone*: The limbs and necks of young children with Down's syndrome are often very floppy. This floppiness is called 'hypotonia', meaning low tone. As a result of this many children and adults with Down's syndrome become tired easily and find it hard to walk long distances.
- *Short stature*: Children with Down's syndrome tend to weigh less than average at birth. Their body length is similarly reduced. During childhood they grow slowly, and their ultimate height in adulthood is generally shorter than would be expected for their family and is usually near the bottom of the normal range.

Diagnosis

A number of tests can be undertaken to screen for Down's syndrome. These tests are offered to all pregnant women, regardless of their age, usually in combination to increase detection rates, while retaining a low false-positive rate:
- *Combined test*: ultrasound scan to measure nuchal translucency plus free beta-hCG and PAPP-A (pregnancy-associated plasma protein A).
- *Quad test*: this test measures maternal serum alpha-fetoprotein, unconjugated estriol, beta hCG, and inhibin-alpha.
- *Intergraded test*: uses measurements from the first-trimester combined test and the second-trimester quad test to yield a more accurate result.

Specific medical problems in Down's syndrome

There are specific medical problems that occur more frequently in people with Down's syndrome, as a result of which all children with Down's syndrome should be offered regular medical review by a paediatric medical team throughout their childhood (Box 128.1).

Prognosis

Over the years there has been a profound change in people's outlook towards individuals with Down's syndrome. The change in parental attitude has in turn resulted in a more positive outlook in terms of the increased competence and achievements of children/young people with Down's syndrome. Affected children should have regular child health surveillance checks so that any specific medical problems can be managed in a timely manner, increasing their quality of life.

Key points
- Down's syndrome is the most common congenital chromosomal disorder.
- The extra chromosome is usually maternal in origin.
- Children with Down's syndrome will have varying degrees of learning disability, and many will attend mainstream school with additional support.

129 Other genetic conditions

Figure 129.1 Phenylketonuria (PKU).

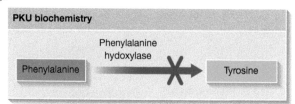

PKU biochemistry

Phenylalanine → [Phenylalanine hydoxylase] ✗ → Tyrosine

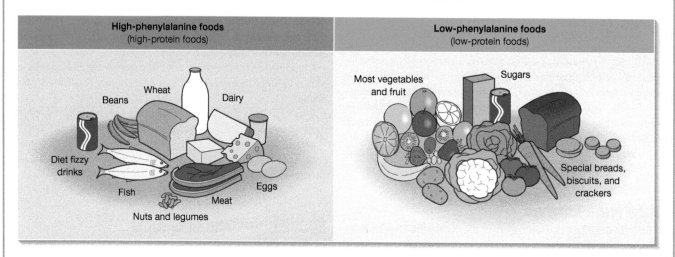

High-phenylalanine foods
(high-protein foods)

Beans, Wheat, Dairy, Diet fizzy drinks, Fish, Nuts and legumes, Meat, Eggs

Low-phenylalanine foods
(low-protein foods)

Most vegetables and fruit, Sugars, Special breads, biscuits, and crackers

Figure 129.2 Main areas of muscle weakness affected by Duchenne muscular dystrophy.

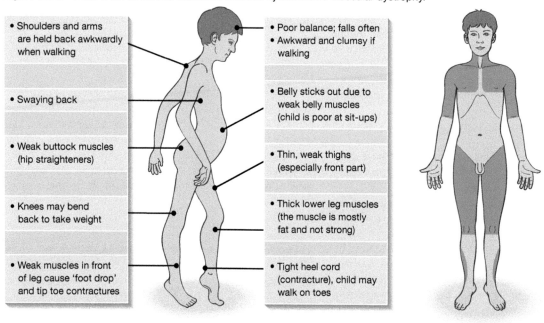

- Shoulders and arms are held back awkwardly when walking

- Swaying back

- Weak buttock muscles (hip straighteners)

- Knees may bend back to take weight

- Weak muscles in front of leg cause 'foot drop' and tip toe contractures

- Poor balance; falls often
- Awkward and clumsy if walking

- Belly sticks out due to weak belly muscles (child is poor at sit-ups)

- Thin, weak thighs (especially front part)

- Thick lower leg muscles (the muscle is mostly fat and not strong)

- Tight heel cord (contracture), child may walk on toes

Phenylketonuria

Phenylketonuria (PKU) is an autosomal recessive human genetic disorder caused by a deficiency of hepatic phenylalanine hydroxylase enzyme activity, which prevents hydroxylation of phenylalanine into tyrosine.

PKU is a common inborn error of amino acid metabolism in Caucasian populations and approximately 1 in 50 is a carrier of a PKU allele. The genetic disorder causes impairment of postnatal brain development, resulting in severe intellectual disability in untreated children.

Phenylalanine is an essential amino acid provided by food that has a key role in the production of other amino acids (Figure 129.1). It is converted to tyrosine, used in the production of neurotransmitters.

How PKU is detected

• Every newborn baby is tested for PKU by taking a blood sample heel prick test measuring the level of phenylalanine.
• Normal range of phenylalanine <120 pmol/L (<2 mg/dL).
• In PKU, blood phenylalanine levels can range from <60 to 7200 pmol/L (1–120 mg/dL), up to 80 times more than the normal level.
• If the baby's blood test results are outside the normal PKU range, they will be retested for confirmation and then immediately put on the standard treatment for PKU, a lifelong restricted diet.

Treatment

In PKU, encouraging adherence to diet includes continuing education, reinforcement, and support from the family and professionals. All dietary proteins are roughly equally rich in phenylalanine, and a suitable diet can therefore be devised only by supplying the bulk of nitrogen as a mixture of amino acids. While it would be possible to mix pure amino acids to obtain such a diet, the costs would render any long-term treatment of even a few cases impossible.

Prognosis

Researchers are studying whether the current standard therapy involving a phenylalanine-restricted diet and meeting phenylalanine targets can still lead to changes in the brain. Some of the evidence gathered involves brain scans. So far, studies show that a large percentage of people with PKU may have some visible brain abnormalities and lifetime phenylalanine levels (the higher the phenylalanine levels, the more brain abnormalities).

Scientific evidence suggests that higher than normal blood phenylalanine levels can reduce the neurotransmitter dopamine in the brain of a person with PKU.

Duchenne muscular dystrophy

Duchenne muscular dystrophy (DMD) is the most common severe childhood form of muscular dystrophy, resulting from a gene mutation in the X-linked *DMD* gene. DMD is a recessive muscle disease that arises as a result of mutations in the gene responsible for dystrophin production, which is involved in maintaining the integrity of sarcolemma. DMD is a severe, progressive disease that affects 1 in 3600–6000 live male births. There is no cure, and management of DMD is limited to glucocorticoids that lengthen ambulation and drugs to treat cardiomyopathy.

Gene replacement

The molecular basis for DMD has been known for over 20 years. Several treatment strategies are under investigation and have shown promise for DMD. Procedures of molecular-based therapies that replace or correct the missing non-dysfunctional dystrophin protein have gained impetus. These approaches include gene replacement with adeno-associated virus, exon skipping with antisense oligo-nucleotides, and mutation suppression with compounds that 'read through' stop codon mutations. Other strategies include cell therapy and surrogate gene products to recompense for the loss of dystrophin. However, attempts to develop gene therapy for DMD have been problematic because of the massive size of the dystrophin gene.

When to suspect DMD

• Presence of Gower's sign in a male child, mainly if the child has a waddling gait. Gower's sign is a medical sign indicating weakness in the proximal muscles, explicitly those of the lower limbs.
• Delayed walking, frequent falls, or difficulty climbing stairs and running.
• Delays in attainment of childhood milestones, such as gross motor functions, walking, running, climbing stairs, and a positive family history of DMD.

Diagnosis

Diagnosis of DMD should be carried out by a neuromuscular specialist who can assess the child clinically and rapidly access and interpret appropriate investigations in the context of the clinical presentation. DMD is typically diagnosed at the age of 5 years, but may be suspected much earlier because of the delays in development milestones. The diagnosis is based on:
• Observation of abnormal muscle function in a male child (Figure 129.2).
• Detection of an increase in serum creatine kinase tested for unrelated conditions.
• Discovery of increased transaminases (aspartate aminotransferase and alanine aminotransferase, which are produced by muscle as well as liver cells). The diagnosis of DMD should therefore be considered prior to a liver biopsy in any child with elevated transaminases.
• Muscle biopsy that demonstrates muscle degeneration, regeneration, isolated 'opaque' hypertrophic fibres, and significant replacement of fat and connective tissue.

Prognosis

Despite the current therapeutic methods under investigation, which are showing great potential for managing DMD, the challenge of finding a cure remains. Corticosteroids characterize the standard of care for treatment of this disease. These classes of drugs can make a change by extending ambulation and delaying or preventing scoliosis. Gene replacement approaches offer the potential for long-term correction.

Key points
• Chromosome disorders are the commonest cause of severe learning disabilities.
• Advances in screening have enabled earlier diagnosis and therefor prompt treatment.
• Children with genetic conditions will require multidisciplinary input from birth to ensure they can live as independently as possible.

Index

Children and Young People's Nursing at a Glance, Second Edition. Edited by Elizabeth Gormley-Fleming and Sheila Roberts.
© 2023 John Wiley & Sons Ltd. Published 2023 by John Wiley & Sons Ltd.

weaning
    CPAP/BiPAP, 217
    incubators, 115
weight, growth measurement, 128–129
weights, traction, 199
well children, observation, 16–17
WETFLAG, 55
wheezing, 18

whey-based formula milk, 125
WHO *see* World Health Organization
World Health Organization (WHO),
    two-step pain management approach,
    160–161
wound healing, 164–165

X-rays, 40–41

young people
    communication, 67
    community children's nurses,
    70–71
    nutritional needs, 120–121
    parental responsibility, 79
    resuscitation, 50–51
    as service users, 139